50 LANDMARK PAPERS

every
Colorectal Surgeon Should Know

There has been an exponential increase in the volume and quality of published research relating to colorectal disease over the last decades. This book identifies the 50 key scientific articles in the field of colorectal disease and colorectal surgery and, through expert reflections and editorial perspectives, explains why these papers are important. Influential contributors who have shaped the practice of modern colorectal surgery comment on the landmark papers that have shaped and defined the specialty.

Among thousands of articles, a small fraction are truly "game changing." Such studies form the foundations of colorectal surgery today, and the selection of papers within this book provides the 50 landmark papers every 21st-century colorectal surgeon needs to know. A commentary to each carefully selected paper explains why these papers are so important, thus providing every surgeon with the foundation of knowledge in this fast-moving area.

This is a valuable reference not only to the established surgeon but also to colorectal surgery residents and trainees, as well as to more experienced surgeons as they continue to learn new techniques and approaches and to improve their knowledge of colorectal disease and treatments. The papers provide an evidence-based resource for those surgeons preparing for professional exams and may inspire clinicians to produce new research.

50 LANDMARK PAPERS

every Colorectal Surgeon Should Know

John R.T. Monson, MD, FRCSI (Hon), FRCSEng, FRCSEd (Hon), FRCS Glas (Hon), FASCRS, FACS

Professor of Surgery, Co-Editor, Diseases of Colon and Rectum
Executive Committee, National
Accreditation Program for Rectal Cancer (NAPRC)
Ridgefield, Connecticut

Lawrence Lee, MD PhD

Colon and Rectal Surgery
McGill University Health Centre
Montreal, QC, Canada

Fergal J. Fleming, MD, MPH, FRCSI, FACS

Associate Professor of Surgery and Oncology,
Director, Surgical Health Outcomes and Research Enterprise (SHORE)
University of Rochester Medical Center,
Rochester, NY

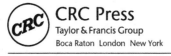

CRC Press
Taylor & Francis Group
Boca Raton London New York

CRC Press is an imprint of the
Taylor & Francis Group, an **informa** business

First edition published 2024
by CRC Press

2385 NW Executive Center Drive, Suite 320, Boca Raton FL 33431
and by CRC Press

4 Park Square, Milton Park, Abingdon, Oxon, OX14 4RN

CRC Press is an imprint of Taylor & Francis Group, LLC

Library of Congress Cataloging-in-Publication Data
Names: Monson, John R. T., editor. | Lee, Lawrence (Fu-Hua Lawrence), editor. | Fleming, Fergal, editor.
Title: 50 landmark papers every colorectal surgeon should know / [edited by] John RT Monson, Lawrence Lee, Fergal Fleming.
Other titles: Fifty landmark papers every colorectal surgeon should know
Description: First edition. | Abingdon, Oxon, OX ; Boca Raton, FL : CRC Press, 2024. | Includes bibliographical references and index.
Identifiers: LCCN 2023051762 (print) | LCCN 2023051763 (ebook) | ISBN 9780367250423 (hbk) | ISBN 9780367202101 (pbk) | ISBN 9780429285714 (ebk)
Subjects: MESH: Colon—urgery | Rectum—surgery | Colorectal Surgery | Review
Classification: LCC RD543.C57 (print) | LCC RD543.C57 (ebook) | NLM WI 650 | DDC 617.5/547—dc23/ eng/20240408
LC record available at https://lccn.loc.gov/2023051762
LC ebook record available at https://lccn.loc.gov/2023051763

ISBN: 9780367250423 (hbk)
ISBN: 9780367202101 (pbk)
ISBN: 9780429285714 (ebk)

DOI: 10.1201/9780429285714

Typeset in Times
by Apex CoVantage, LLC

Contents

Section One   Functional Disorders of the Pelvic Floor

Section Two   Rectal Cancer

Section Three   Hemorrhoids

Section Four   Diverticulitis

Section Five   Inflammatory Bowel Disease

Section Six   Colon Cancer

Section Seven   Anal SCC

Section Eight   Fissure

Section Nine   Anorectal Sepsis

Section Ten   Enhanced Recovery

Preface

There has been an exponential increase in the volume of published research relating to vascular and endovascular surgery over the last few decades. Among the thousands of articles published, a small number are truly "game changing." These may describe a new procedure or surgical approach, evaluate the relative effects of known treatments or techniques, introduce a new classification system, or provide new insights into natural history or disease prognosis. We feel these studies should be familiar to all 21st-century vascular and endovascular surgeons.

It has become increasingly difficult to keep up to date with this growing body of literature. Our goal for this book is to identify and summarize, in a user-friendly format, 50 of these landmark papers. The list has been collated with the help of experts in the field of vascular and endovascular surgery. Although not everyone will agree with all the choices, we think they fulfill the objective of providing an important background for the modern vascular surgeon. We also believe they will provide an essential resource for trainees as they embark on their careers.

The Editors

About the Editors

John R.T. Monson MD, FRCS FASCRS is a colorectal surgeon who trained in Ireland, the United Kingdom and the United States. He served as the Chair of Colorectal Surgery and Digestive Health and Surgery Institute at Advent Health from 2016 until 2024. His areas of expertise include the use of minimally invasive technologies in colorectal cancer treatment, including Transanal Endoscopic Microsurgery (TEMS) laparoscopy and robotic surgery. Dr. Monson is credited with leading the development of laparoscopic colorectal surgery in the United Kingdom. He is a former chair of the UK's National Training Program. His research encompasses a broad range of cancer-related areas including the development of national standards and qualitative assessments of decision making in cancer care. An internationally recognized lecturer and award-winning author of more than 400 peer-reviewed papers and more than 100 book chapters, he is currently coeditor of *Diseases of Colon and Rectum.*

He is a former vice president of the British Association of Surgical Oncology and has served on the Executive Council of the Association of Coloproctology of Great Britain and Ireland. He is a Fellow of the American Society of Colon and Rectal Surgeons and has served in many roles including on their Executive Council and as Chairman of the Research Committee. He was a founding member and vice president of the OSTRiCh Consortium on Rectal Cancer Care, which ultimately became the National Accreditation Program for Rectal Cancer (NAPRC). He is currently a member of the NAPRC Executive Committee. He is a Fellow of all four Royal Colleges of Surgeons – Ireland, England, Edinburgh and Glasgow—and Honorary Fellow of three of the four.

Lawrence Lee MD PhD joined McGill University division of General Surgery as a colon and rectal surgeon in 2017. His main specialty clinical interests relate to the treatment of colorectal neoplasia and inflammatory bowel disease. In particular, Dr. Lee specializes in advanced minimally invasive and endoluminal approaches to the treatment of colorectal disease using flexible endoscopy, transanal endoscopic surgery, and transanal total mesorectal excision (TA-TME). His research interests include health technology assessment and comparative effectiveness research for surgical technologies and innovations, with emphasis on the practice of colorectal surgery. Other areas of research include perioperative assessment and functional and patient-reported outcomes after major abdominal surgery. Dr. Lee completed his General Surgery residency at McGill, during which time he completed an MSc in Epidemiology and a PhD in Healthcare Economics. He then completed a Colon and Rectal Surgery Fellowship at Florida Hospital in Orlando, Florida. He is the recipient of the SAGES Researcher-in-Training award, among other national and international prizes and scholarships for his research and clinical work.

Dr. Lee is a Fellow of the Royal College of Surgeons of Canada and a diplomate of the American Board of Surgery, and holds a specialist certificate from the Collège des Médecins du Québec.

Fergal J. Fleming MB BCh BAO, MD, FRCS is assistant professor of surgery and oncology at the University of Rochester Medical Center. He has been a fellow in the URMC Division of Colorectal Surgery since 2009.

Dr. Fleming was awarded his medical degree from the University College of Dublin, Ireland, in 1998. He is also a Fellow of the Royal College of Surgeons in Ireland. Dr. Fleming's surgical residency included extensive training in general, vascular, and hepatobiliary surgery, as well as dedicated training in colorectal surgery. He was successfully awarded the Intercollegiate Specialist Examination (UK and Ireland) in general surgery with a subspecialty interest in colorectal surgery in 2009. In addition to being licensed to practice medicine in the state of New York, Dr. Fleming is on the Specialist Register of the Irish Medical Council in recognition of his specialist training in the field of surgery.

Throughout his clinical training, Dr. Fleming's academic career flourished with numerous peer-reviewed publications in international journals, as well as distinguished prizes and awards, including a Surgical Research Fellowship in 2002 and the *Irish Journal of Medical Science* Doctor Award, Surgical Section in 2004. He was also awarded a diploma in Cancer Chemoprevention from the National Cancer Institute, Bethesda, Maryland, in 2007.

Contributors

Matthew R. Albert
Advent Health Cancer Institute
Orlando, Florida

Fadwa Ali
UT Southwestern Medical Center
Dallas, Texas

Janet Alvarez
Memorial Sloan Kettering Cancer
    Center,
New York, New York

Allison M. Ammann
University of Cincinnati Medical
    Center,
Cincinnati, Ohio

Christopher T. Aquina
Advent Health Cancer Institute
Orlando, Florida

Motahar Bassam
Kaiser Foundation Hospital Los Angeles
Los Angeles, California

Rishi Batra
University of Nebraska Medical Center
Omaha, Nebraska

Nancy N. Baxter
University of Toronto
St. Michael's Hospital
Toronto, Canada
and
University of Melbourne
Melbourne, Australia

Liliana G. Bordeianou
Massachusetts General Hospital
Boston, Massachusetts

Marylise Boutros
McGill University
Montreal, Canada

William Donald Buie
University of Calgary
Foothills Medical Centre
Calgary, Canada

Elaine M. Burns
Complex Cancer Clinic
St. Mark's, the National Bowel Hospital
London, United Kingdom

Natasha Caminsky
McGill University
Montreal, Canada

Amy M.Y. Cao
Royal Brisbane and Women's Hospital
Queensland, Australia

Manish Chand
University College London
London, United Kingdom

Tyler R. Chesney
University of Toronto
St. Michael's Hospital
Toronto, Canada

William C. Cirocco
Ochsner Health
New Orleans, Louisiana

Kyle G. Cologne
Keck Medicine of USC
Los Angeles, California

Ben Creavin
St. Vincent's University Hospital
Dublin, Ireland

Jacopo Crippa
Humanitas Research Hospital
Milan, Italy

Ian R. Daniels
Royal Devon and Exeter Hospital
Exeter, United Kingdom

Thais Reif de Paula
Lankenau Medical Center
Wynnewood, Pennsylvania

Totadri Dhimal
University of Rochester
Rochester, New York

David W. Dietz
University Hospitals of Cleveland
Cleveland, Ohio

Arman Erkan
Northwell Health
Center for Advanced IBD Care
Manhasset, New York

Cagla Eskicioglu
McMaster University
Ontario, Canada

Erin B. Fennern
St. Luke's Clinic
Boise, Idaho

Alessandro Fichera
Baylor University Medical Center
Texas A&M University
Dallas, Texas

Fergal J. Fleming
Surgical Health Outcomes and Research
   Enterprise (SHORE)
University of Rochester Medical Center
Rochester, New York

James Fleshman
Baylor University Medical Center Dallas
Texas A&M College of Medicine
Dallas, Texas

Charles M. Friel
University of Virginia
Charlottesville, Virginia

Norbert Garcia-Henriquez
Advent Health Cancer Institute
Orlando, Florida

Richard Garfinkle
Mayo Clinic
Rochester, Minnesota

Paolo Goffredo
University of Minnesota
Minneapolis, Minnesota

Ada Graham
University of Chicago Medicine
Chicago, Illinois

Jason F. Hall
Tufts Medical Center
Boston, Massachusetts

Andrew D. Hawkins
University of Virginia
Charlottesville, Virginia

Andrew G. Hill
University of Auckland
Auckland, New Zealand

Emina Huang
UT Southwestern Medical Center
Dallas, Texas

Tracy Hull
Cleveland Clinic
Cleveland, Ohio

Neil Hyman
University of Chicago Medicine
Chicago, Illinois

John T. Jenkins
Complex Cancer Clinic
St. Mark's, the National Bowel Hospital
London, United Kingdom

Carla F. Justiniano
University of Cincinnati Medical Center
Cincinnati, Ohio

Matthew F. Kalady
The Ohio State University Wexner
    Medical Center
Columbus, Ohio

S. Thomas Kang
University of Alabama
Birmingham, Alabama

Deborah S. Keller
Marks Colorectal Surgical Associates
Lankenau Medical Center and
    Lankenau Institute for Medical
    Research
Wynnewood, Pennsylvania

Gregory D. Kennedy
University of Alabama
Birmingham, Alabama

Rory F. Kokelaar
School of Medicine
Swansea University
Swansea, Wales, United Kingdom

Bradley A. Krasnick
The Ohio State University Wexner
    Medical Center
Columbus, Ohio

Sean J. Langenfeld
University of Nebraska Medical Center
Omaha, Nebraska

Lawrence Lee
McGill University Health Centre
Montreal, Canada

Peter Lee
Royal Prince Alfred Hospital
Sydney, Australia

Michael L.R. Lonne
Royal Brisbane and Women's Hospital
Queensland, Australia

Kirk A. Ludwig
Medical College of Wisconsin
Milwaukee, Wisconsin

Anthony R. MacLean
University of Calgary
Calgary, Canada

Robert D. Madoff
University of Minnesota
Minneapolis, Minnesota

John H. Marks
Lankenau Medical Center and Lankenau
    Institute for Medical Research
Wynnewood, Pennsylvania

Justin Maykel
UMass Memorial Medical Center
Worcester, Massachusetts

Tyler McKechnie
McMaster University
Ontario, Canada

John R.T. Monson
National Accreditation Program for
    Rectal Cancer (NAPRC)
Loma Linda University
Florida State University
Professor of Surgery
Ridgefield, Connecticut

Kheng-Seong Ng
The University of Sydney
Sydney, Australia

Bruce Orkin
Digestive Health Institute
Carle Health
Champaign-Urbana, IL

Ana M. Otero-Piñeiro,
Digestive Disease Surgical Institute
Cleveland Clinic
Cleveland, Ohio

Ian M. Paquette
University of Cincinnati Medical Center
Cincinnati, Ohio

Sonia L. Ramamoorthy
University of California
San Diego, California

Timothy J. Ridolfi
Medical College of Wisconsin
Milwaukee, Wisconsin

Tarik Sammour
University of Adelaide
Adelaide, Australia

Niket H. Shah
University of Auckland
Auckland, New Zealand

Ravi Shridhar
Advent Health Cancer Institute
Orlando, Florida

Primal P. Singh
University of Auckland
Auckland, New Zealand

J. Joshua Smith
Memorial Sloan Kettering Cancer
   Center
New York, New York

Michael J. Solomon
The University of Sydney
Sydney, Australia

Antonino Spinelli
Humanitas University Research
   Hospital
Milan, Italy

Christopher J. Steen
Cabrini Monash Department of Surgery
Victoria, Australia

Emily Steinhagen
University Hospitals Cleveland Medical
   Center
Cleveland, Ohio

Andrew R.L. Stevenson
University of Queensland
Queensland, Australia

David B. Stewart
The University of Arizona
Tucson, Arizona

Patricia Sylla
Mount Sinai Health System
New York, New York

Mohamedtaki A. Tejani
Advent Healthcare Group
Orlando, Florida

Larissa Temple
University of Rochester Medical
   Center
Rochester, New York

Eleanor M. Walker
Henry Ford Hospital
Detroit, Michigan

Thomas M. Ward
Massachusetts General Hospital
Boston, Massachusetts

Steven D. Wexner
Cleveland Clinic Florida
Weston, Florida

Desmond Winter
St. Vincent's University Hospital
Dublin, Ireland

Albert M. Wolthuis
University Hospital Gasthuisberg
Leuven, Belgium

Zhaomin Xu
University of Rochester
Rochester, New York

Raymond J. Yap
Cabrini Monash Department of
   Surgery
Victoria, Australia

Dong Yoon
UMass Chan Medical School
Worcester, Massachusetts

CHAPTER 1

Bowel Function after Laparoscopic Posterior Sutured Rectopexy versus Ventral Mesh Rectopexy for Rectal Prolapse: A Double-Blind, Randomised Single-Centre Study

Lundby L, Iversen LH, Buntzen S, Wara P, Høyer K, Laurberg S. The Lancet Gastroenterology & Hepatology.1(4):291–297, 2016

Reviewed by Thomas M. Ward and Liliana G. Bordeianou

Research Question/Objective Myriad procedures have been proposed to treat full-thickness rectal prolapse. This study sought to compare functional symptoms in patients with rectal prolapse who were treated with either laparoscopic posterior sutured rectopexy or laparoscopic ventral mesh rectopexy.

Study Design The study was a single-center, double-blind, randomized trial performed at the Department of Surgery in Aarhus University Hospital in Denmark. It enrolled patients with full-thickness rectal prolapse and randomized them to treatment with either laparoscopic posterior sutured rectopexy or laparoscopic ventral mesh rectopexy. The primary outcome was change in preoperative obstructed defecation syndrome (ODS) score at 1-year postoperative follow-up. Secondary outcomes included the change in patients' preoperative baselines compared to 1-year postoperative follow-up in their Cleveland Clinic constipation scores, Cleveland Clinic fecal incontinence scores, and their colon transit time as measured by ingested radio-opaque markers.

Sample Size A total of 176 patients were assessed for eligibility with 75 patients enrolled from the years 2006 to 2014. Thirty-eight patients were randomized to ventral mesh rectopexy, while the 37 other patients were randomized to posterior suture rectopexy. Thirty-three patients in the ventral mesh rectopexy arm, and 34 in the posterior suture rectopexy arm completed 12-month follow-up.

Follow-Up Study follow-up occurred at 1-year postoperatively, at which time, ODS score, Cleveland Clinic constipation score, Cleveland Clinical fecal incontinence score, and colon transit time were assessed. Additional assessment at 1-year included a clinical examination and defecography.

DOI: 10.1201/9780429285714-1

Inclusion/Exclusion Criteria   Patients were enrolled in the study if they had full-thickness rectal prolapse, as determined by inducible prolapse while straining on a toilet chair in clinic and were deemed suitable for a transabdominal procedure. Exclusion criteria included being a pediatric patient (under 18 years of age), pregnancy or breast-feeding, dementia, psychiatric diseases that would preclude the ability to give informed consent, recurrent rectal prolapse, and the inability to speak or read Danish.

Intervention or Treatment Received   Patients underwent either a laparoscopic posterior suture rectopexy or a laparoscopic ventral mesh rectopexy. The laparoscopic posterior suture rectopexy technique included division of the lateral rectal attachments, full posterior mobilization of the rectum, and suturing of the rectum to the sacral promontory with nonabsorbable sutures. The laparoscopic ventral mesh rectopexy included dissection of the anterior aspect of the rectum, incising the peritoneum to the right of the rectum, suturing of a polypropylene mesh to the distal ventral aspect of the rectum, securing this mesh to the sacral promontory with tacks, and closure of the incised peritoneum to cover the mesh.

Results

Primary Outcome   The ventral mesh rectopexy arm had a mean preoperative ODS score of 9.3, which decreased by 1.97 [95% confidence interval (CI) 0.01 to 3.93] at 1-year follow-up. In comparison, the posterior suture rectopexy arm had a mean pre-operative ODS score of 10.8, which decreased by 2.18 (95% CI −0.14 to 4.49) at 1-year follow-up. There was no difference in the ODS score decrease between the two groups (−0.21, 95% CI −3.19 to 2.78).

Secondary Outcomes   In both arms, the Cleveland Clinic constipation score and fecal incontinence score decreased (functional improvement) at 1-year follow-up. There was no difference in the decrease in either score between the two groups. Colon transit time was affected significantly more in the suture rec-topexy group. The ventral mesh rectopexy group preoperatively took a mean of 2.8 days [standard deviation (SD) 1.5] to pass the radio-opaque markers. Their transit time did not increase when measured at 1-year follow-up. This contrasted with the laparoscopic suture posterior rectopexy, when preoperatively the mark-ers took 2.5 days (SD 1.6) to pass, which increased by 1.39 days (95% CI 0.05 to 2.74) at 1-year follow-up. The suture rectopexy group therefore had 1.11 days (95% CI 0.33 to 1.89) added to their transit timed at 1-year in comparison to the ventral mesh rectopexy.

Defecography was also obtained at 1-year follow-up. The posterior suture rec-topexy group had more occurrences of internal intussusception (53% vs. 28%, $p = 0.04$). There was no difference between patients in each arm when comparing incomplete evacuation (48% in the ventral mesh rectopexy, 43% in the posterior suture rectopexy) at 1 year.

Study Limitations   The first and main study limitation is the patient population. It describes a relatively small sample size, with only 75 patients randomized in the trial with 67 following up at 1 year. Comparison between outcomes is therefore limited due to the lack of power in the trial. It was especially not powered to detect nonfunctional outcomes such as prolapse recurrence. The study's outcomes also describe the functional outcomes for patients at a single institution in Northern Europe, which may not extrapolate to other patient populations. This study is also limited in follow-up, with only 1 year of postoperative outcomes reported.

The study also has limitations regarding surgical technique. The authors do not fully describe their posterior rectopexy technique with respect to the lateral rectal attachments. They do not comment on whether they took one or both stalks and whether they closed the peritoneum after their anchoring sutures.

A last group of limitations involves the surgeons. The results speak to the work of three surgeons, but a closer look at the data shows that one surgeon performed two-thirds of the operations. Another limitation is the experience of the three study surgeons in ventral mesh rectopexy. The three surgeons' combined experience prior to the study was 10 ventral mesh rectopexies. This contrasts with learning curves for laparoscopic ventral mesh rectopexy published in literature, where approximately 25–50 cases were needed until operative proficiency (1, 2).

Relevant Studies   Treatment of rectal prolapse continues to remain an area with no definitive evidence to guide surgeons on the best operative treatment. Prior to this study, additional randomized trials had been done. One was the PROSPER trial, which compared abdominal (posterior suture rectopexy versus sigmoid resection with posterior suture rectopexy) and perineal (Altemeier vs. Delorme) approaches. Ventral mesh rectopexy was not a treatment option in the trial design. The study found no differences in recurrence, bowel function, or quality of life between the treatments (3). This study was also limited by statistical power due to a low sample size and limited follow-up. The Swedish Rectal Prolapse Trial, conducted from 2000 to 2009 with results just published in 2022, similarly showed no difference in recurrence (measured at 3 years in the study) but did show that for all procedures, quality of life improved for patients (4). Like the PROSPER trial, ventral mesh rectopexy was not included as a treatment option in the trial design.

Meta-analyses have also been published looking at the best procedure for treating rectal prolapse. A Cochrane review in 2015, which did not include ventral mesh rectopexy, concluded that recurrence rates between abdominal and perineal procedures were similar but acknowledged a large need for trials with long-term follow-up and adequate power (5). A more recent systemic review and meta-analysis in 2021, which did include ventral mesh rectopexy, showed that the difference between recurrence in suture rectopexy versus ventral mesh rectopexy was not significant (6).

Mesh concerns arise when discussing ventral mesh rectopexy. There have been two larger studies looking at long-term mesh outcomes. One observational study that followed 919 patients found mesh-related complications to occur in 4.6% of patients (7). An additional retrospective review looked at over 2000 patients who had undergone ventral mesh rectopexy and found that 2% of the patients had mesh erosion. Of these patients, 51% needed treatment for minor erosion morbidity (such as local excision of a stitch or mesh), and 40% had major erosion morbidity necessitating an operation for mesh explantation (8).

Lastly, long-term follow-up for the main study was limited. This limited follow-up was partially addressed with a recent publication from the same group, where they published their 6-year follow-up outcomes (9). Recurrence of rectal prolapse did not differ, though the study was not powered to detect such a difference. When looking at functional outcomes, the ventral mesh rectopexy group had a significantly lower mean ODS score (6.52) versus the posterior suture rectopexy group (9.5), $p = 0.01$. They also sent out an additional patient survey that they had not measured preoperatively, the Patient Assessment of Quality of Life (PAC-QoL), where the ventral mesh rectopexy group had a significantly lower (better quality of life) score compared to the suture rectopexy group [mean (95% CI) 0.26 (0.14–0.84) vs. 0.93 (0.32–1.61), $p = 0.01$].

Despite many efforts at both observational and randomized trials, there still exists a lack of quality data to help guide surgeons in treatment of rectal prolapse. This lack of data is not due to a lack of trying. Time and time again, adequate patient accruement in these trials has proven difficult, leading to underpowered studies. An alternative method for studying this pathology is needed, such as a large quality improvement registry that tracks patients' functional outcomes. We have had successful initial efforts at such a registry (10), and we encourage others to enroll their patients in similar efforts, so that we can start to provide the evidence-based treatment to our patients that they deserve.

REFERENCES

1. Mackenzie H, Dixon AR. Proficiency gain curve and predictors of outcome for laparoscopic ventral mesh rectopexy. Surgery. 2014 Jul;156(1):158–67.
2. Pucher PH, Mayo D, Dixon AR, Clarke A, Lamparelli MJ. Learning curves and surgical outcomes for proctored adoption of laparoscopic ventral mesh rectopexy: cumulative sum curve analysis. Surgical Endoscopy. 2017 Mar;31(3):1421–6.
3. Senapati A, Gray RG, Middleton LJ, Harding J, Hills RK, Armitage NCM, et al. PROSPER: a randomised comparison of surgical treatments for rectal prolapse. Colorectal Disease. 2013 Jul;15(7):858–68.
4. Smedberg J, Graf W, Pekkari K, Hjern F. Comparison of four surgical approaches for rectal prolapse: multicentre randomized clinical trial. BJS Open. 2022 Jan 6;6(1):zrab140.
5. Tou S, Brown SR, Nelson RL. Surgery for complete (full-thickness) rectal prolapse in adults. Cochrane Database of Systematic Reviews [Internet]. 2015 [cited 2022 Jul 6];(11).

Available from: www.cochranelibrary.com/cdsr/doi/10.1002/14651858.CD001758.pub3/full?highlightAbstract=rectal

6. Lobb HS, Kearsey CC, Ahmed S, Rajaganeshan R. Suture rectopexy *versus* ventral mesh rectopexy for complete full-thickness rectal prolapse and intussusception: systematic review and meta-analysis. BJS Open. 2021 Jan 8;5(1):zraa037.

7. Consten ECJ, van Iersel JJ, Verheijen PM, Broeders IAMJ, Wolthuis AM, D'Hoore A. Long-term outcome after laparoscopic ventral mesh rectopexy: an observational study of 919 consecutive patients. Annals of Surgery. 2015 Nov;262(5):742–8.

8. Evans C, Stevenson ARL, Sileri P, Mercer-Jones MA, Dixon AR, Cunningham C, et al. A multicenter collaboration to assess the safety of laparoscopic ventral rectopexy. Diseases of the Colon & Rectum. 2015 Aug;58(8):799–807.

9. Hidaka J, Elfeki H, Duelund-Jakobsen J, Laurberg S, Lundby L. Functional outcome after laparoscopic posterior sutured rectopexy versus ventral mesh rectopexy for rectal prolapse: six-year follow-up of a double-blind, randomized single-center study. eClinicalMedicine. 2019 Nov;16:18–22.

10. Cavallaro PM, Vogler SA, Hyman NH, Ky AJ, Savitt LR, Tyler KM, et al. Preliminary report from the pelvic floor disorders consortium: large-scale data collection through quality improvement initiatives to provide data on functional outcomes after rectal prolapse repair. Diseases of the Colon & Rectum. 2021 Aug;64(8):986–94.

CHAPTER 2

Efficacy of Sacral Nerve Stimulation for Fecal Incontinence: Results of a Multicenter Double-Blind Crossover Study

Leroi AM, Parc Y, Lehur P-A, et al. Ann Surg 242(5):662–669, 2005 (1)

Reviewed by Natasha G. Caminsky and Marylise Boutros

Research Question/Objective   Sacral nerve stimulation (SNS) is a promising treatment option for fecal incontinence (FI). A lack of understanding of the mechanism of action and a concern for placebo effect in the context of nonrandomized data motivated the authors to conduct a large, randomized trial to assess the efficacy of a permanent SNS implant for patients with FI.

Study Design   This was a randomized, double-blinded, multicenter crossover trial that took place in France over a 3-year period (2000–2003) assessing the efficacy of SNS for the treatment of refractory FI and (including urgency episodes) in patients with an intact rectum, sphincter, and sacral plexus.

The authors had two primary outcomes of interest: *difference in symptom severity* (as measured by the weekly number of incontinence episodes, the delay for postponing defecation, the weekly number of bowel movements, and the Cleveland Clinic Incontinence Score) and *difference in anal manometry* between the month-long on and off periods. Secondary outcomes included quality of life [QoL, measured using the French version of the American Society of Colon and Rectal Surgeons (ASCRS) Quality of Life Questionnaire for FI (FIQL)] and patients' subjective opinion of whether they felt improvement postimplantation, after each 1-month period, and at the end of the final period.

Sample Size   A formal sample size calculation was not provided.

Follow-Up   Patients completed bowel diaries from the time they were enrolled (prior to implantation of the temporary stimulator) until the end of the final 3-month period (see below). They were asked to record episodes of FI, urgency, delay in postponing defecation (amount of time defecation is delayed, measured categorically), and number of bowel movements per week. At the end of the postimplantation period, after each of the two 1-month periods either in ON or OFF phases (crossover period), and at the end of the final 3-month period, patients were also asked to indicate if they felt they had improved in terms of their symptoms.

DOI: 10.1201/9780429285714-2

Inclusion/Exclusion Criteria Patients were included if they had FI to solid or liquid stools or urgency causing them to remain at home to avoid accidents, at least once per week for at least 3 months and attempts at conservative management had failed. Patients with external anal sphincter damage were included only if this was not thought to be the underlying cause of FI [n = 14/34; (i.e., limited defect, 30° or limited to 1 part (superficial, middle, or deep part) of the external anal sphincter]. Patients were also required to have at least an intact bulbo(clitorido)-cavernosus reflex.

Intervention Patients were first implanted with either (1) a temporary percutaneously placed test stimulation lead or (2) a permanent quadripolar lead (stage 1 SNS) for 8–15 days. Permanent implantation of a stimulator was only performed if the temporary stimulation allowed for 50% reduction in incontinence episodes. Only patients who went on to have a permanent stimulator were randomized.

All patients started with their permanent stimulators ON for 1–3 months (see Figure 2.1 "postimplantation period"), during which time the settings were optimized. Patients were then randomized to a 2-month period where they either (1) had their stimulator ON for 1 month, then OFF for 1 month or (2) had their stimulator OFF for 1 month, then ON for 1 month. All patients then spent a "final period" of 3 months in their setting of choice (ON vs. OFF). If a patient did not have a preferred setting, the stimulator was set to ON.

Results

Sampling A total of 34 patients were recruited and had permanent stimulators implanted; however, 7 exited the trial due to: explantation (3 for unresolved pain and 1 for recurrent infections), insufficient treatment response (n = 1), stroke (n = 1), and no response to follow-up (n = 1) (Figure 2.1). This left 27 patients remaining for randomization. After randomization, 3 patients were removed from the trial for protocol violation (bypassed the study settings by using their handheld programmer either to interrupt start stimulation or to increase or decrease stimulation), leaving 24 patients who completed the entire trial period. One of the 24 patients prematurely crossed over from OFF to ON. There were 19/24 (79.2%) patients who remained in the ON setting during the final period because they either voiced a preference for this setting (n = 18) or had no setting preference (n = 1).

Cohort Demographics Demographics were not provided for the subset of patients who were randomized or for the subset who completed the study. Of the initial cohort of 34 patients, 31 (91.2%) were female and the median age was 57. Most patients had incontinence for ≤5 years (n = 24; 70.6%), and the type of incontinence was most commonly classified as urge incontinence (n = 22; 64.7%). The main causes of incontinence were idiopathic (18; 52.9%) and pudendal neuropathy (14; 41.2%). Six patients (17.6%) had undergone previous surgical procedures for pelvic floor disorders (3 sphincter repair, 2 prolapse repair, and 1 pelvic floor repair), and 14 (41.2%) were found to have sphincter defects on pretreatment ultrasound (7 internal anal sphincter, 7 external anal sphincter).

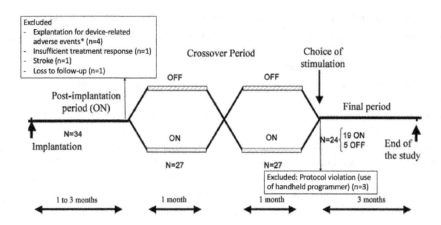

Figure 2.1   Flow diagram of patients through study. (*Source:* Reproduced and annotated with permission from Leroi AM, Parc Y, Lehur PA, Mion F, Barth X, Rullier E, et al. Efficacy of sacral nerve stimulation for fecal incontinence: results of a multicenter double-blind crossover study. Ann Surg. 2005 Nov;242(5):662–669.)

*Device-related adverse events included unresolved pain ($n = 3$) and recurrent infection ($n = 1$).

Outcomes:

1. *Symptom severity*:
   Weekly number of incontinence episodes—There was a significant decrease in median number of FI episodes between ON and OFF periods (1 vs. 2, $p = 0.03$), without evidence of interaction, order, or time effects. There was also a significant decrease in the number of FI episodes from baseline to postimplantation ($p = 0.001$), OFF ($p < 0.05$), and final ($p = 0.005$) periods for the 19 patients who kept their stimulators ON. Of the 19 patients who remained in the ON setting in the final period, 5 (26%) had completely restored continence.
   Weekly number of urgency episodes—There was no difference in the number of urgency episodes between ON and OFF periods or between baseline and OFF periods. There was also no significant difference between baseline and the final period for patients who remained in the ON setting.
   Ability to postpone defecation—There was no difference in the ability to postpone defecation between ON and OFF periods. There was a significant difference in ability to postpone defecation from baseline to all other time points (postimplantation, ON, and OFF periods, $p = 0.01$).
   Weekly number of bowel movements—There was no difference in the number of weekly bowel movements between the ON and OFF periods (10.2 vs. 11.1, $p \geq 0.05$).
   Cleveland Clinic Incontinence Score—There was no significant decrease in the incontinence score between ON and OFF periods (8.5 vs. 10.5, $p = 0.2$); however, there was a significant decrease from baseline to the

postimplantation period (16 vs. 9, $p = 0.0002$). The decrease in incontinence scores between baseline and the ON and OFF periods was statistically significant (90%, $p = 0.0003$ and 76%, $p = 0.001$, respectively). Finally, there was also a significant improvement from baseline to the final period for the patients who remained in the ON setting ($p = 0.0004$). *Anal manometry*—Maximum resting anal pressure was significantly greater in the ON period (50 cm H_2O, $p = 0.02$) and the final period (60 cm H_2O, $p = 0.006$) compared to baseline (40 cm H_2O). There was no significant difference between ON and OFF periods. Maximum squeeze pressure increment was significantly greater in both the ON (53 cm H_2O, $p = 0.004$) and OFF (49 cm H_2O, $p = 0.01$) periods compared to baseline (30 cm, H_2O) and was also significantly improved in the final period compared to baseline (50 cm, H_2O, $p = 0.05$). There were no significant differences between the other manometric measures among the different periods.

2. *QoL (as measured by FIQL)*—Lifestyle, coping/behavior, depression/self-perception, and embarrassment domains all improved significantly between baseline and final values as follows: 1.7 (1–3.8) and 3.2 (1.9–4, $p = 0.001$), 1.5 (1–2.8) and 2.7 (1–4, $p = 0.002$), 2.2 (1–4.1) and 3.6 (1.8–4.2, $p = 0.009$), and 1.3 (1–3) and 2.3 (1–4, $p = 0.002$).

3. *Patients' opinions of whether they felt improved postimplantation*—After completing the ON period, more patients felt they had improved (compared to baseline), compared to when being asked the same question following the OFF period (88.9% vs. 63.0%, $p = 0.02$). After the final period, 17/19 (89.5%) patients who remained in the ON setting felt they had improved compared to baseline ($p = 0.001$).

Complications and mortality: Devices were discontinued in the postimplantation period in 4/34 cases (11.8%; 3 for unresolved pain and 1 for recurrent infection).

Study Limitations This early study on the efficacy of SNS demonstrated that SNS has a positive impact on FI; however, the results still suggest that there is an element of placebo effect. Specifically, when looking at the Cleveland Clinic Score, there is a significant improvement in score postimplantation; however. there is no significant difference between treatment and control groups.

Crossover trials are limited by the risk of aliasing (i.e., carrying over the effect from one treatment period to another). While the authors stated that the significant symptomatic improvement between ON and OFF periods could not be explained by a time effect, there was no washout period between treatment periods. This is even more relevant since certain anal manometry measures were significantly different between periods. The study also states that sphincter damage was an exclusion criterion; however, 14 of the 34 included patients had a sphincter defect. Finally, the short follow-up limits the understanding of the long-term effects of SNS for the treatment of FI from this work.

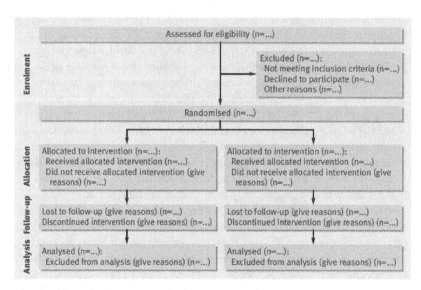

Figure 2.2   CONSORT 2010 flow diagram. (*Source:* Reproduced with permission from Schulz KF, Altman DG, Moher D, the CONSORT Group. CONSORT 2010 Statement: updated guidelines for reporting parallel group randomised trials. BMC Med. 2010 Mar 24;8(1):18.)

The study is also limited by lack of adherence to many elements listed in the CONSORT checklist (2), including lack of a CONSORT diagram (Figure 2.2) that outlines the losses and exclusions (including reason), not stating in the hypothesis that SNS has a placebo effect, lack of trial registration, and not mentioning the allocation ratio, how patients were randomized, how the sample size was calculated *a priori*, or what type of analysis was performed (intention to treat vs. per-protocol). Certain logistics of the study were not described: patient enrollment and bowel diary structure and schedule. The study implied that diaries were used throughout the entirety of the study (6–8 months), whereas typically they are only used for 1–2 weeks in the context of SNS treatment (3). In terms of presenting the results, a table providing the baseline characteristics for each group was not provided (only the initial cohort, prior to randomization, is described) and the effect sizes with the associated intervals was not reported. Finally, the authors did not discuss the generalizability of their study.

Relevant Studies   Since the publication of the study reviewed in this chapter, another crossover study with similar design and sample size was conducted, showing very similar results (4). A large randomized trial was also published in 2010 and demonstrated the efficacy of SNS for FI (5). Other later studies, providing longer follow-up, have also been performed (5–9).

In addition to modulating S3 nerve root impulses, SNS is thought to improve continence by decreasing antegrade colonic motility and increasing retrograde motility (10). Since the publication reviewed in this chapter, other studies have been performed and demonstrated its effectiveness in a broader patient population, namely including patients with low anterior resection syndrome (LARS), incontinence following proctocolectomy and ileal pouch-anal anastomosis, radiation proctitis, and FI caused by sphincter defects up to 120° (11–14).

SNS is not without its complications, including infection (11%), need for revision, lead migration requiring placement, and loss of battery power (13, 15). It also requires two operations (one for efficacy trial and the other to implant a permanent neurostimulator). However, of the treatment options in the middle of the algorithm for the approach to FI (i.e., after conservative management with lifestyle and medication modification and biofeedback and prior to stoma creation), SNS has proven to be the safest and to have the best longevity of results. A study by de Miguel Valencia and colleagues (2022) demonstrated a greater economic burden associated with colostomy versus SNS for FI treatment (16). It is therefore important to continue studying alternative treatments to SNS should it not work for a patient or not be an option to consider in the first place (meets exclusions criteria).

REFERENCES

1. Leroi AM, Parc Y, Lehur PA, Mion F, Barth X, Rullier E, et al. Efficacy of sacral nerve stimulation for fecal incontinence: results of a multicenter double-blind crossover study. Ann Surg. 2005 Nov;242(5):662–9.
2. Schulz KF, Altman DG, Moher D, the CONSORT Group. CONSORT 2010 statement: updated guidelines for reporting parallel group randomised trials. BMC Med. 2010 Mar 24;8(1):18.
3. Carrington EV, Evers J, Grossi U, Dinning PG, Scott SM, O'Connell PR, et al. A systematic review of sacral nerve stimulation mechanisms in the treatment of fecal incontinence and constipation. Neurogastroenterol Motil. 2014 Sep;26(9):1222–37.
4. Kahlke V, Topic H, Peleikis HG, Jongen J. Sacral nerve modulation for fecal incontinence: results of a prospective single-center randomized crossover study. Dis Colon Rectum. 2015 Feb;58(2):235–40.
5. Wexner SD, Coller JA, Devroede G, Hull T, McCallum R, Chan M, et al. Sacral nerve stimulation for fecal incontinence: results of a 120-patient prospective multicenter study. Ann Surg. 2010 Mar;251(3):441–9.
6. Desprez C, Damon H, Meurette G, Mege D, Faucheron JL, Brochard C, et al. Ten-year evaluation of a large retrospective cohort treated by sacral nerve modulation for fecal incontinence: results of a French multicenter study. Ann Surg. 2022 Apr;275(4):735–42.
7. Hull T, Giese C, Wexner SD, Mellgren A, Devroede G, Madoff RD, et al. Long-term durability of sacral nerve stimulation therapy for chronic fecal incontinence. Dis Colon Rectum. 2013 Feb;56(2):234–45.
8. Matzel KE, Lux P, Heuer S, Besendörfer M, Zhang W. Sacral nerve stimulation for faecal incontinence: long-term outcome. Colorectal Dis. 2009 Jul;11(6):636–41.
9. Šlauf P, Vobořil R. Sacral neuromodulation for faecal incontinence—10 years experience and long-term outcomes of a specialized centre. Rozhl Chir. 2021;100(10):475–83.

10. Patton V, Wiklendt L, Arkwright JW, Lubowski DZ, Dinning PG. The effect of sacral nerve stimulation on distal colonic motility in patients with faecal incontinence. Br J Surg. 2013 Jun;100(7):959–68.

11. Ramage L, Qiu S, Kontovounisios C, Tekkis P, Rasheed S, Tan E. A systematic review of sacral nerve stimulation for low anterior resection syndrome. Colorectal Dis. 2015 Sep;17(9):762–71.

12. Johnson BL, Abodeely A, Ferguson MA, Davis BR, Rafferty JF, Paquette IM. Is sacral neuromodulation here to stay? Clinical outcomes of a new treatment for fecal incontinence. J Gastrointest Surg. 2015 Jan;19(1):15–9; discussion 19–20.

13. Thin NN, Horrocks EJ, Hotouras A, Palit S, Thaha MA, Chan CLH, et al. Systematic review of the clinical effectiveness of neuromodulation in the treatment of faecal incontinence. Br J Surg. 2013 Oct;100(11):1430–47.

14. Seifarth C, Slavova N, Degro C, Lehmann KS, Kreis ME, Weixler B. Sacral nerve stimulation in patients with ileal pouch-anal anastomosis. Int J Colorectal Dis. 2021 Sep;36(9):1937–43.

15. Zbar AP. Sacral neuromodulation and peripheral nerve stimulation in patients with anal incontinence: an overview of techniques, complications and troubleshooting. Gastroenterol Rep. 2014 May;2(2):112–20.

16. de Miguel Valencia MJ, Margallo Lana A, Pérez Sola MÁ, Sánchez Iriso E, Cabasés Hita JM, Alberdi Ibáñez I, et al. Economic burden of long-term treatment of severe fecal incontinence. Cir Esp. 2022 Jul;100(7):422–30.

CHAPTER 3

PROSPER: A Randomised Comparison of Surgical Treatments for Rectal Prolapse

Senapati A, Gray RG, Middleton LJ, Harding J, Hills RK, Armitage NC, Buckley L, Northover JM. PROSPER Collaborative Group. Colorectal Dis. 15(7):858–868, 2013

Reviewed by Emily Steinhagen

Research Question/Objective   Rectal prolapse is a surgical problem that is not well understood or described. There are no reliable estimates regarding its prevalence, and the number of procedures performed for prolapse annually is not known. Many different procedures can be used to address prolapse both from the abdominal approach and through perineal procedures. Limited high-quality data are available to compare the risks and benefits of the various procedures for rectal prolapse. A 2008 Cochrane review had only 380 patients in 12 randomized studies[1] with variations in inclusion criteria and procedures performed. The aim of the PROSPER study was to create high-quality evidence comparing procedures for rectal prolapse that include longer follow-up and patient-related outcomes.

Study Design   PROSPER is a multicenter prospective, randomized trial that the authors describe as pragmatic and factorial. Patients could be randomized to either abdominal or perineal surgery and then, within their groups, randomized to either suture rectopexy or resection and rectopexy for the abdominal group and to either the Altemeier or Delorme procedure for the perineal surgery group. Once patients were enrolled, surgeons could opt out at either the first or second randomization and select patients to be in either the abdominal or perineal group but then randomized within that group in the second step of randomization. Randomization was performed electronically, controlling for age, level of incontinence, and preoperative physiologic status. A mentoring system was in place for surgeons who lacked experience with any of the techniques, and a video was provided to assist in training. Abdominal procedures could be performed open or laparoscopically.

The primary outcome was recurrence of prolapse. The other outcomes were inconvenience, bowel function, and quality of life as measured by Vaizey incontinence score[2] and EuroQol Group 5-Dimension Self-Report Questionnaire (EQ-5D).[3] The Vaizey incontinence score ranges from 0 (perfect) to 24 (totally incontinent), and the EQ-5D scores range from −0.59 (worst state) to 1.0 (perfect health). The study design included a follow-up duration of 3 years. The other outcome measures that were collected included morbidity and mortality, overall

DOI: 10.1201/9780429285714-3

bowel function on a 0–100 scale, frequency of bowel motions, straining, incomplete emptying, use of laxatives, suppositories, and enemas, and resource use. The assessments were done by clinicals at 6 weeks, 1 year, and 3 years after surgery. In addition, patients were mailed a modified questionnaire for self-completions. The research team attempted to contact patients by letters and phone if they did not return questionnaires.

The PROSPER study was powered to detect a 5% difference in recurrence, set at 10% versus 5% between the abdominal procedures and perineal procedures; this would have required 950 patients. However, this was later decreased to 300 patients due to slow enrollment. The aim was also revised from comparing recurrences to detecting meaningful difference in quality of life or Vaizey scores. and the new power analysis required 230 patients to detect a 0.37 standard deviation, considered a moderate to small difference with 80% power. The revised recruitment target would only enable detection of large differences in recurrence rates. The analyses were performed on an intention-to-treat basis. Scores on the quality of life measures were analyzed with inclusion of covariant including baseline scores. Recurrence rates were used to create Kaplan–Meier plots that were censored by last follow-up date or form completed or by date of death, withdrawal, or loss of follow-up.

Sample Size   The study enrolled 293 patients over 7 years. They were recruited from 30 centers in the UK, and 1 each in India, Serbia, Spain, and Finland.

Follow-Up   The authors planned to follow the patients at 6 weeks, 1 year, and 3 years with a clinician but had provisions to mail surveys for other patients who did not come for in-person follow-up.

The research team attempted to contact patients by letters and phone if they did not return questionnaires.

Inclusion/Exclusion Criteria   The inclusion criteria for this study was full-thickness rectal prolapse. The protocol states that patients should have a rigid sigmoidoscopy; all other studies are at the discretion of the operating surgeon. No exclusion criteria are noted in the protocol or the manuscript.

Intervention or Treatment Received   There were 49 patients who were randomized in step 1, abdominal versus perineal approach. For the remainder, the surgeon selected the approach and then they were randomized within the approach for step 2 only. For those undergoing perineal procedures, 213 patients were randomized between the Altemeier and Delorme procedures; in the group that underwent abdominal procedures, 78 were randomized between suture and resection rectopexy. Of these 293 randomized patients, 270 underwent surgery and 91% underwent the assigned procedure.

Results Patients who underwent perineal procedures were older and were described as having worse physical status and bowel function preoperatively. The average age for patients who were assigned by their surgeons to abdominal versus perineal procedures was 73 years for perineal procedures and 58 for abdominal procedures. Of the patients who were randomized between abdominal and perineal procedures, the median age was 63.

In terms of recurrences, in the perineal group, the rate of recurrence after Altemeier was 24% compared with 31% for Delorme, but this was not statistically significant (HR 0.81; 95% CI 0.47–1.38, $p = 0.4$). In the abdominal group, recurrence after resection rectopexy was 13% compared with 26% after resection rectopexy; again, this was not statistically significant (HR 0.45; 95% CI 0.14–1.45, $p = 0.2$). When comparing between abdominal and perineal procedures, there were no differences in recurrence between the group; 19% after abdominal procedures compared with 28% after perineal procedures ($p = 0.2$).

For patients who underwent perineal procedures, there were improvements in Vaizey incontinence, bowel function, and EQ-5D scores from baseline to 6 weeks, and this was maintained at 1 and 3 years. The two perineal procedures, Altemeier and Delorme, did not differ in the degree of improvement. The only measure that differed between the two groups was the number of outpatient hospital visits at 6 weeks and 3 years.

Similarly, patients who underwent abdominal procedures had improvements in Vaizey incontinence, bowel function, and EQ-5D scores from baseline to 6 weeks, and this was maintained at 1 and 3 years. No differences were detected between the suture rectopexy and the resection rectopexy groups. The only measure that had a difference between the groups during follow-up was more laxative use in the suture rectopexy group.

When comparing the abdominal procedures to perineal procedures, there were no differences between the groups with all having improvement from baseline in the primary end points. There were a few differences in the secondary end points, with more patients in the abdominal group reporting straining at 1 and 3 years follow-up), more visits by a social worker at 6 weeks, and patients spending more time in a hospital and visiting their general practitioner at 1 year.

Patients who experienced recurrence had much lower EQ-5D scores at 1 year than those who did not (0.23 points; 95% CI 0.10–0.37, $p = 0.0009$).

There were 5 treatment-related deaths in the study; the 4 who died following a perineal procedure (1 each) died of myocardial infarction, chest infection/renal failure, sepsis due to anastomotic leak, and a ruptured aortic aneurysm on postoperative day 2. There was 1 death in the abdominal group; a patient randomized to resection rectopexy who received suture rectopexy had peritonitis and died.

Anastomotic leaks occurred in 4 patients who underwent Altemeier, including 1 who had been randomized to Delorme. Three of the 4 were men from a single center.

Study Limitations   There were significant difficulties in accruing patients to this study, and the initial aims and enrollment targets were modified. Ultimately, while they were able to accrue enough patients to meet the revised target and aims, this limitation prevented the authors from creating the type of high-quality evidence they had hoped to produce that would enable guidance for surgeons who treat rectal prolapse.

Surgical technique was not standardized, and there was no minimum experience required of participating surgeons for each operation. It is possible that surgeons could have performed a procedure that they either never or rarely performed in the context of this trial. This is of particular importance with Altemeier procedure. Though the study initially aimed to compare abdominal to perineal procedures, the design of the study made it possible for the surgeon to select the approach and randomize within it. The groups were different in terms of age and functional status, but other important differences leading to patient selection for each are likely not captured in this dataset.

Recurrence after rectal prolapse surgery was a primary end point in this study but was not well-defined. It could be that mucosal prolapse was considered by some participating clinicians and that self-reporting may have been inaccurate in some cases.

The design of this study was complex and aimed to answer several questions within the same study: recurrence rates and quality-of-life measures were both assessed, and comparisons between and within procedure types were also made. This created a difficult setup for analysis for the study authors.

Relevant Studies   PROSPER was an ambitious study that aimed to provide important clinical guidance in an area with equipoise after many lower-quality studies. Four procedures were included, and the study aimed to randomize patients. However, surgeons were able to specify abdominal or perineal procedures, and their level of comfort with each procedure was not equal. This introduced a significant amount of bias in procedure assignment and potential confounding. However, it does give us more evidence that perhaps there are no clear clinical differences between the many procedures for rectal prolapse.

It is important to recognize that the PROSPER study has high recurrence rates, 24–31% for perineal procedures and 13–26% for abdominal procedures. This is higher than most other studies but may be due to diligent follow-up that is a more accurate assessment than other retrospective studies. On the other hand, it could be due to surgeons performing procedures that are relatively rare for them and that this impacted success. In general, retrospective studies have demonstrated that abdominal approaches have one-fourth the recurrence rates as perineal surgeries, but multiple Cochrane reviews have not found differences when meta-analysis was used.[1,4,5]

Concurrent to the PROSPER study, the Swedish Rectal Prolapse Trial was conducted from 2000 to 2009.[6] Overall, there are striking similarities between the trials both in study design and outcomes. In this randomized, multicenter trial, participants were similarly assigned to either abdominal or perineal surgery and then, within those randomizations, to Delorme or Altemeier or to suture or resection rectopexy. As in PROSPER, the first randomization step was not required to participate; surgeon discretion could be used to assign procedure type. In this study, 134 patients were randomized, and the median follow-up was 2.6 years. The authors noted improvements in Wexner and RAND-36 incontinence scores in all patients but no significant differences between the groups. Recurrence rates between the groups were different between the approaches, but none achieved statistical significance. Similarly, this study had difficulty recruiting their target sample size of 220 patients and was therefore somewhat underpowered. Both these studies underscore the fact that surgeons often have a preference for abdominal or perineal operations for individual patients, even in the absence of evidence to support patient selection.

Subsequent to PROSPER, another Cochrane review in 2015 was published that included three trial types: abdominal compared to perineal approaches (43 patients), rectopexy compared to resection rectopexy (115 patients), and Delorme compared with Altemeier procedure (201 patients).[5] The pooled analysis did not show significant differences in recurrence rates between abdominal and perineal approaches. Others have assessed complication rates after perineal and abdominal procedures for prolapse. Although these rates may be that due to the randomization scheme in PROSPER, surgeon bias about assigning less healthy patients to perineal procedures confirmed the same findings in the retrospective studies that have previously been utilized to draw conclusions on this topic. For example, a study of the National Surgical Quality Improvement Project suggested that the morbidity and mortality of the perineal approach is underestimated and may in fact be higher than abdominal approaches, likely due to patient selection for each approach.[7]

Since PROSPER was designed, the ventral mesh rectopexy (VMR) procedure has become increasingly popular for rectal prolapse. Some prospective trials, such as one with 120 patients that compared VMR with pelvic organ suspension, only followed patients for 6 months but showed no significant differences in function or complications[8] and another comparing suture rectopexy to VMR with 75 patients, again showing no major differences in functional outcomes.[9] There was also a study of 75 patients comparing Delorme, which was the most common perineal procedure in the PROSPER study, to VMR and again was unable to demonstrate superiority of either procedure (Emile). There are even fewer studies that include long-term follow-up to assess recurrence, but again it is difficult to detect differences between techniques.[10] A systematic review that compared posterior rectal dissection and rectopexy to VMR suggested a recurrence rate of 3.4% and a weighted decrease in postoperative constipation rate estimated to be 23% among VMR patients.[11]

While PROSPER was ultimately not successful in achieving its aims in definitively answering the questions about procedure selection for patients with rectal prolapse, it helps create space for the next set of questions about how surgeons and patients decide on a specific procedure.

REFERENCES

1. Tou S, Brown SR, Malik AI, et al. Surgery for complete rectal prolapse in adults. *Cochrane Database of Systematic Reviews*. Epub ahead of print 2008. DOI: 10.1002/14651858. CD001758.pub2.
2. Vaizey CJ, Carapeti E, Cahill JA, et al. Prospective comparison of faecal incontinence grading systems. *Gut*. 1999;44. DOI: 10.1136/gut.44.1.77.
3. EuroQol Group. EuroQol—a new facility for the measurement of health-related quality of life. *Health Policy (New York)*. 1990;16. DOI: 10.1016/0168-8510(90)90421-9.
4. Bordeianou L, Paquette I, Johnson E, et al. Clinical practice guidelines for the treatment of rectal prolapse. *Diseases of the Colon & Rectum*. 2017;60:1121–1131.
5. Tou S, Brown SR, Nelson RL. Surgery for complete (full-thickness) rectal prolapse in adults. *Cochrane Database of Systematic Reviews*. Epub ahead of print 2015. DOI: 10.1002/14651858.CD001758.pub3.
6. Smedberg J, Graf W, Pekkari K, et al. Comparison of four surgical approaches for rectal prolapse: multicentre randomized clinical trial. *BJS Open*. 2022;6. DOI: 10.1093/bjsopen/zrab140.
7. Fang SH, Cromwell JW, Wilkins KB, et al. Is the abdominal repair of rectal prolapse safer than perineal repair in the highest risk patients? An NSQIP analysis. *Diseases of the Colon & Rectum*. 2012;55:1167–1172.
8. Farag A, Mashhour AN, Raslan M, et al. Laparoscopic pelvic organ prolapse suspension (Pops) versus laparoscopic ventral mesh rectopexy for treatment of rectal prolapse: prospective cohort study. *World Journal of Surgery*. 2020;44:3158–3166.
9. Lundby L, Iversen LH, Buntzen S, et al. Bowel function after laparoscopic posterior sutured rectopexy versus ventral mesh rectopexy for rectal prolapse: a double-blind, randomised single-centre study. *The Lancet Gastroenterology and Hepatology*. 2016;1:291–297.
10. Madbouly KM, Mohii AD. Laparoscopic ventral rectopexy versus stapled transanal rectal resection for treatment of obstructed defecation in the elderly: long-term results of a prospective randomized study. *Diseases of the Colon & Rectum*. 2019;62:47–55.
11. Samaranayake CB, Luo C, Plank AW, et al. Systematic review on ventral rectopexy for rectal prolapse and intussusception. *Colorectal Disease*. 2010;12:504–512.

CHAPTER 4

New Operation for Rectal Prolapse

Wells C. Proc R Soc Med. 52(8):602–603, 1959

Reviewed by Steven D. Wexner

Research Question/Objective   Rectal prolapse occurs when the upper rectum descends through the anus. It can involve the entire circumference or part of the rectal wall. It is a common condition that mainly affects older women after childbirth. Since this condition is caused mostly due to anatomical and functional changes in the pelvic floor, the standard treatment of care is surgical repair.[1] Over the years, there have been multiple reports about different surgical techniques. The large number of options and variations in outcomes is attestation to the lack of a panacea operation.[2] In this study, published by Dr. Wells, a surgeon from Liverpool in 1959, he aimed to describe his success rates using a novel surgical technique for the treatment of rectal prolapse, with a polyvinyl alcohol sponge (Ivalon®) used for rectal fixation.[3] It was one of the first descriptions of the use of implantable foreign matter for organ fixation, based on a study conducted at the Mayo Clinic on dogs a few years before by Schofield et al.[4] In that study, the authors induced abdominal wall defects in 7 dogs and used the Ivalon® sponge to close the defect. After 12 weeks, no signs of hernia were seen in all dogs. Based on these encouraging findings, Prof. Wells used the Ivalon® sponge to fix the rectum to the sacrum in patients suffering from rectal prolapse.

Study Design   The study was a letter sent to the Proceedings of the Royal Society of Medicine, the journal of one of the most prestigious and oldest medical societies in the world.[5] In his letter, Prof. Wells retrospectively described and illustrated his experience with 15 procedures in which he used the Ivalon® sponge for rectal fixation. (Figure 4.1).

Sample Size   Prof. Wells mentioned that he had performed this procedure "15 times over a period of 5 years," although it is not clear whether it was done in 15 patients or if the procedure was repeated in certain patients. He stated that "about half" of the patients suffered from recurrent rectal prolapse, although no details about previous surgical procedure were provided in the manuscript.

Follow-Up   There are no data on follow-up of patients, other than reporting "complete resolution" in all patients.

Inclusion/Exclusion Criteria   No inclusion/exclusion criteria were mentioned in the manuscript.

DOI: 10.1201/9780429285714-4

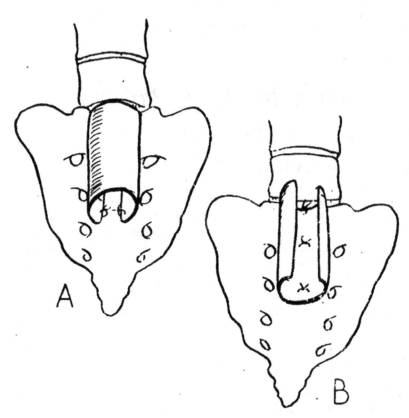

Figure 4.1   (A) Sketch of Ivalon® sponge attached by its free margins to the hollow of the sacrum to form a tunnel. (B) Sketch of Ivalon® sponge attached to the hollow of the sacrum to form a trough.

Intervention or Treatment Received   Surgical repair of rectal prolapse using Ivalon® sponge for rectal fixation.

Results   Prof. Wells reported "complete resolution" of the rectal prolapse in all patients, adding that all patients remained continent following the procedure. Furthermore, he mentioned that, in "two or three" women who also suffered from vaginal prolapse, that did not justify a separate procedure. The latter problem was also resolved after rectal fixation. The author mentioned one patient who required an additional abdominal surgery for unrelated reasons, reporting that the Ivalon® repair was intact with no overlying adhesions. One of the main parts of this report is the detailed description of the procedure, starting with the creation of a flap from the peritoneal covering of the rectum, dissecting along the upper rectum between the prostate/vagina. The rectum is engulfed by the Ivalon® sheet, attaching it first to the sacral promontory and then down to the upper part of the rectum. The rectum is subsequently retracted upward, and the Ivalon® sheet is fixed with sutures. The final step of the procedure includes closing the peritoneal flap to cover the Ivalon® sheet.

Study Limitations This is a retrospective series detailing the experience of a single surgeon with no long-term follow-up and a lack in reporting postoperative outcomes.

Relevant Studies In order to understand the importance of this manuscript, we must closely examine the evidence gathered in regard to rectal prolapse repair prior to the publication of this letter. The author mentioned in the first line of his letter—"I have traced in the literature between 30 and 50 operations for prolapse of the rectum."[3] This statement reflects an issue to which surgeons can still relate, as there remains an abundance of surgical techniques used to treat rectal prolapse.[2] The main reason for this variability is that no technique showed complete resolution without recurrence, and therefore no method reached gold standard status.[6]

Prof. Wells, a prominent surgeon from Liverpool, has endorsed the concept that was first described by Moschowitz in 1912 and was later accepted as the main theory—that rectal prolapse is the result of a sliding hernia of the anterior wall of the rectum at the level of the cul-de-sac of Douglas.[7] Therefore, the peritoneal hernia sac must be opened and the pelvic fascia must be strengthened in order to sustain the rectum in its fixed position. In his letter, Prof. Wells mentions previous attempts by Graham (1942)[8] and Goligher (1958)[9] to repair the sliding pelvis with direct peritoneal sutures. However, Prof. Wells describes this procedure as difficult, which led him to try the use of a "prosthesis"—the Ivalon® sponge.

Looking at the evidence that existed prior to the publication by Prof. Wells, there was only one report about the use of a prosthesis to fix the prolapsed rectum. The Orr procedure, described in 1947 by Dr. Thomas Orr, a surgeon from Kansas City, used strips of fascia lata on both sides of the rectum, fixating it to the dense fascia above the sacral promontory along with obliteration of the cul-de-sac.[10] The report by Prof. Wells is actually one of the earliest descriptions in the use of foreign material as a prothesis, opening the way for the implementation and widespread use of mesh and other products for fixation of the prolapsed rectum. This approach, although using other materials than those used by Prof. Wells, has since become the standard treatment for the majority of patients who undergo surgery for rectal prolapse.

The Wells procedure with the Ivalon® sponge was popular among surgeons until the 1990s when studies showed an increased risk for developing sarcomas in laboratory animals.[11,12] Nonetheless, the few reports about the surgical outcomes of the procedure showed that the recurrence rate was low and that most patients remained continent following the procedure.[13–16]

To conclude, the technique described by Prof. Wells, which can only be performed transabdominally, revolutionized the surgical approach to patients with rectal prolapse. Prior to his accomplished description, rectal prolapse repair was largely a transperineal procedure. Prof. Wells' letter laid the groundwork for the increasing use of transabdominal approaches and protheses for fixation of the rectum, both of which are currently preferred options.

REFERENCES

1. Madiba TE, Baig MK, Wexner SD. Surgical management of rectal prolapse. Arch Surg. 2005;140(1):63–73.
2. Tou S, Brown SR, Malik AI, Nelson RL. Surgery for complete rectal prolapse in adults. Cochrane Database Syst Rev. 2008;(4):CD001758.
3. Wells C. New operation for rectal prolapse. J R Soc Med. 1959;52(8):602–3.
4. Schofield TL, Hallenbeck GA, Grindlay JH, Baldes EJ. Use of polyvinyl sponge in repair of experimentally produced defects in the abdominal wall. Arch Surg. 1954;68(2):191–207.
5. Hunting P. The royal society of medicine. Postgrad Med J. 2005;81(951):45–8.
6. Goldstein SD, Maxwell IV PJ. Rectal prolapse. Clinic Colon Rectal Surg. 2011;24:39–45.
7. Moschcowitz AV. The pathogenesis, anatomy, and cure of prolapse of the rectum. Surg Gynecol Obstet. 1912;15:7–21.
8. Graham RR. Operative repair of massive rectal prolapse. Ann Surg. 1942;115(6):1007–14.
9. Goligher JC. The treatment of complete prolapse of the rectum by the Roscoe Graham operation. Br J Surg. 1958;45(192):323–33.
10. Orr TG. A suspension operation for prolapse of the rectum. Ann Surg. 1947;126(5):833.
11. Walter JB, Chiaramonte LG. The tissue responses of the rat to implanted Ivalon, etheron, and polyfoam plastic sponges. Br J Surg. 1965 Jan;52:49–54.
12. Dukes CE, Mitchley BC. Polyvinyl sponge implants: experimental and clinical observations. Br J Plast Surg. 1962;15:225–35.
13. Vongsangnak V, Varma JS, Watters D, Smith AN. Clinical, manometric and surgical aspects of complete prolapse of the rectum. J R Coll Surg Edinb. 1985;30(4):251–4.
14. Penfold JCB, Hawley PR. Experiences of Ivalon-sponge implant for complete rectal prolapse at St. Mark's Hospital, 1960–70. Br J Surg. 1972;59(11):846–8.
15. Morgan CN, Porter NH, Klugman DJ. Ivalon (polyvinyl alcohol) sponge in the repair of complete rectal prolapse. Br J Surg. 1972;59(11):841–6.
16. Calne RY. Papers [abridged]: Ivalon wrap operation for rectal prolapse. J R Soc Med. 1966;59(2):127–8.

CHAPTER 5

Role of Circumferential Resection Margin Involvement in the Local Recurrence of Rectal Cancer

Adam IJ, Mohamdee MO, Martin IG, Scott N, Finan PJ, Johnston D, Dixon MF, Quirke P. Lancet. 344:707–711, 1994

Reviewed by James Fleshman

Research Question/Objective   The surgical treatment of rectal cancer involves operating in a narrow boney box with numerous critical structures at risk that will affect patient function and well-being. The removal of a rectal cancer for cure was felt to be related only to removing the rectum containing the tumor without regard to the surrounding fat, lymphatics, or embryologic envelope that fills the pelvis outside the rectum itself. This intramesorectal dissection provided protection against injury to genitourinary structures, sacral venous plexus, and sexual nerves. The cost of this protective approach was a high local recurrence rate even after an intended curative resection of a rectal cancer. This is in contradistinction to the resection of colon cancer, which has a very low local recurrence rate because of the ability to perform a wider anatomic resection. The aim of this study was to determine the frequency of resection margin positivity after resection of a rectal cancer and the impact of a positive circumferential resection margin on local recurrence of the tumor and patient cancer-specific survival. The concept was simple, but the controversy surrounding the idea that surgical technique was inadequate was profound. Dr. Phil Quirke and his colleagues reinforced the concept that data based on patient outcomes are essential to determining whether a surgical procedure is successful.

Study Design   The study was a prospective cohort study of all patients undergoing proctectomy for rectal cancer at the Leeds General Infirmary from 1985 to 1990. No preoperative staging other than biopsy-proven adenocarcinoma was mentioned. There was no mention of investigational review board approval. The proctectomy specimen was evaluated by the pathology department in every case using a "bread loaf" transverse slicing technique to produce coronal sections through the fixed rectum and attached mesorectum (1). For the first time, this allowed determination of the distance of the closest tumor cells to the circumferential resection margin at the level of the tumor mass and in the mesorectum proximal to the tumor where involved lymph nodes or tumor deposits might be near the circumferential resection margin. Tumor cells found that 1 mm or less from the circumferential

DOI: 10.1201/9780429285714-5

margin was considered an involved margin. The patients were followed for a minimum of 3 years to determine the frequency of local recurrence and survival.

A multivariate analysis of numerous pathological variables, including circumferential margin positivity, extramural venous invasion [now considered on magnetic resonance imaging (MRI) as prognostic indicator for rectal cancer], tumor thickness, lymph node involvement, histologic grade, lymphatic invasion, apical lymph node positivity, and distal margin positivity, was performed to determine factors that significantly influenced recurrence and survival. Kaplan Meier cancer-specific survival curves were compared to determine differences in survival based on Dukes staging and margin positivity. We are not told the definition of the rectum, the distance of the tumor from the anal verge, or its relationship to the anterior peritoneal reflection to distinguish between colon and rectum.

Sample Size   The number of patients included was not predetermined by sample size calculation for significance. Since this was a prospective cohort study without randomization, the volume of patients with rectal cancer was determined by the incidence of rectal cancer within the local National Health System (NHS) patient population. A total of 190 patients underwent surgical resection of rectal cancer during a 5-year period between 1985 and 1990 at the Leeds General Infirmary, which trained residents with an academic faculty having NHS appointments. The operation was intended for cure (R0 resection) in 141 patients and for palliation in 23 patients in whom obvious tumor was left in the pelvis (R1 resection). The remaining 28 patients were excluded from analysis due to perioperative mortality (11), receiving preoperative or postoperative radiation because this would impact the recurrence rate (14), or loss to follow-up (3).

Follow-Up   Patients were followed for at least 3 years with a median follow-up of 5.3 years (3.0–7.7 years). The patients were not followed with surveillance protocol as they are today but had routine office visits with the surgeon and primary care physicians who only investigated symptoms of recurrence. Only 1 surgeon actively looked for recurrence, and he had the lowest local recurrence rate. One could speculate that he also performed some of the best surgical resections. Survival data were derived from general practitioner notes, and all information was cross-referenced against the Yorkshire Regional Cancer Organization records. Local recurrence was defined as biopsy-proven or radiographic findings of tumor in the pelvis.

Inclusion/Exclusion Criteria   All patients with rectal cancer presenting to the Leeds General Infirmary were considered for inclusion. Patients were excluded if they received radiation before or after surgery. Patients lost to follow-up or who died in the immediate postoperative period were excluded from analysis.

Treatment Received   Rectal cancer was resected with proctectomy with colorectal anastomosis reconstruction (82), abdominoperineal resection with colostomy (95), Hartmann's procedure with colostomy (proctectomy with rectal stump) (9), or transanal local excision (4). No radiation was utilized.

Results The 141 patients treated for cure with R0 resection (no macroscopic tumor left in pelvis) were analyzed separately from the 26 patients who underwent palliative resection (R1). Pathologic positive resection margins were found in 35 of 141 patients resected with R0 operation (25%). Local recurrence occurred in 23 (66%) of those patients. This most likely represents microscopic disease in the mesorectum. Clear pathologic margins after an R0 resection yielded only 9 out of 106 (8%) local recurrence. This most likely represents lymphatic spread to pelvic side wall or drop metastasis. Current literature shows 4% local recurrence after total mesorectal excision with or without neoadjuvant chemoradiotherapy (2). That this markedly reduced the local recurrence rate for patients with a good operation was convincing data to stimulate surgeons all over Europe and eventually the United States to make the change to an embryologic plane dissection of the mesorectum and removal of the rectum within its mesorectal package. It eventually led to education of pathologists in a more standardized evaluation of the rectum and mesorectum with the "breadloafing" technique and of the surgeons to utilize an avascular embryologic plane to retrieve all of the pelvic tissue at risk for rectal cancer spread (3).

Palliative operations, which resulted in macroscopically positive margins (R1), yielded a local recurrence rate of 62% (39 out of 49). However, a palliative resection that resulted in clear pathologic margins yielded only 13% local recurrence. The same principles of pelvic dissection used in resection for cure should therefore apply to palliation since local recurrence leads to a very miserable death.

Survival was adversely affected by positive resection margins for patients with rectal tumors invading through the rectal wall (Dukes B) and tumors with accompanying lymph node metastasis (Dukes C). Surgical clearance of cancer does make a difference. Multivariate analysis confirmed that lymph node involvement with tumor, an infiltrating tumor margin (extramural venous invasion), and circumferential resection margin involvement independently influence poor survival and higher local recurrence. This was the first study to firmly relate local recurrence and poor survival to involved resection margins. Resection margins are related to surgical technique and tumor behavior. We now know that surgical technique with complete mesorectal excision, even if performed minimally invasively, is the major determining factor of success (4).

Limitations The main limitation of this study is the absence of standardization of surgical technique among the 23 different surgeons. However, the issue of technique is the major finding from the study. Fortunately, relating the involvement of the resection margin to technique and to both local recurrence and survival substantiates the importance of surgical technique in the outcome of patients with rectal cancer. Professor R.J. "Bill" Heald taught us that surgeons can improve our resection technique if the embryologic plane outside the mesorectal fat is followed in the pelvic dissection to remove all of the mesorectum and rectum, with the fascial envelope intact (5).

Positive resection margins after a well performed total mesorectal excision may be due to an aggressive tumor invading into the mesorectum toward the mesorectal fascia. This study was not designed to identify those aggressive tumors and their threat to the mesorectal fascia. Photography of the whole mesorectal specimen was not added to the pathologic evaluation until much later. The Leeds pathologists in 1986 suggested poor surgery as a possible cause of local recurrence and produced images of mesorectal violation that indicated no thought to including the fat or lymphatics of the mesorectum in the resected specimen (6). Even so, this study did not comment on the quality of the mesorectal specimen that is now the backbone of pathologic evaluation of a rectal cancer resection specimen, along with the closest circumferential resection margin. Photography and grading of the mesorectal specimen is now considered standard of care in the Commission on Cancer National Accreditation Program for Rectal Cancer (7). The standard technique applied to surgeon training has subsequently been shown in numerous trials to reduce local recurrence to less than 4% and improve the survival for patients with curable rectal cancer.

Documentation of rectal cancer staging, local recurrence, or cancer-related mortality was not performed in this study using present-day methods. Preoperative staging with rectal cancer protocol magnetic resonance imaging is now considered standard of care and will guide the use of neoadjuvant therapy and wider resection of pelvic tissue as needed. Rectal cancer protocol MRI provides a very accurate preoperative look at the depth of tumor invasion, identifies involved lymph nodes and extramural venous invasion within the mesorectum, and guides the decisions for radical resection, neoadjuvant therapy, and warns of threatened circumferential resection margins (8). The absence of this information preoperatively would possibly lead to underestimation of the possibility and impact of positive resection margins. Earlier detection of recurrence might have reduced the associated morbidity and mortality by use of adjuvant chemoradiation and reoperation. Finally, it is interesting to look back knowing the answer, or, in other words, "hindsight" is always clearer.

REFERENCES

1. Quirke P, Durdey P, Dixon MF, Williams NS. Local recurrence of rectal adenocarcinoma due to inadequate surgical resection: histopathological study of lateral tumor spread and surgical excision. Lancet 1986; 2: 996–99.
2. Quirke P, Steele R, Monson J, et al.; MRC CR07/NCIC-CTG Trial Investigators; NCRI Colorectal Cancer Study Group. Effect of the plane of surgery on local recurrence in patients with operable rectal cancer: a prospective study using data from the MRC CR07 and NCIC-CTG CO16 randomized clinical trial. Lancet 2009; 373: 821–28.
3. McFarlane JK, Ryall RDH, Heald RJ. Mesorectal excision for rectal cancer. Lancet 1993; 341: 457–60.

4. Fleshman JW, Branda ME, Sargent DJ, et al. Disease-free survival and local recurrence for laparoscopic resection compared with open resection of stage II to III rectal cancer: follow-up results of the ACOSOG Z6051 randomized controlled trial. Ann Surg. 2019; 269: 589–95.

5. Heald RJ, Ryall RD. Recurrence and survival after total mesorectal excision of rectal cancer. Lancet 1986; i: 1479–82.

6. Quirke P, Dixon MF. How do I do it: the prediction of local recurrence in rectal adenocarcinoma by histopathological examination. Int J Colon Dis. 1988; 3: 579–88.

7. Optimal Resources for Rectal Cancer Care. American College of Surgeons and the Commission on Cancer, National Accreditation Program for Rectal Cancer. July 2020. Facs.org/naprc. Standard 5.10 Photographs of Surgical Specimens, p. 37.

8. Chand M, Siddiqui MR, Brown G. Systematic review of prognostic importance of extramural venous invasion in rectal cancer. World J Gastroenterol. 2016; 22(4): 1721–26.

Preoperative versus Postoperative Chemoradiotherapy for Rectal Cancer

Sauer R, Becker H, Hohenberger W, et al. New England Journal of Medicine. 351(17):1731–1740, 2004

Reviewed by Janet Alvarez and J. Joshua Smith

Research Question/Objective   At the time this study was published, the standard of care for locally advanced rectal cancer consisted of postoperative chemoradiotherapy (CRT). Preoperative CRT became the standard of care after the initial results of this study were published. This chapter will also include the update provided by the study after a median follow-up of 11 years.

Study Design   Rectal cancer patients were randomly assigned to receive postoperative CRT or preoperative CRT. Prerandomization was conducted with a double consent design, which entails obtaining informed consent after the patient was told the result of randomization. This result was disclosed to patients in both groups. The primary end point was overall survival (OS). Secondary end points included disease-free survival (DFS), local and distant recurrence events, postoperative complications, acute and long-term effects, acute and long-term toxic effects, and rates of sphincter preservation.

Sample Size   A total of 823 patients were randomized. Twenty-four patients either withdrew consent to participate or ultimately did not meet inclusion criteria; 799 patients met criteria to be included in the study. Of the remaining patients, 405 were randomly assigned to receive preoperative CRT, and 394 were assigned to the postoperative CRT group.

Follow-Up   During therapy, patients were monitored on a weekly basis for signs of acute toxicity. Long-term effects were assessed at 1, 3, and 5 years. Patients were followed every 3 months for the first 2 years of the study, then every 6 months for 3 years. Median follow-up was 46 months.

Inclusion/Exclusion Criteria   Criteria for patient inclusion were histopathologically confirmed, resectable adenocarcinoma with the inferior margin within 16 cm of the anal verge. Patients were excluded if they had TNM stage I tumors, distant metastases, were older than 75 years of age, had a previous cancer diagnoses other than nonmelanoma skin cancer, had previously received chemotherapy, had previously received radiotherapy to the pelvis, or had contraindications to CRT.

DOI: 10.1201/9780429285714-6

Intervention or Treatment Received   Radiotherapy consisted of a total of 5040 cGy delivered in 28 fractions of 180 cGy, 5 times weekly. During the first and fifth weeks of radiotherapy, fluorouracil was administered as a 120-hour continuous infusion at a dose of 1000 mg/m^2/day. Treatment was identical in both groups except for a 540 cGy boost given to the postoperative CRT group.

Results

Histopathologic Tumor Staging   Of the 415 patients who received preoperative CRT, 33 of them exhibited a pathologic complete response (8%) compared to 0 out of 384 patients (0%) who received postoperative CRT ($p < 0.001$). Of the patients in the preoperative CRT group, 103 of 415 (25%) had positive lymph nodes in the surgical specimen (ypN+) compared to 153 of 384 (40%) of patients in the postoperative CRT group ($p < 0.001$).

Surgical Procedures   194 patients from both groups were determined to require an abdominoperineal resection prior to randomization. Among this group, there was a statistically significant increase in sphincter-preserving surgery performed in patients who received preoperative chemoradiation (45/116, 38%, of patients in the preoperative CRT group versus 15/78, 19%, in the postoperative CRT group, $p = 0.004$). However, the rates of complete resection and sphincter-preserving surgery did not differ between the groups when the full 799 patients were considered.

Morbidity and Toxicity   Rates of grade 3 or 4 acute and long-term toxic effects were lower in patients who received preoperative CRT than those in the postoperative approach ($p = 0.001$ for any acute grade 3 or 4 toxic effect, $p = 0.01$ for any long-term grade 3 or 4 toxic effects). This held true when comparing rates of acute diarrhea ($p = 0.04$) and strictures at anastomotic sites ($p = 0.003$).

OS and DFS   OS for those treated with preoperative CRT was 76% and 74% for those treated postoperatively ($p = 0.80$) The 5-year DFS rate was 68% for the preoperative treatment group and 65% for the postoperative treatment group ($p = 0.32$).

Local and Distant Recurrences   Within the preoperative CRT group of 405 patients, local and distant recurrences occurred in 17 and 99 patients, respectively (4.2% and 24.4%, respectively). Within the postoperative CRT group of 394 patients, local and distance recurrences occurred in 36 and 99, respectively (9.1% and 25.1%). Local recurrences at 5 years were 6% and 13% in the preoperative and postoperative treatment group, respectively ($p = 0.006$). The relative risk of local recurrence in the preoperative treatment group compared to the postoperative treatment group was 0.46 (95% confidence interval, 0.26 to 0.82). The cumulative incidence of distant recurrences at 5 years were 36% and 38% for the preoperative treatment versus postoperative treatment group ($p = 0.84$).

Study Limitations   More patients in the preoperative CRT group had tumors located 5 cm or less from the anal verge compared to the postoperative CRT group (157/405, 38%, in preoperative CRT group versus 117/394, 29%, in the postoperative CRT group, p = 0.008). This difference could have impacted the analysis as tumors closer to the anal verge have different biological potential than tumors farther from the anal verge. For example, Patel et al. demonstrated in a study of 827 patients, on multivariate analysis that patients with tumors 4–6 cm from the anal verge had higher rates of pCR when compared to tumors <4 cm and >8 cm from the anal verge (23.9% of patients vs. 12.3% and 16.6%, respectively, $p = 0.001$) (1). Other factors that may have influenced the outcomes were that 28% of patients in the postoperative group were excluded from receiving postoperative CRT due to either stage I disease or other reasons ($p < 0.001$ for "stage I disease" and "other reasons"). Lastly, the authors noted that the accuracy of endorectal ultrasonography is variable and that this variation ultimately could have altered the accuracy of tumor staging during the time of this study.

Relevant Studies   The German Phase 3 Trial (CAO/ARO/AIO-94) showed that preoperative CRT reduced the rates of local recurrence and acute/long-term toxic effects of treatment (2). The study did not demonstrate benefit relative to long-term survival. The Swedish Rectal Cancer Trial published in 2005 was able to demonstrate improved survival in addition to improvement in local recurrence rates in patients who received preoperative radiotherapy (3); however, it should be noted that this trial utilized short-course radiotherapy (SCRT). Additional randomized clinical trials employing SCRT demonstrated that SCRT before surgery, along with fluorouracil-based adjuvant chemotherapy reduced local recurrence rates (4, 5).

After the German Phase 3 Trial (CAO/ARO/AIO-94) was published, the standard of care for locally advanced rectal cancer (LARC) was established as preoperative radiotherapy with infusional fluorouracil, total mesorectal excision, and adjuvant chemotherapy with fluorouracil (2). Sauer et al. published long-term outcomes after a median follow-up of 134 months, which supported sustained improvement in local recurrence rate using preoperative CRT but no effect relative to OS or distant metastases (6). Rodel et al. went on to explore how to optimize DFS by adding oxaliplatin to the treatment regimen (German CAO/ARO/AIO-04 study), which significantly improved DFS (7) but not OS.

The treatment of rectal cancer has undergone seismic changes since publication of the randomized Phase 3 Trial, CAO/ARO/AIO-94. Initial studies showed the benefits of chemotherapy in the neoadjuvant setting (Capecitabine/Oxaliplatin, mFOLFOX6, or FLOX) as patients had improved treatment response and were more likely to complete their planned chemotherapy (8, 9). Research in the past decade has focused on optimizing the treatment sequence and organ preservation strategies for those who achieve a clinical complete response after neoadjuvant treatment (10–12). Current work has validated the use of a total neoadjuvant therapy (TNT) approach where all treatment is given prior to consideration of TME or organ preservation in certain instances. Table 6.1

summarizes important studies that led to recent changes in the treatment of locally advanced rectal cancer. Fernandez-Martos et al.'s Spanish GCR-3 phase II randomized trial also found better rates of compliance with chemotherapy and lower rates of toxicity without compromising DFS or OS when comparing induction chemotherapy (ICT)/long-course chemoradiotherapy (LCRT) to patients receiving preoperative CRT/adjuvant chemotherapy (13). Fokas et al. (CAO/ARO/AIO-12) studied the effects of upfront LCRT with consolidation chemotherapy (CT) versus induction chemotherapy (ICT) followed by LCRT and found better rates of compliance with CRT and higher pathologic complete response (pCR) rates in the former (14, 15). Garcia-Aguilar et al.'s Organ Preservation in Rectal Adenocarcinoma (OPRA) study, found that patients who were randomized to the LCRT/CT sequence achieved higher clinical complete response rates and subsequently higher 3-year TME-free survival rates than those randomized to the ICT/LCRT approach (53% vs. 41%, $p = 0.01$) without compromising DFS or metastasis-free survival (16). In summary, Fokas et al. and Garcia-Aguilar et al.'s studies showed that LCRT followed by consolidation chemotherapy improved response rates.

In addition to optimizing the treatment sequence, recent studies have included variations in chemotherapeutic options to optimize response and potentially alter oncologic outcomes. Garcia-Aguilar et al.'s TIMING trial showed that LCRT followed by CT in the form of modified FOLFOX6, in addition to lengthening the interval between treatment and surgery, increased the percentage of pCR and improved DFS (17, 18). The PRODIGE trial tested induction chemotherapy using mFOLFIRINOX followed by LCRT and met their primary end point of improving 3-year DFS in the experimental arm and showed a significant improvement in metastasis-free survival (DFS: 76% in the experimental arm vs. 69% in the standard of care arm, $p = 0.034$; MFS: 79% in the experimental arm vs. 72% in the standard of care arm, $p = 0.017$) (19). Rahma et al.'s study used an induction TNT approach in a platform study design in order to test whether Pembrolizumab added to LCRT might improve the neoadjuvant rectal score (NAR) score, which some studies show is an end point associated with DFS and OS. Interestingly, the pCR rate was higher in the pembrolizumab arm; however, the result was not statistically significant (20). Mature oncologic data will likely shed more light on this novel combination therapy.

Studies showing the effect of SCRT versus LCRT have begun to explore the benefits of either in regard to long-term outcomes. The Polish II trial initially showed improved OS in patients receiving a SCRT regimen versus LCRT, but follow-up results did not show superiority with SCRT (OS was 49% for both groups, $p = 0.38$) (21, 22). The RAPIDO trial treated patients either with SCRT/CT in a consolidation TNT approach or with LCRT followed by total mesorectal excision and risk-determined/optional adjuvant chemotherapy and found that the SCRT/CT patient cohort had improved rates of 3-year disease-related treatment failure as well as a doubling in the pCR rate (disease-related treatment

TABLE 6.1 Summary of Important Studies for the Treatment of Rectal Cancer

Study	N	Radiation Length	Treatment Strategy/ Sequence	Outcome Differences	P value	Journal/PMID
Kapiteijn et al[4], 2001	1805	SCRT	Preoperative CRT	2 year OS: 82% 2 year local recurrence: 2.4%	OS: 0.84 LRR: <0.001	New England Journal of Medicine/11547717
			Surgery Alone	2 year OS: 81.8% 2 year local recurrence: 8.2%		
Folkesson et al[3], 2005	908	SCRT	Preoperative CRT	OS: 38% Local recurrence rate: 9%	OS: 0.008 LRR: <0.001	Journal of Clinical Oncology/16110023
			Surgery Alone	OS: 30% Local recurrence rate: 26%		
Chau et al[9], 2006	77	LCRT	Preoperative chemotherapy + preoperative CRT	Radiologic tumor response after CapeOx: 88% Radiologic tumor response after CapeOx/CRT: 97%	NA	Journal of Clinical Oncology/16446339
Sauer et al[6], 2012	799	LCRT	Preoperative CRT	10 year OS: 59.6% DFS: 67.8% 10 year local recurrence rate: 7.1%	OS: 0.85 DFS: 0.65 LRR: 0.048	Journal of Clinical Oncology/22529255
			Postoperative CRT	10 year OS: 59.9% DFS: 68.1% 10 year local recurrence rate: 10.1%		
Rodel et al[7], 2015	1,236	LCRT	Preoperative CRT + and adjuvant 5-FU	3 year DFS: 71.2%	DFS: 0.03	The Lancet Oncology/26189067
			Preoperative CRT + oxaliplatin and adjuvant FOLFOX	3 year DFS: 75.9%		

Study	N	Type	Treatment	Outcomes	Statistics	Journal
Garcia-Aguilar et al[17], 2015	259	LCRT	Preoperative CRT 2, 4, or 6 cycles of mFOLFOX6	(2 cycles of chemo) pCR: 25% (4 cycles of chemo) pCR: 30% (6 cycles of chemo) pCR: 38%	P=0.0036	The Lancet Oncology/26187751
Fernandez-Martos et al[13], 2015	108	LCRT	Preoperative CRT, surgery, postoperative CAPOX	5 year DFS: 64% 5 year OS: 78% 5 year local recurrence: 2% 5 year distant metastasis: 21%	DFS: 0.85 OS: 0.64 LRR: 0.61 DM: 0.79	Annals of Oncology/25957330
			Preoperative CAPOX, preoperative CRT	5 year DFS: 62% 5 year OS: 75% 5 year local recurrence: 5% 5 year distant metastasis: 23%		
Marco et al[18], 2018	211	LCRT	Preoperative CRT 0, 2, 4, or 6 cycles of mFOLFOX6	(0 cycles of chemo) 5 year DFS: 50% (2 cycles of chemo) 5 year DFS: 81 (4 cycles of chemo) 5 year DFS: 86 (6 cycles of chemo) 5 year DFS: 76%	DFS: 0.004	Diseases of the Colon and Rectum/30192323
Cercek et al[8] 2018	628	LCRT	Preoperative CRT, surgery, postoperative chemotherapy	Clinical complete response rate: 21%	NA	Jama Oncology/29566109
			Preoperative CRT and chemotherapy	Clinical complete response rate: 36%		
Fokas et al[14], 2019	306	LCRT	Preoperative chemotherapy followed by CRT	pCR rate: 17%	pCR: <0.001	Journal of Clinical Oncology/31150315
			Preoperative CRT followed by chemotherapy	pCR rate: 25%		

(Continued)

TABLE 6.1   (*Continued*)

Study	N	Radiation Length	Treatment Strategy/ Sequence	Outcome Differences	P value	Journal/PMID
Cisel et al[22], 2019	515	SCRT v LCRT	Preoperative SCRT followed by chemotherapy	8 year OS: 49% DFS: 43%	OS: 0.38 DFS: 0.65	Annals of Oncology/31192355
			Preoperative CRT only	8 year OS: 49% DFS: 41%		
Bahadoer et al[23], 2020	912	SCRT v LCRT	Preoperative SCRT followed by chemotherpy	3 year disease related treatment failure: 23.7%	DRTF: 0.019	The Lancet Oncology/33301740
			Preoperative LCRT +/- postoperative chemotherapy	3 year disease related treatment failure: 30.4%		
Conroy et al[19], 2021	461	LCRT	Preoperative FOLFIRINOX followed by CRT, Postoperative chemotherapy	3 year DFS: 76%	DFS: 0.034	The Lancet Oncology/33862000
			Preoperative CRT, postoperative chemotherapy	3 year DFS: 69%		

Study	N	Comparison	Treatment arms	Outcomes	Statistics	Journal
Rahma et al[20], 2021	137	LCRT	Preoperative FOLFOX followed by CRT + pembrolizumab	Mean NAR score: 11.52 pCR: 31.9%	NAR score: 0.32 pCR: 0.75	JAMA Oncology/34196693
			Preoperative FOLFOX followed by CRT	Mean NAR score: 13.70 pCR: 29.4%		
Fokas et al[15], 2022	306	LCRT	Preoperative chemotherapy followed by CRT	3 year DFS: 73%	DFS: 0.82	JAMA Oncology/34792531
			Preoperative CRT followed by chemotherapy	3 year DFS: 73%		
Jin et al[12], 2022	599	SCRT v LCRT	Preoperative SCRT followed by chemotherapy	3 year DFS: 64.5% 3 year OS: 86.5%	DFS: <0.001 OS: 0.033	Journal of Clinical Oncology/35263150
			Preoperative LCRT	3 year DFS: 62.3% 3 year OS: 75.1%		
Garcia-Aguilar et al[16], 2022	324	LCRT	Preoperative chemotherapy followed by CRT	3 year DFS: 76%	Log rank p DFS: =0.98	Journal of Clinical Oncology/35483010
			Preoperative CRT followed by chemotherapy	3 year DFS: 76%		

Definitions: CRT – chemoradiation, DFS – disease free survival, DM – distant metastasis rate, DRTF – disease related treatment failure, LCRT – long course chemoradiotherapy, LRR – local recurrence rate, NAR – neoadjuvant rectal score, OS – overall survival, pCR – pathologic complete response rate, SCRT – short course radiotherapy, TNT – total neoadjuvant therapy.

failure: 23.7% in the experimental group vs. 30.4% in the standard of care group, $p = 0.019$; pCR: 120/423, 28%, in the experimental group vs. 57/398, 14%, in the standard of care group) (23). Additional studies are warranted to further detect possible outcome differences.

Rectal cancer is undergoing a major change in the paradigms of treatment and will continue to evolve as we discover how to improve patient outcomes, tailor treatments to each patient's specific tumor features and eventually even use de-escalation techniques to lower morbidity.

REFERENCES

1. Patel S, Roxburgh C, Vakiani E, et al. Distance to the anal verge is associated with pathologic complete response to neoadjuvant therapy in locally advanced rectal cancer. *J Surg Oncol*. 2016;114(5):637–641. doi:10.1002/jso.24358
2. Sauer R, Becker H, Hohenberger W, et al. Preoperative versus postoperative chemoradiotherapy for rectal cancer. *N Engl J Med*. 2004;351(17):1731–1740. doi:10.1056/NEJMoa040694
3. Folkesson J, Birgisson H, Pahlman L, Cedermark B, Glimelius B, Gunnarsson U. Swedish rectal cancer trial: long lasting benefits from radiotherapy on survival and local recurrence rate. *J Clin Oncol*. 2005;23(24):5644–5650. doi:10.1200/JCO.2005.08.144
4. Kapiteijn E, Marijnen CAM, Nagtegaal ID, et al. Preoperative radiotherapy combined with total mesorectal excision for resectable rectal cancer. *N Engl J Med*. 2001;345(9):638–646. doi:10.1056/NEJMoa010580
5. Bosset JF, Collette L, Calais G, et al. Chemotherapy with preoperative radiotherapy in rectal cancer. *N Engl J Med*. 2006;355(11):1114–1123. doi:10.1056/NEJMoa060829
6. Sauer R, Liersch T, Merkel S, et al. Preoperative versus postoperative chemoradiotherapy for locally advanced rectal cancer: results of the German CAO/ARO/AIO-94 randomized phase III trial after a median follow-up of 11 years. *J Clin Oncol*. Published online April 23, 2012. doi:10.1200/JCO.2011.40.1836
7. Rödel C, Graeven U, Fietkau R, et al. Oxaliplatin added to fluorouracil-based preoperative chemoradiotherapy and postoperative chemotherapy of locally advanced rectal cancer (the German CAO/ARO/AIO-04 study): final results of the multicentre, open-label, randomised, phase 3 trial. *Lancet Oncol*. 2015;16(8):979–989. doi:10.1016/S1470-2045(15)00159-X
8. Cercek A, Roxburgh CSD, Strombom P, et al. Adoption of total neoadjuvant therapy for locally advanced rectal cancer. *JAMA Oncol*. 2018;4(6):e180071. doi:10.1001/jamaoncol.2018.0071
9. Chau I, Brown G, Cunningham D, et al. Neoadjuvant capecitabine and oxaliplatin followed by synchronous chemoradiation and total mesorectal excision in magnetic resonance imaging–defined poor-risk rectal cancer. *J Clin Oncol*. Published online September 21, 2016. doi:10.1200/JCO.2005.04.4875
10. Smith JJ, Chow OS, Gollub MJ, et al. Organ preservation in rectal adenocarcinoma: a phase II randomized controlled trial evaluating 3-year disease-free survival in patients with locally advanced rectal cancer treated with chemoradiation plus induction or consolidation chemotherapy, and total mesorectal excision or nonoperative management. *BMC Cancer*. 2015;15(1):767. doi:10.1186/s12885-015-1632-z

11. Kim JK, Marco MR, Roxburgh CSD, et al. Survival after induction chemotherapy and chemoradiation versus chemoradiation and adjuvant chemotherapy for locally advanced rectal cancer. *The Oncologist*. 2022;27(5):380–388. doi:10.1093/oncolo/oyac025

12. Jin J, Tang Y, Hu C, et al. Multicenter, randomized, phase III trial of short-term radiotherapy plus chemotherapy versus long-term chemoradiotherapy in locally advanced rectal cancer (STELLAR). *J Clin Oncol*. 2022;40(15):1681–1692. doi:10.1200/JCO.21.01667

13. Fernandez-Martos C, Garcia-Albeniz X, Pericay C, et al. Chemoradiation, surgery and adjuvant chemotherapy versus induction chemotherapy followed by chemoradiation and surgery: long-term results of the Spanish GCR-3 phase II randomized trial. *Ann Oncol*. 2015;26(8):1722–1728. doi:10.1093/annonc/mdv223

14. Fokas E, Allgäuer M, Polat B, et al. Randomized phase II trial of chemoradiotherapy plus induction or consolidation chemotherapy as total neoadjuvant therapy for locally advanced rectal cancer: CAO/ARO/AIO-12. *J Clin Oncol*. Published online May 31, 2019. doi:10.1200/JCO.19.00308

15. Fokas E, Schlenska-Lange A, Polat B, et al. Chemoradiotherapy plus induction or consolidation chemotherapy as total neoadjuvant therapy for patients with locally advanced rectal cancer: long-term results of the CAO/ARO/AIO-12 randomized clinical trial. *JAMA Oncol*. 2022;8(1):e215445. doi:10.1001/jamaoncol.2021.5445

16. Garcia-Aguilar J, Patil S, Gollub MJ, et al. Organ preservation in patients with rectal adenocarcinoma treated with total neoadjuvant therapy. *J Clin Oncol*. 2022;40(23):2546–2556. doi:10.1200/JCO.22.00032

17. Garcia-Aguilar J, Chow OS, Smith DD, et al. Effect of adding mFOLFOX6 after neoadjuvant chemoradiation in locally advanced rectal cancer: a multicentre, phase 2 trial. *Lancet Oncol*. 2015;16(8):957–966. doi:10.1016/S1470-2045(15)00004-2

18. Marco MR, Zhou L, Patil S, et al. Consolidation mFOLFOX6 chemotherapy after chemoradiotherapy improves survival in patients with locally advanced rectal cancer: final results of a multicenter phase II trial. *Dis Colon Rectum*. 2018;61(10):1146–1155. doi:10.1097/DCR.0000000000001207

19. Conroy T, Bosset JF, Etienne PL, et al. Neoadjuvant chemotherapy with FOLFIRINOX and preoperative chemoradiotherapy for patients with locally advanced rectal cancer (UNICANCER-PRODIGE 23): a multicentre, randomised, open-label, phase 3 trial. *Lancet Oncol*. 2021;22(5):702–715. doi:10.1016/S1470-2045(21)00079-6

20. Rahma OE, Yothers G, Hong TS, et al. Use of total neoadjuvant therapy for locally advanced rectal cancer: initial results from the pembrolizumab arm of a phase 2 randomized clinical trial. *JAMA Oncol*. 2021;7(8):1225–1230. doi:10.1001/jamaoncol.2021.1683

21. Bujko K, Wyrwicz L, Rutkowski A, et al. Long-course oxaliplatin-based preoperative chemoradiation versus 5 × 5 Gy and consolidation chemotherapy for cT4 or fixed cT3 rectal cancer: results of a randomized phase III study. *Ann Oncol*. 2016;27(5):834–842. doi:10.1093/annonc/mdw062

22. Ciseł B, Pietrzak L, Michalski W, et al. Long-course preoperative chemoradiation versus 5 × 5 Gy and consolidation chemotherapy for clinical T4 and fixed clinical T3 rectal cancer: long-term results of the randomized Polish II study. *Ann Oncol*. 2019;30(8):1298–1303. doi:10.1093/annonc/mdz186

23. Bahadoer RR, Dijkstra EA, van Etten B, et al. Short-course radiotherapy followed by chemotherapy before total mesorectal excision (TME) versus preoperative chemoradiotherapy, TME, and optional adjuvant chemotherapy in locally advanced rectal cancer (RAPIDO): a randomised, open-label, phase 3 trial. *Lancet Oncol*. 2021;22(1):29–42. doi:10.1016/S1470-2045(20)30555-6

Operative versus Nonoperative Treatment for Stage 0 Distal Rectal Cancer Following Chemoradiation Therapy: Long-Term Results

Habr-Gama A, Perez RO, Nadalin W, et al. Ann Surg. 240(4):711–717, 2004, discussion 717–718

Reviewed by Bradley A. Krasnick and Matthew F. Kalady

Research Question/Objective Multimodality therapy consisting of chemoradiation followed by surgery became standard of care treatment for distal rectal adenocarcinoma by the mid-2000s. After surgical resection, 10–30% of patients were found to have a pathological complete response (ypT0N0 disease).[1,2] Given the known morbidity and mortality after surgery for distal rectal cancer, Dr. Habr Gama and colleagues sought to determine the outcome of patients with a complete clinical response after neoadjuvant chemoradiation, who forego surgery in exchange for a close clinical monitoring protocol. Furthermore, they evaluated how survival compared to that for patients with resected rectal cancer who are found to have no residual disease.

Study Design This study was a single-center prospective cohort study from São Paulo, Brazil. Patients with distal rectal adenocarcinoma were enrolled from 1991 to 2002. Patients were treated with neoadjuvant chemoradiation and evaluated for response to treatment 8 weeks after the completion of neoadjuvant therapy. Patients deemed to have a clinical complete response were then followed on a close observation protocol. The observation group was compared to the surgical resection group who had no residual tumor. The outcome measures included overall survival, disease-free survival, and recurrence.

Sample Size This study screened 256 patients with resectable distal rectal adenocarcinoma. Of these patients, 71 were found to have a clinical complete response (26.8%) and were enrolled in the close observation group (now termed "watch and wait"), while 194 patients were found to have an incomplete response (73.2%) and underwent curative surgical resection. Of these incomplete responders, 22 patients (8.3%) were found to have a pathological complete response.

Follow-Up For patients enrolled in the observation group, mean follow-up was 27.3 months (12–156), with 60 patients (84%) having at least 24 months follow-up. In

DOI: 10.1201/9780429285714-7

those with incomplete response, who underwent surgical resection, mean follow-up was 48 months (12–83), with 18 patients (82%) having at least 24-month follow-up.

Inclusion/Exclusion Criteria   Inclusion criteria consisted of patients presenting with what was deemed resectable rectal adenocarcinoma located 0–7 cm from the anal verge. Exclusion criteria included synchronous distal metastases. In addition, no patients with preoperative T1N0 disease were included in the study. Preoperatively, all patients underwent complete physical exam (PE), digital rectal exam (DRE), proctoscopy, colonoscopy (when possible), chest radiograph (CXR), abdominal and pelvic computed tomography (CT), serum CEA level, and endorectal ultrasound (ERUS, in select cases).

Intervention or Treatment Received   All patients received 5040 cGy of radiation over 6 weeks (5 days/week) with concurrent 5-fluorouracil and folinic acid. At 8 weeks posttreatment, patients underwent repeat complete clinical and radiographical examination (PE, DRE, proctoscopy, colonoscopy if initially obstructed, CXR, CT A/P, CEA, and ERUS in select cases). Any significant residual ulcer or tumor or positive biopsy led to patients being enrolled for proctectomy, while those with no residual disease noted were enrolled in a close observation protocol. This consisted of every 1 month follow-up for 1 year with PE, DRE, proctoscopy, biopsy when able, and CEA. CT A/P, and CXR were done every 6 months for 1 year. After 1 year, patient visits were spaced out to every 2-month follow-up visits for another year, followed by every 6-month follow-up visits during year 3.

Results   This study enrolled 265 total patients, consisting of 71 patients with clinical complete response and 194 with incomplete response.

Observation Group   Of those with a clinical complete response, the mean age was 58.1 years. Mean initial tumor size was 3.7 cm, with a mean distance of 3.6 cm from the anal verge. A total of 22.5% had node-positive disease on preoperative imaging. Of these patients, 2 patients had an endoluminal recurrence (2.8%), of which 1 underwent transanal resection and another underwent brachytherapy. Both had no evidence of disease at >72 months follow-up. A total of 3 patients developed distant metastatic disease (4.2%). Overall recurrence rate was 7%. Five-year overall (OS) and disease-free survival (DFS) for the group were 100% and 92%, respectively.

Resection Group   For those with an incomplete response undergoing proctectomy, a total of 22 patients (8.3%) had pathological complete response on final pathology (ypT0N0). For this group of patients, mean age was statistically similar to the observation group at 53.6 years. Preoperative characteristics were also similar to the observation group, with pretreatment mean tumor size being 4.2 cm, and average tumor distance from the anal verge being 3.8 cm. Node positivity was seen preoperatively in 27.2% of patients. Forty-one percent of patients underwent an abdominoperineal resection (APR), while the rest underwent sphincter-sparing surgery. No perioperative morbidity or mortality was noted in this cohort of 22 patients. Recurrence rate was 13.6%. OS and DFS at 5 years was 88 and 83%, respectively.

Conclusion   Survival was excellent for patients with complete clinical response undergoing observation, as well as those with incomplete response who had no residual disease after proctectomy. For the combined cohort, 10-year OS and DFS were 97 and 84%, respectively. No significant difference was seen between groups in terms of recurrence rate and mortality ($p = 0.2$). Five-year DFS was also similar between groups ($p = 0.09$), while OS was slightly improved in the observation group ($p = 0.01$).

Study Limitations   There are several limitations of the study. This was a single-center study. Patients were enrolled prospectively, but there was no randomization between groups, which introduces some inherent bias in which patients were entered into each arm. Importantly, only patients who had sustained complete tumor regression for at least 12 months were considered stage 0 and entered into the observation group. Thus it appears that those who recurred within the first year were excluded from the study. This would bias toward improved the outcomes of those in the observation group. Despite this, the study does introduce the concept of active surveillance rather than surgical management for clinical responders to neoadjuvant radiation.

Follow-up did differ slightly between groups, with a mean of 27.2 follow-up months in the observation group and 48 months in the resection group. The shorter mean follow-up in the observation group may not capture all recurrences. Nevertheless, the authors do note that over 80% of recurrences occur in the first 2 years posttreatment.[3]

Other limitations are inherent to the time period of the study (patients accrued from 1991 to 2002). Preoperative MRI was not the standard of care at the time and thus was not done. In addition, radiation was given differently than it is in the modern era, with now outdated anterior-posterior and lateral fields being utilized, as opposed to modern-day 3D conformal or intensity-modulated radiation therapy. Despite these limitations, this was some of the earliest data that complete clinical response after chemoradiation can lead to durable survival.

Relevant Studies   Prior to this study, the idea of chemoradiation without surgery for rectal cancer was extremely controversial. Historically, proctectomy was done as first-line treatment, with adjuvant chemoradiation following surgical recovery. Approaches began to slowly change with the completion of several trials. In 1990, the Swedish group published data, demonstrating decreased local recurrence when radiotherapy was given in the neoadjuvant setting for rectal cancer.[4] This led to the randomized Swedish Rectal Cancer Trial, which showed superiority of radiotherapy prior to surgical resection compared to postoperatively.[5] Just prior to the initial Swedish study, Washington University in St. Louis published their data on improved outcomes after neoadjuvant radiation for rectal cancer, and multiple centers began publishing consistent data.[6–9] In 1998 Dr. Habr Gama's group published data demonstrating a 30.5% complete response rate after upfront chemoradiation followed by surgery for low rectal cancer.[1] The following year, the MD Anderson Cancer Center published a 27% rate of pathological complete response, and this was quickly followed by a similar complete response rate seen at Duke University.[2,10] This excitement for neoadjuvant chemoradiation culminated in the randomized German Rectal Cancer Trial, published in *The New England Journal of Medicine* in 2004, demonstrating decreased local recurrence and higher rates of sphincter-sparing surgery with initial long-course chemoradiation for rectal cancer—further strengthening the role of neoadjuvant chemoradiation for at least T3 or node-positive rectal cancer.[11] In the same month as this publication, Dr. Habr Gama published her work showing durable clinical complete response after neoadjuvant chemoradiation and observation for distal rectal cancer.[12]

Prior to Dr. Habr Gama's publication in 2004, the idea of nonsurgical treatment for rectal cancer was not considered a viable option for rectal cancer. Dr. Habr Gama published additional data in 2009 and then in 2013, whereby she treated low rectal cancer patients with long-course chemoradiation, followed by additional cycles of 5-fluorouracil and leucovorin.[13,14] At a minimum 12-month follow-up, an initial 68% clinical complete response rate was noted, with a sustained 57% clinical complete response.[14] Around the same time, two European institutions reported their promising results using a "watch-and-wait" type of protocol after neoadjuvant chemoradiation.[15,16]

More recently, several trials have built on Dr. Habr Gama's work, further supporting the watch-and-wait paradigm, as well as the concept of chemoradiation and chemotherapy being given entirely in the neoadjuvant setting (i.e., total neoadjuvant therapy, TNT). In 2021, the randomized RAPIDO trial was published in *The Lancet Oncology* and demonstrated that the addition of neoadjuvant chemotherapy (CAPOX or FOLFOX) after chemoradiation, was superior to chemotherapy given in the adjuvant setting, with decreased locoregional treatment failure and with higher rates of complete pathological response.[17] The PRODIGE 23 study out of France also demonstrated enhanced outcomes with a TNT regimen, as opposed to chemoradiation, then surgery, followed by adjuvant chemotherapy.[18] More recently, Dr. Garcia Aguilar and colleagues published results of the randomized Phase II organ preservation for rectal cancer (OPRA) trial that showed TNT yields significant complete clinical response rates and successful nonoperative management.[19] In the OPRA trial, chemoradiation followed by consolidation chemotherapy was slightly more effective than induction chemotherapy followed by neoadjuvant chemoradiation in terms of complete clinical response. The 53% sustained clinical complete response rate at 3-year follow-up shown in OPRA mirrors the impressive results seen by Dr. Habr Gama more than a decade earlier. To learn more about the nonoperative management of rectal cancer, the International Watch & Wait Database (IWWD) was established with multiple institutions from various countries. This dataset has demonstrated that the overwhelming majority of locoregional failures occur within the first 3 years after therapy and, more recently, that patients with a near complete response can be safely monitored and in many cases will convert into clinical complete responders.[20-22]

The field of rectal cancer is rapidly changing. Multiple trials are actively underway to further elucidate the best treatments and treatment sequences that will result in complete clinical responses and better rectal cancer outcomes. Dr. Habr Gama's "radical" work published in 2004 laid the foundation and spurred an entire new line of protocols and study. The pioneering work that was initially met with skepticism has been further supported with other studies and has proven to withstand the test of time. TNT and nonoperative management have recently been included in treatment algorithms for rectal cancer by the National Comprehensive Cancer Network.[23]

REFERENCES

1. Habr-Gama A, de Souza PM, Ribeiro UJ, et al. Low rectal cancer: Impact of radiation and chemotherapy on surgical treatment. *Dis Colon Rectum*. 1998;41(9):1087–1096. doi: 10.1007/BF02239429.
2. Janjan NA, Khoo VS, Abbruzzese J, et al. Tumor downstaging and sphincter preservation with preoperative chemoradiation in locally advanced rectal cancer: The M. D. Anderson cancer center experience. *Int J Radiat Oncol Biol Phys*. 1999;44(5):1027–1038. doi: 10.1016/s0360-3016(99)00099-1.
3. Kraemer M, Wiratkapun S, Seow-Choen F, Ho YH, Eu KW, Nyam D. Stratifying risk factors for follow-up: A comparison of recurrent and nonrecurrent colorectal cancer. *Dis Colon Rectum*. 2001;44(6):815–821. doi: 10.1007/BF02234700.
4. Pahlman L, Glimelius B. Pre- or postoperative radiotherapy in rectal and rectosigmoid carcinoma. Report from a randomized multicenter trial. *Ann Surg*. 1990;211(2):187–195. doi: 10.1097/00000658-199002000-00011.
5. Swedish Rectal Cancer Trial, Cedermark B, Dahlberg M, et al. Improved survival with preoperative radiotherapy in resectable rectal cancer. *N Engl J Med*. 1997;336(14):980–987. doi: 10.1056/NEJM199704033361402.
6. Kodner IJ, Shemesh EI, Fry RD, et al. Preoperative irradiation for rectal cancer. Improved local control and long-term survival. *Ann Surg*. 1989;209(2):194–199. doi: 10.1097/00000658-198902000-00010.
7. Minsky BD, Cohen AM, Kemeny N, et al. Enhancement of radiation-induced downstaging of rectal cancer by fluorouracil and high-dose leucovorin chemotherapy. *J Clin Oncol*. 1992;10(1):79–84. doi: 10.1200/JCO.1992.10.1.79.
8. Chari RS, Tyler DS, Anscher MS, et al. Preoperative radiation and chemotherapy in the treatment of adenocarcinoma of the rectum. *Ann Surg*. 1995;221(6):778–786. doi: 10.1097/00000658-199506000-00016.
9. Stryker SJ, Kiel KD, Rademaker A, Shaw JM, Ujiki GT, Poticha SM. Preoperative "chemoradiation" for stages II and III rectal carcinoma. *Arch Surg*. 1996;131(5):514–519. doi: 10.1001/archsurg.1996.01430170060012.

10. Onaitis MW, Noone RB, Hartwig M, et al. Neoadjuvant chemoradiation for rectal cancer: Analysis of clinical outcomes from a 13-year institutional experience. *Ann Surg.* 2001;233(6):778–785. doi: 10.1097/00000658-200106000-00007.

11. Sauer R, Becker H, Hohenberger W, et al. Preoperative versus postoperative chemoradiotherapy for rectal cancer. *N Engl J Med.* 2004;351(17):1731–1740. doi: 10.1056/NEJMoa040694.

12. Habr-Gama A, Perez RO, Nadalin W, et al. Operative versus nonoperative treatment for stage 0 distal rectal cancer following chemoradiation therapy: Long-term results. *Ann Surg.* 2004;240(4):711–718. doi: 10.1097/01.sla.0000141194.27992.32.

13. Habr-Gama A, Perez RO, Sabbaga J, Nadalin W, Sao Juliao GP, Gama-Rodrigues J. Increasing the rates of complete response to neoadjuvant chemoradiotherapy for distal rectal cancer: Results of a prospective study using additional chemotherapy during the resting period. *Dis Colon Rectum.* 2009;52(12):1927–1934. doi: 10.1007/DCR.0b013e3181ba14ed.

14. Habr-Gama A, Sabbaga J, Gama-Rodrigues J, et al. Watch and wait approach following extended neoadjuvant chemoradiation for distal rectal cancer: Are we getting closer to anal cancer management? *Dis Colon Rectum.* 2013;56(10):1109–1117. doi: 10.1097/DCR.0b013e3182a25c4e.

15. Maas M, Beets-Tan RGH, Lambregts DMJ, et al. Wait-and-see policy for clinical complete responders after chemoradiation for rectal cancer. *J Clin Oncol.* 2011;29(35):4633–4640. doi: 10.1200/JCO.2011.37.7176.

16. Dalton RSJ, Velineni R, Osborne ME, et al. A single-centre experience of chemoradiotherapy for rectal cancer: Is there potential for nonoperative management? *Colorectal Dis.* 2012;14(5):567–571. doi: 10.1111/j.1463-1318.2011.02752.x.

17. Bahadoer RR, Dijkstra EA, van Etten B, et al. Short-course radiotherapy followed by chemotherapy before total mesorectal excision (TME) versus preoperative chemoradiotherapy, TME, and optional adjuvant chemotherapy in locally advanced rectal cancer (RAPIDO): A randomised, open-label, phase 3 trial. *Lancet Oncol.* 2021;22(1):29–42. doi: 10.1016/S1470-2045(20)30555-6.

18. Conroy T, Bosset J, Etienne P, et al. Neoadjuvant chemotherapy with FOLFIRINOX and preoperative chemoradiotherapy for patients with locally advanced rectal cancer (UNICANCER-PRODIGE 23): A multicentre, randomised, open-label, phase 3 trial. *Lancet Oncol.* 2021;22(5):702–715. doi: 10.1016/S1470-2045(21)00079-6.

19. Garcia-Aguilar J, Patil S, Gollub MJ, et al. Organ preservation in patients with rectal adenocarcinoma treated with total neoadjuvant therapy. *J Clin Oncol.* 2022;40(23):2546–2556. doi: 10.1200/JCO.22.00032.

20. Temmink SJD, Peeters KCMJ, Bahadoer RR, et al. Watch and wait after neoadjuvant treatment in rectal cancer: Comparison of outcomes in patients with and without a complete response at first reassessment in the international watch & wait database (IWWD). *Br J Surg.* 2023;110(6):676–684. doi: 10.1093/bjs/znad051.

21. van der Valk MJM, Hilling DE, Bastiaannet E, et al. Long-term outcomes of clinical complete responders after neoadjuvant treatment for rectal cancer in the international watch & wait database (IWWD): An international multicentre registry study. *Lancet.* 2018;391(10139):2537–2545. doi: 10.1016/S0140-6736(18)31078-X.

22. Fernandez LM, Sao Juliao GP, Figueiredo NL, et al. Conditional recurrence-free survival of clinical complete responders managed by watch and wait after neoadjuvant chemoradiotherapy for rectal cancer in the international watch & wait database: A retrospective, international, multicentre registry study. *Lancet Oncol.* 2021;22(1):43–50. doi: 10.1016/S1470-2045(20)30557-X.

23. Benson AB, Vebook AP, Al-Hawary MM, et al. NCCN clinical practice guidelines in oncology: Rectal cancer. www.nccn.org. Updated 2022. Accessed 12/2/22.

CHAPTER 8

Preoperative Radiotherapy Combined with Total Mesorectal Excision for Resectable Rectal Cancer

Kapiteijn E, Marijnen CA, Nagtegaal ID, Putter H, Willem H, Steup WH, Wiggers T, Rutten HJ, Pahlman L, Glimelius B, van Krieken JH, Leer JW, van de Velde CJ: Dutch Colorectal Cancer Group. N Engl J Med. 345(9):638–646, 2001

Reviewed by Patricia Sylla and Motahar Bassam

Research Question/Objective   Improving outcomes through better local disease control is the holy grail in rectal cancer surgery. The use of sharp instead of blunt dissection to achieve total mesorectal excision (TME) has led to improved survival.[1] The role of radiotherapy combined with a standardized total mesorectal excision surgical technique for rectal cancer required further clarity. The aim of this study was to provide a 2-year follow-up regarding the combined effect of preoperative radiotherapy and total mesorectal excision in patients with resectable rectal cancer. This was defined as overall survival, local/distant recurrence, overall recurrence, as well as morbidity and mortality.

Study Design   This study was a prospective, randomized trial conducted among 108 different hospitals across the Netherlands, Sweden, other parts of Europe, and Canada. Between January 1996 and December 1999, patients were enrolled and randomly assigned by a central office to treatment either with radiotherapy followed by surgery with total mesorectal excision or with surgical TME alone. Quality control measures concerning radiotherapy, surgery, and pathologic examination were only applied in the Netherlands. Surgeons there watched instructional videos and attended workshops and symposia, and they were monitored by trained instructor surgeons in accordance with strict, controllable quality demands. Pathologists were trained to identify mesorectal spread using the Quirke et al.[2] protocol, and the results of each exam were reviewed by supervising pathologists and a quality manager. In Sweden, the standardized national standard for the technique of TME and pathologic examination was followed. At all the other participating centers, the quality of treatment was ensured prior to start of the trial through visits from the research group.

Sample Size   In total, 1861 patients were randomly assigned to either preoperative radiotherapy followed by TME (924 patients) or TME alone (937 patients). Most of the patients were from Dutch hospitals (1530 patients), some from Swedish

DOI: 10.1201/9780429285714-8

hospitals (228 patients), and the rest from other parts of Europe and Canada (103 patients). Ultimately, 1805 patients were included in the analysis: 897 patients in the radiotherapy and surgery group, 908 patients in surgery alone group. Patients were randomized based on stratification by center and expected type of operation.

Follow-Up   There was a mean follow-up period of 2 years (24.9 months). Surviving eligible patients underwent clinical evaluation every 3 months in the first year, followed by annual visits thereafter for at least 2 years, including annual liver imaging and endoscopy. Results were reported based on the 2-year follow-up, which was achieved for 54% of patients.

Inclusion/Exclusion Criteria   Adult patients with good performance status (WHO ≤ 2) and histologically confirmed adenocarcinoma of the rectum with inferior margin ≤ 15 cm from the anal verge, as measured by flexible endoscopy and below a level of S1–2, were included. The patient's tumor had to be clinically resectable, which was defined as mobile without evidence of adjacent organ invasion. Exclusion criteria included patients with tumors that were locally resected/resectable transanally; previously treated rectal cancer; synchronous distant metastases; emergency operation; hereditary polyposis disease; previous pelvic treatment with chemotherapy, immunotherapy, or radiotherapy.[3]

Intervention or Treatment Received   In accordance with the participating hospital medical ethics committees, informed consent was obtained then the patients were randomly assigned to each group. Patients randomized to the preoperative radiotherapy arm underwent short-course radiation (5 Gy/day × 5 days) followed by standard TME within 10 days of starting treatment. Radiotherapy volume targets included the primary tumor site and mesentery with the vascular supply containing the perirectal, presacral, and internal iliac (up to S1/S2 junction) lymph node basins. Surgery using techniques of low anterior resection or abdominoperineal resection (APR) with standard TME ensuring complete resection of the entire mesorectal envelope using precise, sharp dissection. Pathologic examination also included molecular biology studies and residual tumor classification. Patients with R1 (infiltration < 1 mm from resection margin, spillage during the operation, or positive cytology) and R2 (residual locoregional or distant disease) underwent adjuvant therapy (chemotherapy, radiotherapy, or chemoradiotherapy).

Results   Of the 1805 total patients included, 1653 underwent curative resection. Fifty-seven patients had macroscopically complete local resection, and 95 patients were found to have distant metastases at the time of surgery.

In the radiotherapy followed by surgery group, 29 patients did not undergo preoperative radiotherapy due to withdrawal of informed consent (11 patients), metastases (8 patients), physical impossibility (5 patients), sigmoid carcinoma (3 patients), carcinoma *in situ* (1 patient), and second cancer (1 patient). Preoperative radiotherapy was discontinued in 14 patients. Long-course radiotherapy was given to 7 patients for locally advanced tumor and to 1 patient for inability to tolerate surgery. The interval between the first day of radiotherapy and surgery exceeded 10 days in 110 patients. There were also minor violations in the radiotherapy protocol: in 127 patients, the upper border of the treatment field was at the level of S1–2 instead of the sacral promontory, and 161 patients undergoing an APR did not have the perineum included in the treated volume.

In the surgery alone group, 8 patients had advanced local tumors treated with long-course preoperative radiotherapy, and 3 patients withdrew informed consent.

Patient and Tumor Characteristics Patients were similar with regard to median age (65 years in radiotherapy followed by surgery, 66 years in surgery alone, $p = 0.79$) and gender (64% male). There was no significant difference in tumor location. Most were in the midrectum (5.1–10 cm from the anal verge): 43% in the radiotherapy followed by surgery group, 40% in the surgery alone group; followed by the upper rectum (10.1–15 cm from the anal verge): 30% in the radiotherapy followed by surgery group and 31% in the surgery alone group; and the lower rectum (<5 cm from the anal verge): 27% in the radiotherapy followed by surgery group and 29% in the surgery alone group. Less than 1% of each group had unknown tumor locations.

The types of resections were similar as well. Most patients underwent low anterior resection (65% in the radiotherapy followed by surgery group and 67% in the surgery alone group, $p = 0.12$). Pathologic staging results were also similar. In the radiotherapy followed by surgery group, 1% was stage 0, 30% stage I, 28% stage II, 33% stage III, 7% stage IV, and <1% stage unknown; in the surgery alone group 2% stage 0, 27% stage I, 27% stage II, 36% stage III, 7% stage IV, and 2% stage unknown ($p = 0.53$).

Morbidity and Mortality Patients assigned to radiotherapy followed by surgery had more operative blood loss (1000 mL vs. 900 mL, $p < 0.001$). In those who underwent APR, patients who underwent preoperative radiotherapy had higher rates of perineal complications compared with surgery alone (26% vs. 18%, $p = 0.05$).

Overall Survival and Recurrence There was no significant difference in the rate of overall survival at 2 years (82% in patients who underwent radiotherapy followed by surgery vs. 81.8% in those who underwent surgery alone, $p = 0.84$). Local recurrence rates were almost 3.5 times higher in the surgery alone group (8.2% vs. 2.4%, $p > 0.001$) with univariate analysis showing a hazard ratio for local recurrence of 3.4 (95% CI 2.1–5.7). Other predictors of local recurrence were TNM stage ($P < 0.001$) and location of the tumor ($p = 0.003$) with subgroup analyses showing a significant reduction in local recurrence in patients who had tumors ≤5 cm from anal verge ($p = 0.05$) and 5.1–10 cm from anal verge ($p < 0.001$).

There was no significant difference in distant (14.8% radiotherapy followed by surgery, 16.8% surgery alone, $p = 0.87$) and in overall recurrence rates (16.1% radiotherapy followed by surgery, 20.9% surgery alone, $p = 0.09$).

Study Limitations Logistically, the study was limited by a lack of control and training in standard TME for surgeons located throughout all the participating hospitals outside the Netherlands (331 patients). This may have contributed to higher rates of local recurrence rates seen in the surgery alone group.
In addition, a short follow-up duration of just 2 years and low follow-up rate of 54% at 2 years may have hindered the group's ability to capture differences in recurrence and overall survival.

Relevant Studies Although combination radiotherapy and surgery had been studied by others,[4] the Dutch Colorectal Cancer Group was the first to publish a prospective, randomized trial of patients who underwent standardized TME as part of their treatment. They published extensively on this cohort, including risk factors for anastomotic failure, acute side effects and complications after preoperative radiotherapy, a 6-year follow-up and a 12-year follow-up on their patients.[5-8] In their latest report of 12-year median follow-up, they continued to demonstrate a significant reduction in local recurrence (5% radiotherapy followed by surgery, 11% surgery alone, $p < 0.0001$) without a difference in distant recurrence (25% radiotherapy followed by surgery, 28% surgery alone, $p = 0.21$) and overall survival (48% radiotherapy followed by surgery, 49% surgery alone, $p = 0.86$).

REFERENCES

1. MacFarlane JK, Ryall RD, Heald RJ. Mesorectal excision for rectal cancer. *Lancet*. 1993;341(8843):457–460. doi:10.1016/0140-6736(93)90207-w
2. Quirke P, Durdey P, Dixon MF, Williams NS. Local recurrence of rectal adenocarcinoma due to inadequate surgical resection: histopathological study of lateral tumour spread and surgical excision. *Lancet*. 1986;2:996–999.
3. Kapiteijn E, Kranenbarg EK, Steup WH, et al. Total mesorectal excision (TME) with or without preoperative radiotherapy in the treatment of primary rectal cancer: prospective randomised trial with standard operative and histopathological techniques. *Eur J Surg*. 1999;165:410–420.
4. Swedish Rectal Cancer Trial, Cedermark B, Dahlberg M, et al. Improved survival with preoperative radiotherapy in resectable rectal cancer [published correction appears in N Engl J Med 1997 May 22;336(21):1539]. *N Engl J Med*. 1997;336(14):980–987. doi:10.1056/NEJM199704033361402
5. Marijnen CA, Kapiteijn E, van de Velde CJ, et al. Acute side effects and complications after short-term preoperative radiotherapy combined with total mesorectal excision in primary rectal cancer: report of a multicenter randomized trial. *J Clin Oncol*. 2002;20(3):817–825. doi:10.1200/JCO.2002.20.3.817
6. Peeters KC, Tollenaar RA, Marijnen CA, et al. Risk factors for anastomotic failure after total mesorectal excision of rectal cancer. *Br J Surg*. 2005;92(2):211–216. doi:10.1002/bjs.4806

7. Peeters KC, Marijnen CA, Nagtegaal ID, et al. The TME trial after a median follow-up of 6 years: increased local control but no survival benefit in irradiated patients with resectable rectal carcinoma. *Ann Surg.* 2007;246(5):693–701. doi:10.1097/01.sla.0000257358.56863.ce

8. van Gijn W, Marijnen CA, Nagtegaal ID, et al. Preoperative radiotherapy combined with total mesorectal excision for resectable rectal cancer: 12-year follow-up of the multicentre, randomised controlled TME trial. *Lancet Oncol.* 2011;12(6):575–582. doi:10.1016/S1470-2045(11)70097-3

Effect of the Plane of Surgery Achieved on Local Recurrence in Patients with Operable Rectal Cancer: A Prospective Study Using Data from the MRC CR07 and NCIC-CTG CO16 Randomised Clinical Trial

Quirke P, Steele R, Monson J, Grieve R, Khanna S, Couture J, O'Callaghan C, Myint AS, Bessell E, Thompson LC, Parmar M, Stephens RJ, Sebag-Montefiore D. Lancet. 7:373(9666):821–828, 2009

Reviewed by Michael L.R. Lonne, Amy M.Y. Cao, and Andrew R.L. Stevenson

Research Question/Objective Local recurrence rates in operable rectal cancer were historically variable and unacceptably high. The aims of this study were threefold: to determine whether circumferential resection margin (CRM) involvement was a prognostic factor for local recurrence, whether the plane of surgery achieved was an independent risk factor for local recurrence, and whether preoperative radiotherapy led to greater reduction in local recurrence when a poorer plane of surgery was achieved.

Study Design This study was a prospective cohort study using data from the Medical Research Council (MRC) CR07 and NCIC-CTG CO16 trial, which was an international randomized controlled trial (RCT) in 80 centers across 4 countries comparing short-course preoperative radiotherapy to upfront surgery with selective postoperative chemoradiotherapy (1). Surgical specimens were assessed for both involvement of the CRM (defined as tumor equal to or less than 1 mm from the CRM) and for the plane of surgery achieved (mesorectal, intramesorectal, or muscularis propria plane). (See Table 9.1.) Pathologists received training in the grading of the specimen, dissection, and reporting using the TNM version 5 proforma. The primary outcomes were 3-year local recurrence rates and disease-free survival.

Sample Size The initial MRC CR07 and NCIC-CTG CO16 trial enrolled 1350 patients between March 1998 and August 2005. A total of 1156 patients underwent standardized pathological assessment and were included in this study.

Follow-Up Patients were followed up at 3, 6, 9, and 12 months and then every 6 months up to 3 years, and yearly thereafter. Local recurrence was defined as positive biopsy, imaging, or CEA if imaging was equivocal.

DOI: 10.1201/9780429285714-9

TABLE 9.1 Definitions of Specimen Grading

Grade	Dissection Plane		Definition
3	Mesorectal	Good plane of surgery achieved; complete	Intact mesorectum with only minor irregularities of a smooth mesorectal surface; no defect deeper than 5 mm; no coning; and smooth CRM on slicing
2	Intramesorectal	Moderate plane of surgery achieved; nearly complete	Moderate bulk to mesorectum, with irregularities of the mesorectal surface; moderate distal coning; muscularis propria not visible with the exception of levator insertion and moderate irregularities of CRM
1	Muscularis propria	Poor plane of surgery achieved; incomplete	Little bulk to mesorectum with defects down onto muscularis propria; very irregular CRM; or both

Inclusion/Exclusion Criteria   All patients who underwent standardized pathological assessment were included. Inclusion criteria were patients with resectable histologically confirmed rectal adenocarcinoma (defined as distal tumor less than 15 cm from the anal verge on rigid sigmoidoscopy) with no evidence of metastasis on liver ultrasound or computed tomography (CT) and plain chest X-ray. Patients were excluded if they were not fit for all treatments or had previous malignant disease. There were no age limitations.

Intervention or Treatment Received   All patients underwent standardized pathological assessment to determine involvement of the CRM and the plane of the surgery achieved by the surgeon. Surgeons were encouraged to use a total mesorectal excision technique, but this was not mandated in the protocol, and no formal training was provided. Patients received adjuvant or neoadjuvant therapy as per-protocol with selective postoperative chemoradiotherapy in the case of an involved CRM. All analyses were intention to treat.

Results

Demographics   Median age was 65 years. Majority of patients were male (72%) with WHO performance status 0 (80%); 564 (48.8%) were allocated to preoperative short-course radiotherapy and 592 (51.2%) to selective chemoradiotherapy.

Effect of Circumferential Margin Status   An involved CRM was associated with increased 3-year local recurrence (HR 0.32 95% CI 0.16–0.63, $p = 0.001$) and reduced 3-year disease-free survival (HR 0.19, 95% CI 0.13–0.28, $p < 0.001$). However, this difference did not persist on multivariate analysis.

An involved CRM was significantly associated in univariate analysis with the procedure performed [abdominoperineal resection (APR) 16%, anterior resection 7%, $p < 0.0001$], tumor position (distal extent 0–5 cm 15%; 5–10 cm 9%; 10–15 cm 9%, $p = 0.004$), higher T stage ($p < 0.0001$), nodal stage ($p < 0.0001$) and tumors with an anterior component (involved 13%; not involved 7%, $p = 0.001$). In multivariate analysis, T stage, N stage, and anterior tumor position remained independent risks for an involved CRM.

Effect of Plane of Surgery   Of the 1156 specimens assessed, 604 (52%) were in the mesorectal plane, 398 (34%) in the intramesorectal plane, and 154 (13%) in the muscularis propria plane, with no significant difference in the plane of surgery achieved between the two treatment groups. The plane of surgery achieved was strongly associated with 3-year local recurrence rates with 4% in the mesorectal plane, 7% intramesorectal plane, and 13% muscularis propria plane ($p = 0.0039$). There was a similar trend for 3-year disease-free survival that did not reach significance. Similar to CRM positivity, the plane of surgery achieved improved during the trial period but was worse in patients who underwent APR compared to an anterior resection ($p < 0.001$). There was no association between plane of surgery and TNM stage or lymph node yield.

Effect of Short-Course Radiotherapy   When patients received both short-course preoperative radiotherapy and surgery within the mesorectal plane, local recurrences were almost completely abolished (1% at 3 years), as shown in Table 9.2.

Study Limitations   This was a cohort study of the effect of surgical plane on local recurrence using results from a published RCT. Randomization of surgical technique in this context would be difficult.

Whilst pathologists were trained in the assessment of the specimens, surgeons were not provided with training on dissection in the mesorectal plane. However, as noted by the authors, the quality of the dissection improved over the trial period.

Overall and longer-term survival rates were not explored in this study. Whether the reduction in local recurrence translated to improved overall survival was unclear.

Relevant Studies   This was the first study to provide high-quality evidence that the plane of surgery achieved was one of the most important independent risk factors for local recurrence. Furthermore, the plane of surgery was determined by the "ability of the surgeon to stay in the mesorectal plane" and not by an advancing TNM stage.

Since this study, several studies have reported on the effect of the surgical plane on rectal cancer outcomes with variable results. In 2012 a meta-analysis showed a decreased risk of local recurrence when an optimal dissection in the mesorectal plane was achieved (2). In 2015, the PROCARE study showed an improved disease-free survival when surgery was in the mesorectal plane though no

TABLE 9.2   Effect of Treatment on Local Recurrence and Disease-Free Survival

Effect of Treatment	3-Year Local Recurrence	P-Value	3-Year Disease-Free Survival	P-Value
Circumferential resection margin (CRM)	Positive CRM 17% Negative CRM 6% (HR 0.32; 95% CI 0.16–0.63)	0.001	Positive CRM 50% Negative CRM79% (HR 0.19; 95% CI 0.13–0.28)	<0.001
Plane of surgery	Mesorectal 4% Intramesorectal 7% Muscularis propria 13%	0.004	Mesorectal 79% Intramesorectal 75% Muscularis propria 70%	0.14
Radiotherapy	Preoperative short course: 10.6% Selective postoperative chemoradiotherapy: 4.4% (HR 0.39; 95% CI 0.27–0.58)	<0.001	Preoperative short course: 77.5% Selective postoperative chemoradiotherapy: 71.5% (HR 0.76; 95% CI 0.62–0.94)	0.013

reduction in local recurrence was demonstrated (3). In 2018, Kitz et al. used data from the Phase III CAO/ARO/AIO-04 RCT, which confirmed the findings of the MRC CR07 trial with a significant association in multivariate analysis between plane of surgery and local recurrence (4). Both studies also found that surgeons' assessments of the quality of the TME were less reliable, confirming the role of expert pathological assessment in the grading of TME.

Assessment of the grade of TME has now become a core component of the International Collaboration on Cancer Reporting dataset from which the colorectal structured histopathology reports are based (5). It is used as a surrogate for the quality of rectal surgery and is a key outcome measure in many RCTs comparing surgical techniques (6). The AlaCaRT Trial comparing laparoscopic to open resection for rectal cancer used a composite of complete mesorectal excision, clear CRM, and distal resection margin to define a successful surgical resection (7). Similar definitions were used in the Z6051 Trial and in a recent RCT on laparoscopic and transanal TME by Liu et al. (8, 9). Notably, these more recent trials showed far greater proportions of patients having a complete mesorectal excision, with 77–92% compared to this historic rate of 56% (2).

The outcomes of this study support Heald's theory that most local recurrences were failures of surgical technique and highlight the completeness of the TME as a critical metric when reporting and comparing outcomes for rectal cancer.

REFERENCES

1. Sebag-Montefiore D, Stephens RJ, Steele R, Monson J, Grieve R, Khanna S, et al. Preoperative radiotherapy versus selective postoperative chemoradiotherapy in patients with rectal cancer (MRC CR07 and NCIC-CTG C016): a multicentre, randomised trial. Lancet. 2009;373(9666):811–20.
2. Bosch SL, Nagtegaal ID. The importance of the pathologist's role in assessment of the quality of the mesorectum. Curr Colorectal Cancer Rep. 2012;8(2):90–8.
3. Leonard D, Penninckx F, Laenen A, Kartheuser A. Scoring the quality of total mesorectal excision for the prediction of cancer-specific outcome. Colorectal Dis. 2015;17(5):O115–22.
4. Kitz J, Fokas E, Beissbarth T, Ströbel P, Wittekind C, Hartmann A, et al. Association of Plane of total mesorectal excision with prognosis of rectal cancer: secondary analysis of the CAO/ARO/AIO-04 phase 3 randomized clinical trial. JAMA Surg. 2018;153(8):e181607.
5. Loughrey MB, Brown I, Burgart LJ, Cunningham C, Flejou JF, Kakar S, et al. Nagtegaal ID Colorectal Cancer Histopathology Reporting Guide. Sydney: International Collaboration on Cancer Reporting, 2020.
6. Maslekar S, Sharma A, Macdonald A, Gunn J, Monson JR, Hartley JE. Do supervised colorectal trainees differ from consultants in terms of quality of TME surgery? Colorectal Dis. 2006;8(9):790–4.
7. Stevenson AR, Solomon MJ, Lumley JW, Hewett P, Clouston AD, Gebski VJ, et al. Effect of laparoscopic-assisted resection vs open resection on pathological outcomes in rectal cancer: the ALaCaRT randomized clinical trial. JAMA. 2015;314(13):1356–63.
8. Fleshman J, Branda M, Sargent DJ, Boller AM, George V, Abbas M, et al. Effect of laparoscopic-assisted resection vs open resection of stage II or III rectal cancer on pathologic outcomes: the ACOSOG Z6051 randomized clinical trial. JAMA. 2015;314(13):1346–55.
9. Liu H, Zeng Z, Zhang H, Wu M, Ma D, Wang Q, et al. Morbidity, mortality, and pathologic outcomes of transanal versus laparoscopic total mesorectal excision for rectal cancer short-term outcomes from a multicenter randomized controlled trial. Ann Surg. 2023;277(1):1–6.

CHAPTER 10

Defunctioning Stoma Reduces Symptomatic Anastomotic Leakage after Low Anterior Resection of the Rectum for Cancer: A Randomized Multicenter Trial

Matthiessen P, Hallbook O, Rutegard J, Simert G, Sjodahl R. Ann Surg. 246(2):207–214, 2007

Reviewed by Albert M. Wolthuis

Research Question/Objective   After the introduction of total mesorectal excision (TME) as the surgical technique to treat mid- and low rectal cancer, high morbidity and mortality rates remained a problem. Symptomatic anastomotic leak rate was estimated to be between 1% and 24%, with the associated risk of mortality between 6% and 22%. The central aim of this study was to evaluate the impact of a defunctioning stoma to reduce the rates of symptomatic anastomotic leakage. A clinical definition of anastomotic leakage was used: peritonitis caused by leakage from any staple line, rectovaginal fistula, and pelvic abscess without radiological signs of leakage.

Study Design   This was a prospective multicenter randomized controlled trial in all Swedish hospitals performing rectal cancer surgery. In 1999 all 65 hospitals were asked to participate, but only 21 hospitals provided patients for the randomized trial. However, to assess and eliminate selection bias, data from randomized patients (included in the study) were compared to data from nonrandomized patients, obtained from the Swedish Rectal Cancer Registry. The primary outcome was symptomatic anastomotic leakage. Secondary outcome measures included postoperative morbidity and outcome regarding reversal of the defunctioning stoma.

Sample Size   To detect a decrease in symptomatic anastomotic leak rate from 15% to 7.5%, with a statistical power of 80% and a level of significance at 5%, 220 patients were required. This study screened 821 potential participants and enrolled 234 patients into the study who met inclusion and exclusion criteria. Of this sample, 116 patients underwent a defunctioning stoma, and 118 did not receive a stoma.

Follow-Up   Patients were followed during their hospital stay, at 1 and at 12 months after TME. When a defunctioning stoma was created, the patient was assessed at the time of reversal, and 12 months thereafter.

DOI: 10.1201/9780429285714-10

Inclusion/Exclusion Criteria   Criteria for patient inclusion in this randomized study were based on preoperative and intraoperative information. Preoperative inclusion criteria were biopsy-proven rectal adenocarcinoma ≤15 cm from the anal verge measured with a rigid rectoscope, age ≥18 years, informed consent, with the ability to understand the study information, and estimated survival >6 months. Intraoperative criteria were anastomosis ≤7 cm above the anal verge, negative air leak test, intact anastomotic stapler rings, and absence of major adverse intraoperative events. Exclusion criteria were not described in this study.

Intervention or Treatment Received   If patients met preoperative and intraoperative inclusion criteria, randomization was performed intraoperatively, after construction and testing of the anastomosis, by opening a sealed envelope. Of note, both loop ileostomy and loop colostomy were accepted as defunctioning stoma.

Results

Primary End Point   A total of 587 patients were not randomized, leaving 234 randomized to stoma ($n = 116$) and no stoma ($n = 118$). The majority of patients with a defunctioning stoma had a loop ileostomy ($n = 112$, 96.6%). The total rate of symptomatic anastomotic leakage was 19.2% (45 of 234 patients). In patients with a defunctioning stoma, the symptomatic leak rate was 10.3% (12 of 116), compared with 28% (33 of 118) of those without defunctioning stoma (odds ratio = 3.4, 95% confidence interval, 1.6–6.9, $P<0.001$).

Secondary End Point

- In this study, reoperations were used as a surrogate marker to assess postoperative morbidity. Reoperation rate was 8.6% in patients with a stoma versus 25.4% in patients without a stoma ($p < 0.001$). A total of 30 patients in the no stoma group underwent a reoperation, and 25 had a laparotomy with creation of a defunctioning loop stoma.
- At a median of 5 months, 86.2% of patients with a defunctioning stoma had their stoma reversed. Overall, 16 patients did not have their stoma reversed. Progressive liver metastasis and poor anorectal function were the main reasons to keep any kind of stoma. In the group of patients with a defunctioning stoma and leakage, 7 out of 12 patients were stoma free at median follow-up of 42 months. In the group of patients without a defunctioning stoma, 25 were reoperated with creation of a loop ileostomy, and 3 were reoperated with a permanent colostomy. Overall, 11 out of 25 patients (44%) had their stomas reversed after a median of 10 months.

Other Findings   In this trial, different types of anastomoses (J-pouch 43.6%, side-to-end 38.9%, and end-to-end 16.2%, unspecified 1.3%) were made, but this had no impact on anastomotic leak rates. Overall, the median hospital stay was 11 days.

Hospital stay was significantly shorter in patients who did not have a defunctioning stoma. Also, when scheduled and unscheduled leakages were taken into account, hospital stay was shorter in the no stoma group. Early mortality in the present study was low. The 30-day mortality was 0.4% (1 of 234) and after elective reversal of a defunctioning stoma 0.9% (1 of 111). Of note, after a median follow-up of 42 months, stoma rate was similar: 13.8% of the initially defunctioned patients still had a stoma (of any kind), compared with 16.9% of those not defunctioned.

Study Limitations   Overall, only 28.5% of patients that underwent a TME were randomized. The most frequent reasons for nonrandomizing patients were serious intraoperative adverse events (28%), absence of patient consent (25%), anastomosis >7cm above the anal verge (18%), and advanced stage IV and/or T4 cancer (10%). Although the majority of patients had a loop ileostomy (112 out of 116), defunctioning loop colostomies were also allowed in this study. Clinical outcomes between loop ileostomy and loop colostomy are considered to be different and could have had a small impact on study results. In this cohort of patients, preoperative radiotherapy was given to 81% of patients randomized to stoma, compared to 77% of patients randomized to no stoma. Moreover, only 55% of patients underwent radiotherapy in the group that was not randomized ($p < 0.001$). Stratification to radiotherapy as a risk factor for anastomotic leak might have been better to reduce bias. Regarding anastomotic leak as an outcome parameter, radiological leaks without symptoms were not included in the present study. These subclinical leaks are known to be the reason to not reverse the stoma and could have had an impact on study findings.[1] In the present study, postoperative morbidity was not really measured, and this could also be considered a study limitation.

Relevant Studies   The rationale to perform this trial in that period was clear. With the introduction of a standardized technique to treat rectal cancer by means of TME, not only oncological outcome but also surgical outcome could be studied in a more structured way. At that moment, the way to perform a low double-stapled anastomosis was established, but patients and surgeons still faced dreadful complications. Anastomotic leak was estimated to happen in about 12% of cases and could also occur in patients without any risk factors.[2,3] Moreover, when anastomotic leak was present, the associated risk of postoperative mortality increased to between 6% and 22%.[2] Therefore, it was often a point of discussion whether to perform a defunctioning stoma in order to mitigate the clinical impact of symptomatic anastomotic leak. Previously, one randomized trial including only 38 patients showed no decreased leak rates, but it showed that a defunctioning colostomy prevented most of the severe infective complications of an anastomotic leak.[4] Another trial on 50 patients, who underwent low anterior resection, showed a clinical leak rate of 4% in the colostomy group versus 12% in the noncolostomy group, respectively. However, the authors stated that a loop colostomy was inconvenient and costly and that most patients could be spared a temporary colostomy.[5] With this in mind, the Swedish surgeons set up a randomized controlled trial to really answer the question whether a defunctioning stoma could decrease symptomatic anastomotic leaks. With some of the study limitations as just discussed, the present study found a clear argument in favor of a defunctioning stoma to decrease symptomatic leaks. A number of systematic reviews including retrospective and prospective data corroborated these findings and showed that a stoma clearly decreased the clinical consequences of an anastomotic leak.[6–9] However, it has been shown that overall anastomotic leak rate was not different between groups.[6]

With the data from the present randomized trial, the authors published 3 other studies regarding costs, anorectal function, and risk of permanent stoma.[10–12] They found that defunctioning stoma was more expensive than no stoma, despite the reduced costs associated with a reduced frequency of anastomotic leakage. An unexpected finding was that after 5 years, the number of days with any stoma did not differ between groups. Although the final rate of stomas (30%) was lower in the group of patients initially randomized to no stoma, they had a longer median time with a stoma (839 days vs. 196 days, respectively), explaining the similar rate of total number of days with a stoma.[10] At longer follow-up, a temporary stoma might have had an impact on anorectal function, although the incidence of low anterior resection syndrome was similar in the stoma and no-stoma groups.[11] In more recent years, 3 other randomized trials investigating the role of defunctioning stoma after low anterior resection have been published.[13–15] Findings of these trials are in line with the results of the present trial. Strong recommendations were made for the use of loop ileostomy in patients at risk, such as low anastomosis (<6 cm) and male patients. Recommendation to defunction a low anastomosis to avoid symptomatic leak and poor outcome still stands today. As such, results of this revolutionary trial are actual, although the debate is still ongoing.

REFERENCES

1. Borstlap WAA, Westerduin E, Aukema TS, et al. Anastomotic leakage and chronic presacral sinus formation after low anterior resection: results from a large cross-sectional study. Ann Surg. 2017;266(5):870–77.
2. Rullier E, Laurent C, Garrelon JL, et al. Risk factors for anastomotic leakage after resection of rectal cancer. Br J Surg. 1998;85(3):355–8.
3. Matthiessen P, Hallböök O, Andersson M, et al. Risk factors for anastomotic leakage after anterior resection of the rectum. Colorectal Dis. 2004;6(6):462–9.
4. Pakkastie TE, Ovaska JT, Pekkala ES, et al. A randomized study of colostomies in low colorectal anastomoses. Eur J Surg. 1997;163(12):929–33.
5. Graffner H, Fredlund P, Olsson SA, et al. Protective colostomy in low anterior resection of the rectum using the EEA stapling instrument. A randomized study. Dis Colon Rectum. 1983;26(2):87–90.
6. Hüser N, Michalski CW, Erkan M, et al. Systematic review and meta-analysis of the role of defunctioning stoma in low rectal cancer surgery. Ann Surg. 2008;248(1):52–60.
7. Tan WS, Tang CL, Shi L, Eu KW. Meta-analysis of defunctioning stomas in low anterior resection for rectal cancer. Br J Surg. 2009;96(5):462–72.
8. Chen J, Wang DR, Yu HF, et al. Defunctioning stoma in low anterior resection for rectal cancer: a meta-analysis of five recent studies. Hepatogastroenterology. 2012;59(118):1828–31.

9. Gu WL, Wu SW. Meta-analysis of defunctioning stoma in low anterior resection with total mesorectal excision for rectal cancer: evidence based on thirteen studies. World J Surg Oncol. 2015;13:9.

10. Floodeen H, Hallböök O, Hagberg LA, Matthiessen P. Costs and resource use following defunctioning stoma in low anterior resection for cancer—a long-term analysis of a randomized multicenter trial. Eur J Surg Oncol. 2017;43(2):330–36.

11. Gadan S, Floodeen H, Lindgren R, Matthiessen P. Does a defunctioning stoma impair anorectal function after low anterior resection of the rectum for cancer? A 12-year follow-up of a randomized multicenter trial. Dis Colon Rectum. 2017;60(8):800–6.

12. Gadan S, Floodeen H, Lindgren R, et al. What is the risk of permanent stoma beyond 5 years after low anterior resection for rectal cancer? A 15-year follow-up of a randomized trial. Colorectal Dis. 2020;22(12):2098–2104.

13. Chude GG, Rayate NV, Patris V, et al. Defunctioning loop ileostomy with low anterior resection for distal rectal cancer: should we make an ileostomy as a routine procedure? A prospective randomized study. Hepatogastroenterology. 2008;55(86–87):1562–7.

14. Thoker M, Wani I, Parray FQ, Khan N, Mir SA, Thoker P. Role of diversion ileostomy in low rectal cancer: a randomized controlled trial. Int J Surg. 2014;12(9):945–51.

15. Mrak K, Uranitsch S, Pedross F, et al. Diverting ileostomy versus no diversion after low anterior resection for rectal cancer: a prospective, randomized, multicenter trial. Surgery. 2016;159(4):1129–39.

Preoperative Magnetic Resonance Imaging Assessment of Circumferential Resection Margin Predicts Disease-Free Survival and Local Recurrence: 5-Year Follow-Up Results of the MERCURY Study

Taylor FGM, Quirke P, Heald RJ, et al. J Clin Oncol. 32(1):34–43, 2014

Reviewed by Eleanor M. Walker and Ian R. Daniels

Research Question/Objective   This study was conducted to assess the outcome in terms of overall survival, disease-free survival, and local recurrence rate of rectal cancer patients who had undergone an MRI scan at their initial staging. The MRI was performed to determine the relationship between the depth of invasion of the tumor and the mesorectal fascia, whose envelop is the embryological limit of the hind gut and the principle plane of dissection for a total mesorectal excision (TME), i.e., the circumferential resection margin (CRM). This study compared the clinical outcomes between AJCC TNM staging and MRI CRM prediction prior to treatment.

Study Design   This is a case series of patients who had been enrolled in the MERCURY Study (Magnetic rEsonance and Rectal Cancer eURopean equivalence studY), which had a minimum 5-year follow-up to determine the relationship between pretreatment MRI-predicted CRM status and their disease outcome following treatment, with a minimum 5-year follow-up.

Sample Size   The original MERCURY study recruited 729 rectal cancers from 11 centers to determine the correlation of depth of invasion beyond the bowel wall between the MRI scan and corresponding histological whole-mount section. Published in 2006, this had determined that a mesorectal fascial clearance of >1 mm on MRI predicted an intact circumferential resection margin. The MERCURY Study included standardized radiological and pathological proforma-based reporting with workshops for the clinicians using validated MRI images and histological samples. This study comprised 374 patients who had complete data (MRI staging, surgery, histopathology, and 5-year follow-up data) from 477 who had undergone surgical treatment+/−preoperative therapy.

Follow-Up   Minimum 5-year (median 62 months).

DOI: 10.1201/9780429285714-11

Inclusion/Exclusion Criteria   MRI-staged prediction of potential CRM involvement.

Intervention/Treatment Received   Prior to 2000 the use of preoperative therapy was largely based upon clinical examination (per rectal digital assessment), CT scanning, and endorectal ultrasound scanning to predict the AJCC TNM stage. Variations in oncological regimes to improve outcome ranged from the German preoperative versus postoperative long-course radiotherapy (LRT) studies, the short-course radiotherapy (SRT) trials performed in Sweden and the UK/European (MRC-CR07), and the preoperative chemoradiotherapy (CRT) trials at the time. The MERCURY Study was designed to determine the depth of extramural invasion and the diagnostic accuracy of high-resolution MRI scanning to predict curative resection.

Results   Of the 374 patients who were followed up, 216 (57.8%) underwent primary surgery based upon MRI CRM prediction, and 158 received a preoperative (neoadjuvant) strategy (LRT 53, SRT 47, CRT 55, chemotherapy alone 3). The MRI prediction of margin positivity pretreatment was 53%, the negative predictive value being 94%, with an overall accuracy of 87% in this cohort.

The surgery performed included 288 (77%) undergoing an anterior resection versus 86 (23%) undergoing an APE. Overall specimen quality by visual meso-rectal grading was graded as intact mesorectum 233 (62.3%), intramesorectal 67 (17.9%), just the muscularis propria 20 (5.3%), with 54 (14.5%) unknown.

During follow-up, 159 patients died, with rectal-cancer-specific deaths being 108 (68%). Local recurrence was identified in 14 (3.7%), local and distant recurrence in 22 (5.9%), and distant recurrence alone in 93 (25%), with 51 (13.6%) cases having deaths from other/unknown causes.

In those with MRI-predicted CRM involvement, 50% developed recurrence, with a 5-year overall 5-year survival in those with MRI-prediction CRM clear of 62.2% compared to 42.2% with MRI-prediction CRM involved ($P = 0.01$). The 5-year disease-free survival was 67.2% versus 47.3% ($P = 0.003$). The MRI-predicted CRM involvement remained significant for poor DFS on multivariate analysis.

For all analyses [univariate (UV) and multivariate (MV)], the outcomes for an involved margin were worse for an APE compared to an anterior resection with hazard ratios for local recurrence (LR) being UV = 2.14 ($P < 0.05$), MV = 2.95 ($P < 0.01$); for disease-free survival (DFS) UV = 1.34, MV = 1.24; and for overall survival UV = 1.14, MV 1.34 ($P < 0.05$). This was supported by further data on the preoperative tumor site (position and height above the anal verge).

Overall, the LR rate was small (9.6%) in the whole group, but if MRI predicted that there would be CRM involvement, local recurrence was 20% and 27% in histopathologically confirmed cases compared to 7% if MRI predicted clear assessed on either modality.

The relationship to LR demonstrated a hazard ratio of 3.50 (95% CI 1.53–8.00, $P < 0.05$) between MRI CRM prediction rates and that overall high-resolution MRI preoperative predicted assessment of CRM status was superior to the AJCC TMN staging in prediction of outcome. The implication is that preoperative treatment selection should be based upon MRI prediction of CRM status at patient presentation.

Study Limitations   In the MERCURY Study the use of preoperative therapy was recorded although not standardized between the recruiting centers. However, all units agreed that MRI prediction of CRM involvement would be used as a policy for offering preoperative therapy (based upon local treatment policy). Follow-up was similarly determined by local protocols with the diagnosis of recurrence either biopsy confirmed or with radiological evidence of disease progression and with radiological evidence of distant metastases being recorded as a rectal-cancer-specific death. With the surgery being performed from 2001 to 2004, there was subsequent focus on the performance of the APE leading to the development of the extralevator approach (elAPE) and the emphasis of continued audited MRI and histological evidence of surgical specimen quality. One of the challenges faced with the introduction of MRI treatment planning was the influence on the choice or not of preoperative therapy, and it was considered unethical to withhold the MRI staging prediction and to randomize between clinical and MRI staging. There was no comparison to endorectal ultrasound and the use of preoperative therapy in T3 or node-positive-predicted disease; however, with these high-risk factors it was recognized that these would likely be more advanced tumors. With the different preoperative therapies used, this potentially impacted both differences in tumor "down-staging" and overall survival. However, subsequent clinical trials and recognition of the potential for nonoperative management of complete clinical/radiological responders would still maintain the significance of the initial relationship between tumor spread, the recognition on MRI of extramural vascular invasion (EMVI) and mesorectal fascia, and potential surgical circumferential margin. Further surgical advancement with the "Beyond TME" would reduce involved margins as the MRI offers a "surgical road map" determined by the relationship between tumor and mesorectal fascia/circumferential resection margin.

Relevant Studies   The relationship between the outcome for rectal cancer and local recurrence was first articulated in the 1980s by the histopathologist Phil Quirke (1), and the description of the detail of optimal surgical technique focusing on the importance of total mesorectal excision (TME) was described by R.J. "Bill" Heald. This demonstrated that an intact mesorectal excision containing the tumor, local deposits, and lymph nodes could dramatically reduce local recurrence rates if a clear circumferential margin were achieved (2). Strategies to reduce the risk of local recurrence and improve outcome were focused on the use of preoperative oncological therapies versus postoperative therapy, the different radiotherapy regimes

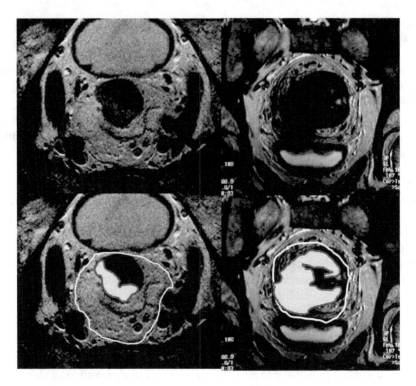

Clear Margin   Involved Margin

Figure 11.1   Mesorectal fascia (potential CRM) outlined by the white boundary and extent of tumour in light grey and demonstration in the lower right image of where tumour extent and CRM meet, i.e. an involved margin as compared to the lower left image, i.e. CRM clear.

[short-course (SRT) and long-course radiotherapy (LRT)], and the recognition that preoperative therapy with the addition of chemotherapy improved outcome (3–5).

The demonstration of the mesorectal fascia on high-resolution thin-section MRI scans was first described in 1999 (6) and the recognition of high-risk factors on MRI in 2003 (7). Combining these elements through the multidisciplinary team meeting was aimed at eliminating the involved circumferential resection margin (8). The standardization of the MRI technique and reporting, along with improvements in histopathological assessment including the visual standard of mesorectal specimen, would further improve outcome (9–11).

Replication of the "triumpherate of steps"—high-resolution MRI scanning to aid MDT decision making for selection of treatment, optimal (TME) surgery, and histopathological audit with comparison between the MRI staging and histological outcome—was the foundation of the MERCURY Study performed across 11 European centers (12, 13) and the basis of this follow-up study.

The data presented in this paper supported the focus on areas for further improvement. The recognition that there were differences in (local) recurrence and survival between anterior resections and abdominoperineal excisions led to improvements in the MRI assessment (14), the surgical technique employed (15), and the importance of determining the surgical strategy prior to "knife to skin" using MRI to direct the surgical operative technique (16).

This paper added to the body of evidence for MDT decision making and for optimization of preoperative oncological therapies to "down-stage/-size" tumors prior to surgery and formed the basis of support for the development of "watch-and-wait" policies in those patients with a complete clinical/radiological response to their preoperative therapy. This watch-and-wait policy following preoperative therapy and complete tumor response, as first described by Angelita Habr-Gama in 2004, has been validated by MRI scanning and with MRI-directed care and has become accepted international practice (17, 18).

Further developments from the MERCURY Study library of scans and histology demonstrated the importance of recognizing the prognostic significance of extramural vascular invasion and the targeted preoperative strategies that we now employ (19).

The importance of this paper is that it supported the original premise of the MERCURY Study, emphasized the value of MDT-directed care, demonstrated low levels of local recurrence with optimal MRI-directed surgery and continued improvement in survival. Twenty years after the original MERCURY Study was commenced, and 30 years after the recognition of the importance of the mesorectal fascia, this paper confirmed the value of MRI in future study design and principally the importance of the circumferential resection margin.

REFERENCES

1. Quirke P, Durdey P, Dixon MF, et al. Local recurrence of rectal adenocarcinoma due to inadequate surgical resection: histopathological study of lateral tumour spread and surgical excision. Lancet. 1986;2:996–999.
2. Heald RJ, Ryall RD. Recurrence and survival after total mesorectal excision for rectal cancer. Lancet. 1986;1:1479–1482.
3. Swedish Rectal Cancer Trial. Improved survival with preoperative radiotherapy in resectable rectal cancer. N Engl J Med. 1997;336:980–987.
4. Chau I, Brown G, Cunningham D, et al. Neoadjuvant capecitabine and oxaliplatin followed by synchronous chemoradiation and total mesorectal excision in magnetic resonance imaging-defined poor-risk rectal cancer. J Clin Oncol. 2006;24(4):668–674.
5. Sauer R, Becker H, Hohenberger W, et al. Preoperative versus postoperative chemoradiotherapy for rectal cancer. N Eng J Med. 2004;351:1731–1740.
6. Brown G, Richards CJ, Newcombe RG, et al. Rectal carcinoma: thin-section MR imaging for staging in 28 patients. Radiology. 1999;211(1):215–222.

7. Brown G, Radcliffe AG, Newcombe RG, et al. Preoperative assessment of prognostic factors in rectal cancer using high-resolution magnetic resonance imaging. Br J Surg. 2003;90:355–364.

8. Brown G, Burton S, Daniels IR, et al. MRI directed multidisciplinary team preoperative treatment strategy: the way to eliminate positive circumferential margins? Br J Cancer. 2006;94(3):351–357.

9. Brown G, Daniels IR, Richardson C, et al. Technique and trouble-shooting in high spatial resolution thin slice MRI for rectal cancer. Br J Radiol. 2005;78:245–251.

10. Quirke P, Steele R, Monson J, et al. Effect of the plane of surgery achieved on local recurrence in patients with operable rectal cancer. A prospective study using data from the MRC CR07 and NCIC-CTG C016 randomised clinical trial. Lancet. 2009;373:821–828.

11. Nagdetaal ID, van de Velde CJ, van der Worp E, et al. Macroscopic evaluation of rectal cancer specimen: clinical significance of the pathologist in quality control. J Clin Oncol. 2002;20:1729–1734.

12. MERCURY Study Group. Extramural depth of tumour invasion at thin-section MR in patients with rectal cancer: results of the MERCURY study. Radiology. 2007;243:132–139.

13. MERCURY Study Group. Diagnostic accuracy of preoperative magnetic imaging in predicting curative resection of rectal cancer: prospective observational study. BMJ. 2006;333:779.

14. Salerno GV, Daniels IR, Moran BJ, et al. Magnetic resonance imaging prediction of an involved circumferential resection margin in low rectal cancer. Dis Colon Rectum. 2009;52:632–639.

15. Holm T, Ljung A, Häggermark T, et al. Extended abdominoperineal resection with gluteus maximus flap reconstruction of the pelvic floor for rectal cancer. Br J Surg. 2007;94:232–238.

16. West NP, Finan PJ, Anderin C, et al. Evidence of the oncological superiority of cylindrical abdominoperineal excision for low rectal cancer. J Clin Oncol. 2008;26:3517–3522.

17. Habr-Gama A, Perez RO, Nadalin W, et al. Operative versus nonoperative treatment for stage 0 distal rectal cancer following chemoradiation therapy: long-term results. Ann Surg. 2004;240(4):711–717.

18. Chadi SA, Malcolmson L, Ensor J, et al. Factors affecting local regrowth after watch and wait for patients with a clinical complete response following chemoradiotherapy in rectal cancer (InterCoRe consortium): an individual participant data meta-analysis. Lancet Gastroenterol Hepatol. 2018;3(12):825–836.

19. Smith NJ, Barbachano Y, Norman AR, et al. Prognostic significance of magnetic resonance imaging-detected extramural vascular invasion in rectal cancer. Br J Surg. 2008;95(2):229–236.

Effect of Laparoscopic-Assisted Resection vs Open Resection of Stage II or III Rectal Cancer on Pathologic Outcomes: The ACOSOG Z6051 Randomized Clinical Trial

Fleshman J, Branda M, Sargent DJ, et al. JAMA. 314(13):1346–1355, 2015

Reviewed by Tyler R. Chesney and Nancy N. Baxter

Research Question/Objective   High-quality total mesorectal excision (TME) is central to curative-intent rectal cancer treatment, and the surgical technique is known to affect the quality of surgical resection. Therefore, ensuring that similar-quality TME could be obtained through a laparoscopic approach was essential. Due to the known benefits of a laparoscopic approach in terms of short-term recovery, a noninferiority approach was taken. The primary aim of this study was to investigate whether laparoscopic resection for stage II/III rectal cancer was not importantly worse than conventional open resection based on the pathologic assessment of surgical resection.

Study Design   This was a multicenter randomized parallel-group nonblinded noninferiority clinical trial conducted in Canada and the United States. The primary outcome was a novel composite outcome defined by the authors as "successful resection" combining pathological assessment of distal margin (>1 mm between tumor and cut edge), circumferential resection margin (>1 mm between tumor and inked margin), and plane of mesorectal excision quality (intact mesorectal envelope with no more than 5 mm deep defect rated as complete or near complete). The authors chose the noninferiority margin for pathologic surgical success at 6% based on clinical relevance derived from medical oncology trials.

Sample Size   This study randomized 486 patients to either laparoscopic or open rectal resection with 243 patients in each study arm. After withdrawals, 225 received open surgery as randomized (222 in final analysis due to 3 having improper consent), and 240 received laparoscopic surgery as randomized with 27 of these being converted to open surgery intraoperatively. The recruitment goal based on predetermined power calculation was 240 per arm.

Follow-Up   The primary outcome of pathologic surgical success was assessed postoperatively in all patients included for final analysis.

DOI: 10.1201/9780429285714-12

Secondary outcomes of operative time, blood loss, incision length, analgesia use, complications, and length of stay were available for all analyzed patients. Longer-term secondary outcomes of disease-free survival, local recurrence, and quality of life were not available for this report.

Inclusion/Exclusion Criteria   Eligible patients were at least 18 years old with clinically stage II or III rectal cancer treated with neoadjuvant chemoradiotherapy/radiotherapy alone with body mass index no more than 34 and Eastern Cooperative Oncology Group performance score less than 3. Exclusion criteria included T4 tumors, prior pelvic cancer within 5 years, psychiatric or addiction disorder affecting adherence, American Society of Anesthesiologists classification IV or V, or contraindication to laparoscopy.

Intervention Received   Patients underwent laparoscopic or open rectal resection based on randomization using standard TME approaches. Surgeons were instructed to perform proximal vascular ligation, splenic flexure mobilization, and sharp dissection in the plane outside the mesorectal fascia with a 5 cm distal transection margin for upper rectal tumors, and transection below the mesorectum for middle and low rectal tumors. Abdominoperineal resection was used if the tumor was not separable from the pelvic floor or anal sphincter. Robotic resection was allowable in the laparoscopic arm. Hand assistance was allowable in the laparoscopic arm if this was used for the upper abdominal dissection, and only laparoscopic instruments were used for pelvic dissection. In the laparoscopic arm, 14% had robotic and 17% had hand assistance. In the open arm, laparoscopic mobilization of the proximal colon and vessel ligation were allowable if the pelvic dissection was accomplished entirely with hand instruments and hand retraction. Surgeons were credentialed before patient enrollment. Credentialing included submission of an unedited laparoscopic video and 20 operative reports for both open and laparoscopic resection.

Results

Study Population and Intervention   A total of 486 patients were randomized. In the open arm, 222 were included in final analysis; 21 of the initially randomized patients were not in the final analysis due to withdrawal, improper consent, metastases, refusing open surgery, or choosing surveillance without surgery. In the laparoscopic arm, 240 were included in final analysis of which 27 (11%) were converted to open surgery; 3 of the initially randomized patients were not in the final analysis due to withdrawal. Overall, 77% underwent low anterior resection with the majority receiving diverting ileostomy and 23% abdominoperineal resection. Conversion to open surgery was required for safe completion of rectal dissection (12), due to locally advanced disease found at surgery (4), as the result of complications at surgery (4), to complete anastomosis safely (4), and adhesions (3). Demographics were balanced between groups. About half had low rectal tumors, and mean distance from anal verge was 6 cm in both groups. Almost 60% were stage III disease.

Primary Outcome   The primary analysis was a modified intention-to-treat analysis, meaning patients randomized to laparoscopy but converted to open were analyzed with the laparoscopy arm. The rate of successful resection was 81.7% (95% CI 76.8 to 86.6) in the laparoscopic group and 86.9% (95% CI 82.5 to 91.4) in the open group with a difference of −5.3% (1-sided 95% CI −10.8 to ∞) and *p*-value for noninferiority of 0.41. An additional per-protocol analysis was done, meaning patients randomized to laparoscopy but converted to open were analyzed with the open arm; per-protocol analysis is standard for noninferiority trials. The results were consistent with a difference of −5.3% (1-sided 95% CI −10.8 to ∞) and *p*-value for noninferiority of 0.41. Because the 1-sided 95% confidence interval included the noninferiority margin of 6%, the results are inconclusive regarding noninferiority of laparoscopic compared to open rectal resection for this composite pathologic outcome of successful resection. While not designed to evaluate differences in secondary outcomes, surgical conduct, postoperative stay, and postoperative complications were similar between groups, and operative time was longer in the laparoscopic group by 45 minutes on average.

Study Limitations   The authors used a novel composite pathologic outcome. The association of this composite surrogate outcome, as opposed to the individual end points that comprise the composite, to patient-relevant outcomes such as local recurrence, disease-free survival, and overall survival was not known, and these outcomes are not available in this report. The noninferiority margin was selected by the authors based on medical oncology trials, but the method used to make this selection was not elaborated, so the meaning of this threshold is unknown. The authors do not explicitly report any study limitations.

Relevant Studies   While investigating whether laparoscopy is not worse than conventional open technique for rectal resection is conceptually straightforward, establishing that a new treatment is not importantly worse than a conventional treatment requires a noninferiority trial design.[1] An important element of noninferiority design is the selection of the noninferiority margin, which sets the maximum accepted loss in efficacy for the new treatment to be considered not importantly worse.[1] Selecting this margin should consider trade-offs including other benefits of the new technique in a rigorous way, and for patient-oriented outcomes this should incorporate the preferences of patients.[2]

Acknowledging the importance of the noninferiority margin, a Delphi consensus study was conducted to establish acceptable noninferiority margins for the pathological outcomes of rectal cancer resection.[3] Notably, a consensus noninferiority margin for the "successful resection" composite outcome could not be reached. A noninferiority meta-analysis of all 14 randomized clinical trials comparing laparoscopic to open rectal resection was reported using these consensus-based noninferiority margins.[4] In this synthesis, laparoscopy was noninferior to open surgery for rectal cancer for all pathologic outcomes including circumferential resection margin, distal resection margin, and plane of mesorectal excision.

As noted, these pathological outcomes are surrogates for more patient-oriented outcomes including recurrence and disease-free survival. The subsequent report of the longer-term outcomes from this ACOSOG Z6051 trial identified no difference in 2-year disease-free survival, locoregional recurrence, or distant recurrence.[5] Similar longer-term results were found across the other randomized clinical trials examining open versus laparoscopic surgery for rectal cancer. Three-year disease-free survival of laparoscopic surgery was not inferior to open surgery in the COREAN trial, and these results persisted at 10 years.[6,7] At 3 years, disease-free and overall survival are similar between open and laparoscopic surgery in the COLOR II trial.[8] At 5 years, there were no differences between open and laparoscopic surgery in overall survival, disease-free survival, and recurrence in the CLASICC trial.[9] The ALaCaRT trial shared trial design elements with ACOSOG Z6051, and there were no differences between laparoscopy and open surgery in disease-free and overall survival at 2 years.[10] A meta-analysis of survival outcomes across randomized clinical trials comparing laparoscopic and open rectal cancer surgery confirms that laparoscopic surgery is not worse than open surgery on these patient-oriented outcomes.[11] In conclusion, the ACOSOG Z6051 provided an important examination of pathologic outcomes comparing laparoscopic to open rectal cancer surgery. With further trials and long-term follow-up, laparoscopy surgery is now a standard approach for eligible rectal cancers.

REFERENCES

1. Acuna SA, Dossa F, Chesney TR. Improving the reporting of non-inferiority trials by incorporating non-efficacy benefits: not all non-inferiority trials are created equal. *Eur J Epidemiol.* 2021;36(11):1097–1101.
2. Acuna SA, Chesney TR, Baxter NN. Incorporating patient preferences in noninferiority trials. *JAMA.* 2019;322(4):305–306.
3. Acuna SA, Chesney TR, Amarasekera ST, Baxter NN. Defining non-inferiority margins for quality of surgical resection for rectal cancer: a Delphi consensus study. *Ann Surg Oncol.* 2018;25(11):3171–3178.
4. Acuna SA, Chesney TR, Ramjist JK, Shah PS, Kennedy ED, Baxter NN. Laparoscopic versus open resection for rectal cancer: a noninferiority meta-analysis of quality of surgical resection outcomes. *Ann Surg.* 2019;269(5):849–855.
5. Fleshman JW, Branda ME, Sargent DJ, Boller AM, et al. Disease free survival and local recurrence for laparoscopic resection compared to open resection of stage II-III rectal cancer: follow up results of the ACOSOG Z6051 randomized controlled trial. *Ann Surg.* 2019;269(4):589.
6. Jeong SY, Park JW, Nam BH, et al. Open versus laparoscopic surgery for mid-rectal or low-rectal cancer after neoadjuvant chemoradiotherapy (COREAN trial): survival outcomes of an open-label, non-inferiority, randomised controlled trial. *Lancet Oncol.* 2014;15(7):767–774.

7. Park JW, Kang SB, Hao J, et al. Open versus laparoscopic surgery for mid or low rectal cancer after neoadjuvant chemoradiotherapy (COREAN trial): 10-year follow-up of an open-label, non-inferiority, randomised controlled trial. *Lancet Gastroenterol Hepatol.* 2021;6(7):569–577.

8. Bonjer HJ, Deijen CL, Abis GA, et al. A randomized trial of laparoscopic versus open surgery for rectal cancer. *N Engl J Med.* 2015;372(14):1324–1332.

9. Jayne DG, Thorpe HC, Copeland J, Quirke P, Brown JM, Guillou PJ. Five-year follow-up of the Medical Research Council CLASICC trial of laparoscopically assisted versus open surgery for colorectal cancer. *Br J Surg.* 2010;97(11):1638–1645.

10. Stevenson AR, Solomon MJ, Brown CS, et al. Disease-free survival and local recurrence after laparoscopic-assisted resection or open resection for rectal cancer: the Australasian laparoscopic cancer of the rectum randomized clinical trial. *Ann Surg.* 2019;269(4):596–602.

11. Kong M, Chen H, Shan K, Sheng H, Li L. Comparison of survival among adults with rectal cancer who have undergone laparoscopic vs open surgery: a meta-analysis. *JAMA Netw Open.* 2022;5(5):e2210861. doi:10.1001/jamanetworkopen.2022.10861

The Evolution of Pelvic Exenteration Practice at a Single Center: Lessons Learned from over 500 Cases

Koh CE, Solomon MJ, Brown KG, Austin K, Byrne CM, Lee P, Young JM. Dis Colon Rectum 60(6):627–635, 2017

Reviewed by Ben Creavin and Desmond Winter

Research Question/Objective   The evolution of pelvic exenteration has seen a dramatic improvement in morbidity along with standardization of surgical approaches and terminology. The aim of this study was to evaluate the journey pelvic exenteration has gone on in a single high-volume exenterative center. Its goal was to present an update on lessons learned over the exenterative program, how they overcame them, recommend surgical techniques to improve outcomes, and give advice on how to prevent and deal with morbidity and quality of life issues.

Study Design   This was a special article of the exenterative program in a single center. There was no study design or review guidelines.

Sample Size   While the title states lessons learned from over 500 exenterations, this was a review article with no sample size.

Follow-Up   The study examines the exenterative program from 1991 to 2016. No specific patient follow-up is stated.

Inclusion/Exclusion Criteria   No inclusion or exclusion criteria were stated.

Intervention or Treatment Received   Included commentary was based on patients undergoing pelvic exenteration and mainly focused on new surgical approaches.

Results

The authors present a concise review of the exenterative program in the Royal Prince Alfred Hospital in Sydney. They have included a timeline of the evolution of this center along with seminal papers published from the group over the years. They divided the main body of the text into developing the program, patient factors, surgical techniques, morbidity, and future prospective.

   DOI: 10.1201/9780429285714-13

Development of a Pelvic Exenteration Service   This article gives a concise breakdown of the evolution of the service in table form. Essentially, the initial policy was focused on the safety of this approach and providing a multidisciplinary approach to surgery. They started with central resections and developed a compartmental approach over time. This compartmental approach was further developed to include higher and wider techniques in line with patient needs and utilized cross-disciplinary expertise. Over time, the exenterative numbers increased due to the safety of the approach, and the center broadened and extended programs to include comprehensive preoperative assessment and postoperative rehabilitation. This led to support from medical administration and meticulous documentation to demonstrate the outcomes of this approach.

Patient Selection   Pelvic exenteration is reserved for resectable disease with curative intent, with MRI being the crucial modality in determining resectability. Palliative measures are contentious due to morbidity but are used in fungating or fistulating disease or when intractable pain is present. Oligometastatic disease is resectable if no progression on neoadjuvant therapy. Systemic failures are seen more frequently than local recurrence due to delays in pelvic exenterative patients undergoing adjuvant therapy.

Novel Surgical Techniques

1. *Compartmental approach*—Multidisciplinary collaboration is paramount to pelvic exenteration due to the challenges of extra-anatomical dissection. A compartmental approach divides the pelvis into compartments and removes structures *en bloc* to prevent margin involvement. Specific procedures, such as sacrectomy, are recommended for recurrent tumors near the sacral periosteum.

2. *Novel pelvic side wall approaches*—Pelvic side wall disease is challenging; however, the use of preoperative MRI, CT angiograms, and venograms along with specific surgical techniques results in R0 resection rates of 66.5%. Surgery involves a layered approach, with mobilization of the ureters, iliac arteries and veins, and deep neuromuscular structures. The internal iliacs act as a fixation point allowing mobilization of surrounding structures. Involvement of vasculature may require wider resection and reconstruction to achieve improved oncological outcomes. Venous compression may lead to collateral formation resulting in a reduced need for venous reconstruction.

3. *Novel anterior dissection techniques*—Two novel approaches are adopted for cystoprostatectomy. Firstly, a more radical surgical approach including excision of the anterior pelvic soft tissue is described, including the urogenital diaphragm and membranous urethra. This reduces bleeding as it allows better control of the dorsal venous complex. The second approach involves a more radical *en bloc* resection of the pubic ramus or symphysis to achieve negative margins. Reconstruction of the pubic symphysis can be done with internal fixation or a 2-layeered mesh. The penis can be reattached to the periosteum of the pubic bone if complete mobilization was required.

4. *Novel sacral approaches*—Modifications to staged abdominosacral resection have been seen, with low sacrectomy, anterior table sacrectomies, and posterior first approach now used with similar outcomes. High and low sacrectomy R0 rates are similar when curative intent is the objective; however, neurological morbidity is higher with high sacrectomy. Perineal wound issues are common due to radiation effects and devascularization of flaps. Autologous myocutaneous flaps such as vertical rectus abdominus flaps are preferred due to reduced morbidity. Biological mesh and gluteal-based flaps are used less frequently with sparse data on outcomes.

Surgical Outcomes and Morbidity   The oncological superiority of pelvic exenteration over palliation or chemoradiotherapy is well established, with surgical mortality of 1–2% in specialized centers. Morbidity is seen in 20–80% of previous publications, with septic complications commonest. Implementation of 5 days of intravenous antibiotics, parenteral nutrition, and drain monitoring with creatinine at days 1 and 5 all helping to reduce the impact of morbidity and allow early reintervention if required. Early recognition of urine leaks is important as early surgical reintervention can reduce length of stay. Furthermore, ureteric stents, nephrostomies, and catheters can all allow natural decompression of the conduit, with interventional drainage of urinomas to reduce sepsis. Meticulous audit and data collection are important to implement exenteration services. Randomized trials are needed to refine practice, and guidelines would be welcome.

Quality of Life Outcomes   Previously described harshly as "mutilation" surgery, the early quality of life reports were not well-documented; however, large research studies have allowed insight into this topic. Patients who undergo pelvic exenteration have a quick recovery, with baseline quality of life achieved in 3–6 months postoperatively. Furthermore, compared to nonexenteration patients, quality of life was better at 6–9 months due to disease progression in the latter group. Improvements in quality of life are due to the multidisciplinary approach.

Future Directions   While surgical and oncological outcomes improve, focus has shifted to what should be resected and to the costs to society and quality of life. Chemotherapy, immunotherapy, and targeted therapies are being explored to improve outcomes. Three-dimensional printing and reconstructive prosthetics are being used to improve MRI planning and bridge nerve resection segments. Gynecological exenterations are evolving along with pelvic connective tissue malignancies. Focus of research is now on graft techniques, wound healing, and reconstruction methods to prevent complications such as fistula and obstruction.

Study Limitations   While this is a comprehensive article, it is limited by its review nature. There were no guidelines used to structure the review, and no study design was presented. It was a commentary of a single-center exenterative program, making its level of evidence low.

The focus of this article was examining novel approaches to dealing with certain aspects of pelvic exenteration. Even though the authors do comment that detailed description of the various surgical approaches is beyond the scope of the paper, the reviewers feel a little more detail or diagrammatic representation of these approaches would add to the article and would help readers have a single resource to refer to for surgical approaches. The authors do include a timeline with dates of articles that can direct readers to specific articles dealing with the various approaches.

Relevant Studies   Pelvic exenteration has seen a dramatic change over the years with improved oncological outcomes seen with more extensive resections. The use of flap reconstruction and bone resection has seen a dramatic rise in use over the last 10–15 years, with a significant improvement in R0 resections seen in high-volume centers (1). Negative resection margins in the region of 80% have been quoted with mortality rates of 1.5% seen (2). Median survival, too, has increased with an R0 resection equating to 43-month median survival; however, nodal disease and an involved margin have been noted as poor predictors of survival (2, 3). Neoadjuvant therapy is associated with improved survival; however, more postoperative complications, readmission, and radiological interventions are associated with it (1, 2).

The boundaries for oligometastatic disease are continually being tested, with simultaneous resection for liver metastasis being feasible. However, only a quarter of surgeons would undertake a simultaneous resection currently (4). The results of simultaneous resections are promising, with excellent R0 resection margins being achieved in the primary and liver, with 30-day mortality of 1.6% and major morbidity of 32% (5). Five-year survival for R0 resections are in the region of 55% compared to 20% in non-R0 resections. Induction chemotherapy has been advocated as first-line treatment, with a diverting stoma utilized in symptomatic disease (5).

Minimally invasive techniques are being used in highly selective cases of pelvic exenteration. Laparoscopic exenteration is associated with a shorter length of stay and reduced morbidity compared to its open counterpart. However, it must be highlighted that tumor and patient factors play into selection and should only be used in select cases (6). Robotic platforms are also being used with low conversion rates, similar morbidity, and equivalent oncological outcomes (7).

A recent PelvEx collaborative paper assessed the minimum standard required for a pelvic exenterative practice. This detailed paper gives concise definitions of the 7 intrapelvic compartments, which helps define the topography of the tumor, predict involved structures, and plan curative surgery (8). The center requires all specialties to be present, from surgical teams, physios, and psychologists. A dedicated MDT is required to discuss all cases to aid in identifying which case will require certain specialties, with specialized templates for standardized documenting all discussed at the MDT (8). The paper details baseline preoperative workup for patients in terms of staging, anesthetic input, and prehabilitation for patients, which has a big influence on patient outcomes (8, 9). Furthermore, detailed surgical approaches along with reconstructive methods are presented. Bladder and bone reconstructions can be challenging; however, this paper breaks down the various bone reconstructions and gives tips with regard to what needs reconstruction and how reconstruction can be achieved (8).

REFERENCES

1. PelvEx C. Changing outcomes following pelvic exenteration for locally advanced and recurrent rectal cancer. BJS Open. 2019;3(4):516–20.
2. The PelvEx C. Surgical and survival outcomes following relvic exenteration for locally advanced primary rectal cancer: results from an international collaboration. Annals of Surgery. 2019;269(2).
3. The PelvEx C. Factors affecting outcomes following pelvic exenteration for locally recurrent rectal cancer. British Journal of Surgery. 2018;105(6):650–7.
4. PelvEx C. Management strategies for patients with advanced rectal cancer and liver metastases using modified Delphi methodology: results from the PelvEx Collaborative. Colorectal Disease. 2020;22(9):1184–8.
5. PelvEx C. Simultaneous pelvic exenteration and liver resection for primary rectal cancer with synchronous liver metastases: results from the PelvEx Collaborative. Colorectal Disease. 2020;22(10):1258–62.
6. Srinivasaiah N, Shekleton F, Kelly ME, Harji D, Malietzis G, Askari A, et al. Minimally invasive surgery techniques in pelvic exenteration: a systematic and meta-analysis review. Surgical Endoscopy. 2018;32(12):4707–15.
7. Chang TP, Chok AY, Tan D, Rogers A, Rasheed S, Tekkis P, et al. The emerging role of robotics in pelvic exenteration surgery for locally advanced rectal cancer: a narrative review. J Clin Med. 2021;10(7).
8. PelvEx C. Minimum standards of pelvic exenterative practice: PelvEx Collaborative guideline. British Journal of Surgery. 2022;109(12):1251–63.
9. PelvEx C. Perioperative management and anaesthetic considerations in pelvic exenterations using Delphi methodology: results from the PelvEx Collaborative. BJS Open. 2021;5(1):zraa055.

CHAPTER 14

Neoadjuvant (Chemo)Radiotherapy with Total Mesorectal Excision Only Is Not Sufficient to Prevent Lateral Local Recurrence in Enlarged Nodes: Results of the Multicenter Lateral Node Study of Patients with Low cT3/4 Rectal Cancer

Ogura A, Konishi T, Cunningham C, Garcia-Aguilar J, Iversen H, Toda S, Lee IK, Lee HX, Uehara K, Lee P, Putter H, van de Velde CJH, Beets GL, Rutten HJT, Kusters M: Lateral Node Study Consortium. J Clin Oncol. 1;37(1):33–43, 2019

Reviewed by Kheng-Seong Ng and Michael J. Solomon

Research Question/Objective Despite improvements in the surgical management of rectal cancer over the past decades, local recurrence (LR) following rectal cancer surgery remains a challenging problem. Lateral LR (LLR), i.e., recurrence in the lateral pelvic compartment(s), accounts for a large proportion of these, especially in low rectal cancers where lateral lymph node spread is well-documented.

Traditionally, there has been an "East–West divide" in the management of lateral lymph nodes (LLNs) for rectal cancer. The Western approach has been to achieve local control with preoperative (chemo)radiotherapy (CRT) to sterilize the lateral pelvic compartment, resulting in CRT followed by TME as a standard treatment of clinical stage II/III rectal cancer. By contrast, TME with prophylactic lateral lymph node dissection (LLND) has been adopted by the East. Similar LR rates observed between the two approaches have provided a justification for Western surgeons to rely on CRT for lateral nodal control, which obviates the morbidity and long-term genitourinary dysfunction associated with LLND.

Contemporary evidence, however, has questioned the adequacy of CRT to prevent LLR. In patients with enlarged lateral LNs (LLNs) who undergo CRT followed by TME, LLR accounts for more than one-half of LR in some series, with an almost linear relationship between nodal size and LLR demonstrable. Moreover, distant metastases are documented in only approximately one-half of these patients, suggesting that LLR should be regarded as a locoregional failure potentially preventable by optimized surgery (i.e., LLND).[1,2]

DOI: 10.1201/9780429285714-14

This study therefore aimed to ascertain the outcomes of patients with enlarged LLNs managed by CRT plus TME and to assess whether the addition of LLND could decrease rates of LLR.

Study Design   This study was a retrospective multicenter study of patients who underwent resection for cT3/4 low rectal cancer between 2009 and 2013. Most patients received neoadjuvant radiotherapy, with or without chemotherapy. This was followed by TME surgery, and LLND was performed according to local practice.

Pretreatment MRIs of all patients were re-reviewed to ascertain LLN status. This was based on the largest LLN identified, for which both long-axis (LA) and short-axis (SA) measurements, as well as site (internal iliac, external iliac, or obturator), were recorded. The presence of malignant features was also noted.

The primary outcome measure was time to LR, which was categorized as either lateral, presacral, anastomotic, anterior, or perineal. Secondary outcomes included distant recurrence and cancer-specific survival. The associations between these outcome measures and LLN status, as well as other standard clinicopathological variables, were assessed by Cox regression.

Sample Size   Overall, 1216 patients from across 12 hospitals in 7 countries were included.

Follow-Up   Patient follow-up was performed according to local practice. The median follow-up duration after surgery was 56.5 months (IQR 55.0–58.1).

Inclusion/Exclusion Criteria   Patients with low rectal cancer (within 8 cm from the anal verge on MRI) were included. Exclusion criteria included the absence of appropriate pretreatment imaging, presence of distant metastases at initial staging, or a noncurative resection.

Intervention or Treatment Received   Treatment strategies for individual patients were determined by a multidisciplinary approach. Data relating to CRT regimens were retrieved. It was confirmed that, generally, both the obturator and internal iliac compartments were in the standard irradiated fields.

While all patients underwent TME following CRT, LLND was variably practiced across participating centers and according to heterogeneous indications. In some cases, only sampling ("cherry-picking") of a suspected LLN was performed. A formal LLND was defined as complete clearance of lymphatic tissue from the lateral compartment (both internal iliac and obturator areas). One center performed LLND on all patients, irrespective of LLN size (i.e., prophylactic LLND). Other centers performed LLND selectively based on imaging appearance of LLN, but criteria for LLND varied between centers.

Results   Of the 1216 patients included, at least 1 visible LLN was detected in 703 patients (57.8%) on pretreatment MRI. The majority of these were in the obturator compartment (63.7%). The median size of the largest LLN was 7.0 mm in LA, and 5.0 mm in SA. Most patients underwent either a low anterior resection or abdominoperineal excision of the rectum. LLND was performed in only 11.7% (n = 142) of patients, which resulted in 35 patients with pathologically positive LLNs.

A total of 108 patients developed LR. Of these, over one-half were diagnosed in the lateral compartment. The 5-year overall LR rate was 10.0%, and the 5-year LLR rate was 5.5%. A relationship between increasing LLN size and higher LLR rates was demonstrated in this study. On the argument that an LLR rate of 20% was considered too high, a decision was made to select an SA cutoff value of 7 mm on pretreatment MRI for further analyses.

A total of 192 patients (16%) had LLNs with SA ≥7 mm on pretreatment MRI. These patients had significantly higher 5-year rates of LLR (15.0%) and overall LR (19.2%) compared with patients with smaller LLNs. These findings persisted on multivariable analysis, and patients with LLNs ≥7 mm in SA had a significantly higher risk of lateral (HR 2.060, 95% CI 1.017–4.173) and overall LR (HR 2.010; 95% CI 1.157–3.495).

After LLND, 5-year lateral and overall LR rates were significantly lower in patients with LLNs with SA ≥7 mm compared with patients who did not undergo LLND (5.7 vs. 19.5% and 5.7 vs. 25.6%, respectively). Pathologically involved LLNs were found in approximately over one-half of patients with LLNs with SA ≥7 mm who underwent LLND.

Study Limitations   This study was limited by its retrospective and multi-institutional nature, which led to heterogeneity in patients and treatments. There was therefore variability in the way patients were selected for LLND and in the surgical technique by which LLND was performed. While efforts were made to standardize the re-evaluation of imaging (including both pre- and posttreatment scans), inter-observer agreement could have been better established through blinded double interpretation of scans or central review of imaging.

Relevant Studies   The results of this study form an important contribution to the growing body of literature that suggests neoadjuvant CRT is insufficient for sterilization of potentially involved LLNs in patients in low rectal cancer and that LLND is indicated to achieve local control in these circumstances.

Preceding this study, some of the earliest data postulating the inadequacy of neoadjuvant CRT in managing LLNs were borne from case series in "the East." Kim et al. (2008) analyzed the outcomes of 366 patients with low rectal cancer, all of whom received CRT and TME without LLND; LR was recorded in 7.9% of patients, of which the majority (82.7%) of cases were LLRs.[1] Kim et al.

(2015) investigated 900 patients in an attempt to determine which patients might benefit from LLND; in that series, LR was diagnosed in 7.2%, of which two-thirds were LLRs, and LLN SA measurement was significantly associated with recurrence-free survival and overall survival.[2] These studies spurred discussions regarding the role of LLN size as an important criterion by which patients could be selected for LLND.

The rate of pathologically proven positive LLNs in clinically suspicious nodes after CRT + TME + LLND was the subject of a recent systematic review.[3] Nodal metastases were identified after LLND in up to 61% of cases. In cases where suspicious LLNs responded to CRT, the rate of involved nodes was between 0 and 20.4%, but between 25.0 and 83.3% of persistent LLNs were found to be pathologically involved. This disparity in outcomes between "responsive" and "non-responsive" LLNs spawned interest in the use of *post*treatment imaging to guide LLN management.

Several studies from Japan,[4] South Korea,[5,6] and North America,[7] have suggested a posttreatment LLN SA measurement ≥5 mm to be an appropriate cutoff for which LLND should be performed. It should be noted, though, that pathologically proven metastases in responsive LLNs measuring <5 mm have been reported in as high as 20% of patients in one series.[4] Kim et al. (2020) found that the addition of LLND resulted in a significant reduction in LR in both "responders" (i.e., SA <5mm post CRT) and "non-responders" (i.e., those with persisting nodes, SA ≥5 mm post CRT).[5] In keeping with this, Ogura et al. (2019), in a large multinational lateral node consortium publication, suggested that LLNs measuring on SA <4 mm posttreatment could be managed nonoperatively, as no episodes of LLRs were recorded in patients with LLNs measuring <4 mm on SA post-CRT.[8]

Numerous meta-analyses have been performed investigating the benefits of LLND for rectal cancer, each with different outcome measures, inclusion criteria, and time period inclusion. Improved LLR-free survival has been shown in several meta-analyses,[9–11] whereas survival advantage has been more difficult to prove. Yet, while a clear survival benefit has not been shown for LLND following CRT and TME, it should be remembered that LLR is associated with significant morbidity, often resulting in ureteric and intestinal obstruction, severe pain, fistula formation, and poor quality of life. Management of LLR is complex, often requiring exenterative surgery with its attendant morbidity and functional implications. Therefore, the role of LLND in rectal cancer patients with enlarged LLNs following CRT and TME to reduce LLR seems justified. Prospective studies are required to determine evidence-based protocols by which patients are best selected for LLND.

REFERENCES

1. Kim TH, Jeong SY, Choi DH, et al. Lateral lymph node metastasis is a major cause of locoregional recurrence in rectal cancer treated with preoperative chemoradiotherapy and curative resection. *Ann Surg Oncol* 2008; **15**(3): 729–37.
2. Kim MJ, Kim TH, Kim DY, et al. Can chemoradiation allow for omission of lateral pelvic node dissection for locally advanced rectal cancer? *J Surg Oncol* 2015; **111**(4): 459–64.
3. Atef Y, Koedam TW, van Oostendorp SE, Bonjer HJ, Wijsmuller AR, Tuynman JB. Lateral pelvic lymph node metastases in rectal cancer: a systematic review. *World J Surg* 2019; **43**(12): 3198–206.
4. Akiyoshi T, Matsueda K, Hiratsuka M, et al. Indications for lateral pelvic lymph node dissection based on magnetic resonance imaging before and after preoperative chemoradiotherapy in patients with advanced low-rectal cancer. *Ann Surg Oncol* 2015; **22 Suppl 3**: S614–20.
5. Kim MJ, Chang GJ, Lim HK, et al. Oncological impact of lateral lymph node dissection after preoperative chemoradiotherapy in patients with rectal cancer. *Ann Surg Oncol* 2020; **27**(9): 3525–33.
6. Oh HK, Kang SB, Lee SM, et al. Neoadjuvant chemoradiotherapy affects the indications for lateral pelvic node dissection in mid/low rectal cancer with clinically suspected lateral node involvement: a multicenter retrospective cohort study. *Ann Surg Oncol* 2014; **21**(7): 2280–7.
7. Malakorn S, Yang Y, Bednarski BK, et al. Who should get lateral pelvic lymph node dissection after neoadjuvant chemoradiation? *Dis Colon Rectum* 2019; **62**(10): 1158–66.
8. Ogura A, Konishi T, Beets GL, et al. Lateral nodal features on restaging magnetic resonance imaging associated with lateral local recurrence in low rectal cancer after neoadjuvant chemoradiotherapy or radiotherapy. *JAMA Surg* 2019; **154**(9): e192172.
9. Yang X, Yang S, Hu T, et al. What is the role of lateral lymph node dissection in rectal cancer patients with clinically suspected lateral lymph node metastasis after preoperative chemoradiotherapy? A meta-analysis and systematic review. *Cancer Med* 2020; **9**(13): 4477–89.
10. Fahy MR, Kelly ME, Nugent T, Hannan E, Winter DC. Lateral pelvic lymphadenectomy for low rectal cancer: a META-analysis of recurrence rates. *Int J Colorectal Dis* 2021; **36**(3): 551–8.
11. Law BZY, Yusuf Z, Ng YE, Aly EH. Does adding lateral pelvic lymph node dissection to neoadjuvant chemotherapy improve outcomes in low rectal cancer? *Int J Colorectal Dis* 2020; **35**(8): 1387–95.

CHAPTER 15

Transanal Total Mesorectal Excision: Why, When, and How

Penna M, Cunningham C, Hompes R. Clin Colon Rectal Surg. 30(5):339–345, 2017

Reviewed by Justin Maykel and Dong Yoon

Research Question/Objective   Transanal total mesorectal excision (taTME) is a minimally invasive technique developed to overcome inherent challenges of a rectal cancer operation while adhering to the tenets of total mesorectal excision (TME). Combining various aspects of existing transanal surgical techniques, taTME allows for low rectal TME dissection from a novel vantage point ("bottom-up") and bypasses the challenges of the transabdominal approach ("top-down"). After its success in the first patient in 2010, taTME has gained significant interest in the surgical community for its potential to improve oncologic resection. This study reviews the benefits, indications, and technical details of taTME.

Study Design   Review.

Sample Size   Not applicable.

Follow-Up   Not applicable.

Inclusion/Exclusion Criteria   Not applicable.

Intervention or Treatment Received   TaTME use mainly in the context of rectal cancer.

Results   Precise dissection in the TME plane has shown to improve oncologic resection quality and local recurrence rates for rectal cancer. However, open transabdominal dissection in the pelvis is hampered by poor visualization and limited mobility due to the small, rigid working space of the pelvis. These challenges are compounded for distal rectal dissections, resulting in positive circumferential resection margins in up to 22% of cases. Despite advances in minimally invasive surgery, laparoscopic and robotic transabdominal approaches have failed to definitively improve pathologic resection outcomes; in fact, some evidence suggests inferiority. TaTME has been shown to provide clearer visualization and allow for a more precise dissection to result in higher oncologic specimen quality while maintaining comparable perioperative morbidity rates.

DOI: 10.1201/9780429285714-15

Indications for taTME require considerations of both patient and surgeon factors. TaTME may be indicated for both benign (including inflammatory bowel disease, familial polyposis syndromes) and malignant diseases requiring precise proctectomy of the mid- to distal rectum. Factors that pose challenges for the transabdominal approach, including male gender, visceral obesity, utilization of neoadjuvant radiation, and low tumor requiring precise distal resection margin placement, are indications for the taTME approach.

Additionally, taTME is an advanced technique combining components of various specialized transanal techniques, including transanal endoscopic microsurgery (TEM), transanal minimally invasive surgery (TAMIS), and intersphincteric dissection. Therefore, a surgeon's mastery of these techniques is a prerequisite. As with all new techniques, learning experience in simulation, participation in training courses, and mentor guidance during the early phases of the learning curve are highly recommended.

TaTME is most commonly performed in a synchronous fashion with both transabdominal "top-down" and transanal "bottom-up" components. The transabdominal component (open or minimally invasive) proceeds in the usual fashion and includes descending colon mobilization, vascular ligation, and splenic flexure mobilization. The transanal component can be performed simultaneously with two operating teams.

The five critical steps of the procedure are distal purse string placement, full-thickness rectotomy, TME dissection, specimen extraction, and anastomosis. Using a transanal platform, such as the GelPOINT Path, and laparoscopic instruments, a watertight purse string closure of the rectum 1 cm distal to the tumor using a 2–0 or 0 monofilament suture is performed to allow for tumor exclusion and maintenance of pneumorectum. A monopolar electrocautery is then used to perform a circumferential full-thickness rectotomy distal to the purse string closure. A high-flow insufflation/ventilation system (e.g., AirSeal) is essential to maintaining a stable operating field and while preventing smoke from obscuring visualization.

Initial dissection is started off the midline and typically in the order of posterior, anterior, and lateral sides. Careful and meticulous attention to the correct plane of dissection is essential to prevent injury to surrounding structures and dissecting into the mesorectum itself. The dissection continues cephalad to meet the transabdominal field, typically anteriorly at the anterior peritoneal reflection. Once free, the specimen can be extracted transanally or, more commonly, transabdominally. A coloanal anastomosis is then performed in hand-sewn or stapled fashion, the latter of which requires a double purse string technique. The study compares various anastomotic techniques.

Study Limitations   Not applicable.

Relevant Studies   Since its inception in 2010, the taTME technique has been refined by various pioneering surgeons.[1,2] The importance of the five critical steps just listed cannot be overstated, as each component has large pitfalls. The retrograde dissection plane is novel even for experienced surgeons, and surgeon preparation and training are absolute prerequisites for the procedure.[3]

A few additional notes regarding the technique are worth mentioning. Both purse string placement and rectotomy can be guided by circumferentially marking the rectal mucosa with electrocautery at the desired level prior to each step.[2] This prevents spiraling of the purse string or dissection. Using a 0 prolene suture allows for synching down on the purse string knot to ensure a watertight closure. During the rectotomy, the rectum often appears thicker than expected, especially after neoadjuvant chemoradiation. Some recommend starting the dissection posteriorly,[1] while others recommend starting anteriorly where the rectal wall is thinnest and the TME plane can immediately be entered.[2]

Dissection in the correct plane is crucial to avoid inadvertent injuries to surrounding structures, including the urethra. While the anterior dissection is typically the most challenging in the top-down approach, the transanal view and angle significantly facilitates this portion. A rare complication during dissection is CO_2 embolism related to the high-flow CO_2 insufflation required to maintain pneumopelvis in a small operative field. The incidence of CO_2 embolism is reported to be 3.8% and manifests as a sudden decrease in O_2 and end-tidal CO_2 followed by rapid cardiovascular collapse.[4] By maintaining a high index of suspicion, this complication can be managed with minimal morbidity with immediate desufflation, repositioning in Trendelenberg and left lateral decubitus position, and providing hemodynamic support.

Prior to this study, multiple case series showed feasibility, perioperative safety, and favorable pathologic outcomes after taTME for rectal cancer.[5] The international taTME registry published its short-term outcomes of the first 720 cases.[6] Conversion to transabdominal approach occurred in 2.8% of cases. Incorrect plane dissection occurred in 7.8% with resultant urethral injury rate of 0.7%. Postoperative mortality and morbidity were 2.4% and 32.6%, respectively, with an anastomotic leak rate of 6.7%. Pathologic evaluation showed an R0 resection rate of 97.3%. This study concluded that taTME had acceptable perioperative outcomes and appears to be an effective and oncologically safe technique.

Another more recent series from a high-volume institution including 79 patients showed favorable perioperative outcomes with 1.3% conversion rate and no urethral injury.[7] Patients had consistent short lengths of stay (4 days, IQR 4–5 days) and a postoperative morbidity rate of 13.9%, with an anastomotic leak rate of 3.8%. The rate of composite optimal pathologic specimen (i.e., complete or nearly complete TME specimen, negative circumferential and distal resection margins) was 94.9%. With increased experience over time, patients undergoing taTME in high-volume specialized centers appear to have excellent perioperative and pathologic outcomes.

TaTME has been compared to laparoscopic TME. A large meta-analysis in 2020 compared outcomes of 495 taTME and 547 laparoscopic TME cases for mid- to low rectal cancer.[8] TaTME had lower but nonsignificant conversion rates (3.2% vs. 8.8%, $p = 0.09$), similar intraoperative complication rates and lower postoperative morbidity rates (34% vs. 41%, $p = 0.01$). Positive CRM rates were significantly lower in taTME (4% vs. 8.8%, $p = 0.01$) while positive DRM rates were similar (1.4% in both). A systemic review in 2021 assessing oncologic outcomes after taTME and laparoscopic TME reported similar local recurrence rates (2.1% vs. 3.1%, $p = 0.71$), distant metastasis (7.1% vs. 13.3%, $p = 0.23$), 2-year disease-free survival (RR 1.01, $p = 0.86$), and overall survival (RR 1.04, $p = 0.25$).[9] TaTME may have improved perioperative outcomes while maintaining similar pathologic and mid-term oncologic outcomes when compared to laparoscopic TME.

There is evidence for concern with taTME use in rectal cancer. In 2020, a Norwegian nationwide audit showed high rates of local recurrence as well as significantly higher postoperative morbidity and mortality rates compared to the retrospective laparoscopic TME cohort, leading to a nationwide moratorium on taTME.[10] Though possibly limited by patient selection and technique learning curve, this study questions the oncologic outcomes following taTME.

Ultimately, additional conclusive evidence for the role of taTME is needed. Currently there are two ongoing randomized controlled trials that compare taTME to laparoscopic TME. The COLOR III trial is designed as a superiority study and plans to enroll 1098 patients with mid- to low rectal cancer in a 2 taTME to 1 laparoscopic TME ratio.[11] The GRECCAR 11 trial is a noninferiority designed study with an anticipated 266 patients with T3 low rectal cancers.[12] Completion and follow-up data from these trials are eagerly awaited to solidify the role of taTME in rectal cancer.

REFERENCES

1. Maykel JA. Laparoscopic Transanal Total Mesorectal Excision (taTME) for Rectal Cancer. J Gastrointest Surg. 2015 Oct;19(10):1880–1888.
2. Albert M, Lee L. Tips and Tricks. Clin Colon Rectal Surg. 2020 May;33(3):173–179.
3. McLemore EC, Lavi P, Attaluri V. Learning Transanal Total Mesorectal Excision. Clin Colon Rectal Surg. 2020 May;33(3):168–172.
4. Harnsberger CR, Alavi K, Davids JS, et al. CO2 Embolism Can Complicate Transanal Total Mesorectal Excision. Tech Coloproctol. 2018 Nov;22(11):881–885.
5. Ma B, Gao P, Song Y, et al. Transanal Total Mesorectal Excision (taTME) for Rectal Cancer: A Systematic Review and Meta-Analysis of Oncological and Perioperative Outcomes Compared with Laparoscopic Total Mesorectal Excision. BMC Cancer. 2016 Jul 4;16:380.

6. Penna M, Hompes R, Arnold S, et al. TaTME Registry Collaborative. Transanal Total Mesorectal Excision: International Registry Results of the First 720 Cases. Ann Surg. 2017 Jul;266(1):111–117.

7. Maykel JA, Hahn SJ, Beauharnais CC, et al. Oncologic Outcomes After Transanal Total Mesorectal Excision for Rectal Cancer. Dis Colon Rectum. 2022 Jun 1;65(6):827–836.

8. Aubert M, Mege D, Panis Y. Total Mesorectal Excision for Low and Middle Rectal Cancer: Laparoscopic versus Transanal Approach–a Meta-Analysis. Surg Endosc. 2020 Sep;34(9):3908–3919.

9. Alimova I, Chernyshov S, Nagudov M, et al. Comparison of Oncological and Functional Outcomes and Quality of Life After Transanal or Laparoscopic Total Mesorectal Excision for Rectal Cancer: A Systematic Review and Meta-Analysis. Tech Coloproctol. 2021 Aug;25(8):901–913.

10. Wasmuth HH, Faerden AE, Myklebust TÅ, et al. Transanal Total Mesorectal Excision for Rectal Cancer Has Been Suspended in Norway. Br J Surg. 2020 Jan;107(1):121–130.

11. Deijen CL, Velthuis S, Tsai A, et al. COLOR III: A Multicentre Randomised Clinical Trial Comparing Transanal TME versus Laparoscopic TME for Mid and Low Rectal Cancer. Surg Endosc. 2016 Aug;30(8):3210–3215.

12. Lelong B, de Chaisemartin C, Meillat H, et al. French Research Group of Rectal Cancer Surgery (GRECCAR). A Multicentre Randomised Controlled Trial to Evaluate the Efficacy, Morbidity and Functional Outcome of Endoscopic Transanal Proctectomy versus Laparoscopic Proctectomy for Low-Lying Rectal Cancer (ETAP-GRECCAR 11 TRIAL): Rationale and Design. BMC Cancer. 2017 Apr 11;17(1):253.

CHAPTER 16

Reappraisal of the 5 Centimetre Rule of Distal Excision for Carcinoma of the Rectum: A Study of Distal Intramural Spread and of Patients' Survival

Williams NS, Dixon MF, Johnston D. Clin Colon Rectal Surg. 30(5):330–345, 2017

Reviewed by S. Thomas Kang and Gregory D. Kennedy

Research Question/Objective Traditional teaching in curative resection of colon and rectal tumors necessitate distal resection margin (DRM) of 5 cm in order to (1) eradicate the tumor and (2) prevent recurrence. With introduction of new surgical devices and techniques such as staplers and coloanal anastomosis, patients who would have otherwise required permanent ostomies have now been able to undergo sphincter-preserving operations even in low-lying rectal cancers. Nonetheless, if one were to be dogmatic about the "5 cm distal margin," then it would become inevitable for patients to be subjected to abdominoperineal resection (APR). The aim of the study was to discern whether it would be feasible for the specimen to have less than a 5 cm distal margin, and if so what would be the smallest safe margin allowed.

Study Design There were two parts to this retrospective study. In Part I, the authors sought to delineate the exact distance of spread of a tumor using 50 consecutive APR specimens containing rectal carcinoma. Each resection was performed for biopsy-proven rectal carcinoma whose distal edge was 5–10 cm from the anal verge as confirmed on digital rectal exam as well as sigmoidoscopy. Each specimen was received fresh and fixed in a standardized manner in formalin and an outline of the rectum prepared to notate the locations of the tumor, lymph nodes, and vasculature. The specimens were then prepared into strips to classify the tumor using Dukes criteria as well as to study the exact distal spread of the malignancy.

In Part II, the authors reviewed clinical and pathological records of all rectal carcinoma patients who underwent anterior resection over a 10-year period from 1958 to 1968. After excluding those without necessary clinical records and those who had undergone palliative resection, 79 patients were included in survival analysis. Those 79 patients were then further divided into those with gross distal margin of 4 cm or less and those with distal margin of 5–9 cm.

DOI: 10.1201/9780429285714-16

Sample Size   The study had two separate sample sizes. In Part I were 50 consecutive APR specimens from curative-intent operations.

In Part II were 79 patients undergoing anterior resection performed with curative intent.

Follow-Up   5 years

Inclusion/Exclusion Criteria   In both Parts I and II, those specimens included in the study were from resections done with curative intent.

In Part II, 126 patients who underwent anterior resection for rectal cancer were included. Of those, 115 had regular follow-up records. Out of the 115, 19 were excluded for inadequate pathology documentation, leaving 96 patients. Of those, 17 had undergone palliative resection; thus 79 patients who had undergone curative resection with sufficient clinical records were included.

Intervention/Treatment Received   Not applicable

Results

Part I   Distal intramural spread was present in 24% (12) of the specimens and absent in 76% (38). The distal spread ranged from 0.5 to 5 cm and was 1 cm or less in 14% of the specimens, drawing attention to the fact that about 90% of patients had no distal intramural spread or spread of less than 1 cm. Only 10% (5) of the samples demonstrated a distal spread of more than 1 cm, and 3 of those samples had a spread of greater than 2 cm; all 5 had poorly differentiated Dukes grade C. Not all distal spread was contiguous with the lower edge of the tumor with satellite microscopic involvement—separate from the actual tumor—being observed in 4 patients, all with poorly differentiated Dukes grade C carcinoma.

A total of 12 tumors with distal intramural presence spread by direct extension through the lymphatics present in the submucosal layer. Of the 12, 10 were available for follow-up analysis as 1 died postoperatively, and the other was lost to follow-up. Eight of 10 had recurrence, and 6 of those 8 died within 3 years of operation. Seven of the 8 patients had distant recurrence, mainly in the liver and lung; the site of recurrence in the eighth patient was unclear from the records. If a patient's tumor had even a 0.5 cm distal intramural spread and Dukes grade C, metastasis was almost certain.

Part II   The patients were divided into those with shorter than 5 cm distal margin and those with distal margin of 5 cm or more: 61% (48) of patients had distal margin clearance of <5 cm (mean 2.8 cm, Group I), and 39% (31) of patients had a distal clearance margin of 5 cm or more (mean 6.5 cm, Group II). Patient characteristics, such as age (61 vs. 58, Group I vs. Group II), sex, and distance of tumor from anal verge (10.6 cm vs. 11.4 cm, Group I vs. II), were similar in both groups. In terms of tumor grade, 54% in Group I and 23 % in Group II had Dukes grade C tumors.

Operative mortality in both groups were similar with 6% in Group I versus 6.5% in Group II, as well as overall rate of anastomotic leak proven on contrast enema, endoscopy, or digital exam (54% vs. 52%, Group I vs. II, respectively, no clinical significance). Corrected 5-year survival was 77% and 65% in Group I and Group II, respectively. With regard to postoperative mortality, 15% (7) of patients in Group I and 10% (3) of patients in Group II passed away within 5 years of operation due to recurrent disease and/or metastasis. All but 2 patients who passed away had Dukes stage C carcinoma.

Study Limitations   Several limitations exist for this paper.

The retrospective nature of the study prohibits study of local and distant rectal cancer recurrence in those who had achieved less than 5 cm distal margin; for example, a prospective trial would allow researchers to look at varying distal resection margins and respective outcomes. We also do not have clinical information regarding preoperative local staging of each tumor, which we now know plays an important role in rectal cancer treatment. Professor Heald's 1982 paper demonstrated a dramatic decrease in local recurrence with excision of the meso-rectum in rectal cancer operations. The authors of the study do not comment on the quality of the mesorectal excision in the 50 specimens examined in Part I of the paper.

The authors concluded in Part II that those in Group I had a higher proportion of Dukes Class C tumors compared to patients in Group II. Despite having a shorter distal margin compared to Group II, those in Group I had a higher corrected 5-year survival as well as similar operative mortality, anastomotic leak rate, and distant metastasis. Except for the difference in distal margin, all other factors were not found to be statistically significant. However, the rate of local recurrence was 15% in Group I compared to 10% in Group II. While this may not have statistical significance, it may be clinically significant and may in fact—contrary to the authors' conclusion—have a detrimental effect on the patients' quality of life as in the right setting, those patients would need close monitoring and may require another operation.

Relevant Studies   The concept of necessitating a wide margin in colon resection originated in the early 1900s. The thought was that, despite the gross mucosal appearance, the tumor likely extends into the submucosal space with a wider base.[1,2]

This teaching was upheld in later years when in 1954, Grinnell reported distal intramural spread of up to 4 cm in over 10% of potentially curative rectal resections, further putting an emphasis on the need for the "5-cm rule."[3]

This idea began to be challenged when Quer et al. reported a 1% incidence of distal spread of 1.5 cm or more. Based on the findings, the authors recommended a distal resection margin of 2.5 cm in well- or average-differentiated tumors versus a 6 cm clearance with poorly differentiated carcinomas.[4] Including this paper, the "5-cm rule" was challenged time and time again by numerous researchers who sought to justify a shorter distal resection margin by looking at recurrence.[5–8]

The treatment algorithm for rectal cancer has changed drastically since publication of this paper. The question of "How much distal margin is sufficient?" becomes paramount especially when considering sphincter preservation.[9] Since Heald's groundbreaking paper describing total mesorectal excision (TME)[10] that drastically reduced local recurrence, the advent of preoperative chemoradiotherapy further pushed the boundaries for DRM.[11] Rutkowski et al. reported a noninferior oncologic outcome of 1 cm DRM in those patients who had neoadjuvant chemoradiation in low rectal cancer.[12]

In more recent years, the idea of watch and wait has gained traction in those patients with complete clinical response (cCR) after neoadjuvant chemoradiotherapy. Given this radical concept published in 2004 by Dr. Habr-Gama,[13] in carefully selected patients, the era of organ preservation as a guideline-supported option does not seem far off.

REFERENCES

1. Handley W.S.: The surgery of the lymphatic system. Br. Med. J. 1910;1:922–8.
2. Cole P.P.: The intramural spread of rectal carcinoma. Br. Med. J. 1913;1:431–3.
3. Grinnell R.S.: Distal intramural spread of carcinoma of the rectum and rectosigmoid. Surg. Gynecol. Obstet. 1954;99:421–30.
4. Quer E.A., Dahlin D.C. and Mayo C.W.: Retrograde intramural spread of carcinoma of the rectum and rectosigmoid. Surg. Gynecol. Obstet. 1953;96:24–30.
5. Wilson S.M. and Beahrs O.H.: The curative treatment of carcinoma of the sigmoid, rectosigmoid, and rectum. Ann. Surg. 1976;183:556–65.
6. Lofgren E.P., Waugh J.M. and Dockerty M.B.: Local recurrence of carcinoma after anterior resection of the rectum and the sigmoid. Arch. Surg. 1957;74:825–38.
7. Copeland E.M., Millar L.D. and Jones R.S.: Prognostic factors in carcinoma of the colon and rectum. Am. J. Surg. 1968;116:875–81.
8. Williams N.S., Dixon M.F. and Johnston D. Reappraisal of the 5 centimetre rule of distal excision for carcinoma of the rectum: a study of distal intramural spread and of patients' survival. Br. J. Surg. 1983;70:150–4.
9. Pollett W.G. and Nicholls R.J. The relationship between the extent of distal clearance and survival and local recurrence rates after curative anterior resection for carcinoma of the rectum. Ann. Surg. 1983;198:159–63.
10. Heald R.J. A new approach to rectal cancer. Br. J. Hosp. Med. 1979;22:277–81.
11. Park I.J. and Kim J.C.: Adequate length of the distal resection margin in rectal cancer: from the oncological point of view. J. Gastrointest. Surg. 2010;14:1331–37.

12. Rutkowski A., Bujko K., Nowacki M.P. et al.: Distal bowel surgical margin shorter than 1 cm after preoperative radiation for rectal cancer: is it safe? Ann Surg. Oncol. 2008;15:3124–31.
13. Habr-Gama A., Perez R.O., Nadalin W., et al.: Operative versus nonoperative treatment for stage 0 distal rectal cancer following chemoradiation therapy. Ann. Surg. 2004;240:711–18.

CHAPTER 17

Recurrence and Survival after Total Mesorectal Excision for Rectal Cancer

Heald RJ, Ryall RD. Lancet. 1(8496):1479–1482, 1986

Reviewed by Paolo Goffredo and Robert D. Madoff

Research Question/Objective   The primary aim of this study was to report oncologic outcomes of patients with rectal carcinomas undergoing total mesorectal excision (TME), a novel technique devised by R.J. "Bill" Heald. TME focused on sharp dissection in the anatomic embryologic planes of the visceral mesentery of the rectum with the goal to decrease the high rates of local recurrence, a major unresolved problem of rectal surgery until TME's widespread adoption. In addition, the advent of circular staplers the 1980s deeply impacted the practice of colorectal surgeons by providing the ability to perform low rectal anastomoses (1). In order to preserve bowel continuity, surgeons had to defy the reigning dogma of the 5 cm surgical margin. A secondary hypothesis of this paper was that a reduction of the bowel wall margin to preserve the sphincters was safe when TME was performed.

Study Design   This was a single surgeon series from the Colorectal Research Unit in Basingstoke, United Kingdom, between July 1978 and January 1986. Tumor recurrence was determined by clinical suspicion or "significant" increases of the carcinoembryonic antigen (CEA) level on two or more occasions.

Sample Size   During the study period, a total of 188 patients with rectal cancers were evaluated. Of those, 30 did not undergo an anterior resection due to no procedure being performed (2) or other surgical management, including abdominoperineal resection (21), Hartmann's procedure (3), laparotomy and/or colostomy (2), and local excision (2). Among the 158 anterior resections, 8 were not performed by Professor Heald, and 35 were of palliative intent, defined as visible metastatic or residual local disease. These exclusions left a final cohort of 115 patients.

Follow-Up   Study follow-up included an office postoperative visit within the first month and then every 3–4 months for 2 years, 6 months for a further 3 years, and yearly thereafter. Serum CEA was checked at each visit.

Inclusion/Exclusion Criteria   All patients referred for rectal cancer during the study time were screened for inclusion. Exclusion criteria were (1) not having an anterior resection, (2) being operated on by a surgeon other than Professor Heald, and (3) undergoing palliative surgery.

DOI: 10.1201/9780429285714-17

Intervention or Treatment Received   All patients underwent a complete TME with sharp scissors dissection and separate high ligation of the inferior mesenteric vessels. The middle rectal vessels were divided as far from the cancer margins as possible. When allowed by the position of the tumor, a small rectal stump was preserved. A right-angled clamp was placed across this bowel remnant, which was then thoroughly irrigated, prior to stapling to the previously mobilized colon.

Results

Postoperative Morbidity and Mortality   The postoperative mortality was 2.6% (3 out of 115 patients). Postoperative complications were not reported.

Local Recurrence   Out of 115 patients, only 3 (2.6%) experienced local recurrence with the cumulative risk at 5 years of 3.7%. One patient had both local and distant recurrence and died of disease 7 months later. The second patient had an anastomotic breakdown followed by a presacral recurrence treated with radiotherapy. The third patient developed a pararectal nodule 2 years postoperatively and was managed with the implantation of radioactive gold grains. In contrast, the rate of local failure in those who underwent a palliative resection was 34%.

Survival and Recurrence   Overall survival for the curative cohort was 70%, while the disease-free survival was 87%. Life tables were constructed from the last date when the status of every patient was known, incorporating a predictive factor from those patients who had not yet reached the 5-year follow-up time. The "corrected" survival rate at 5 years was 87.5%, and the disease-free survival was 81.7%. Negative prognostic factors were poor differentiation, advanced tumor staging, and extramural vascular invasion. However, height of the tumor/anastomosis and length of the surgical margins were not associated with survival.

Study Limitations   This is a single-surgeon series including only patients undergoing surgery with curative intent and without controls for comparison, limiting the generalizability of the results. There is no description of the demographic and clinical characteristics of the cohort, such as age, gender, and comorbidities, which are all relevant prognostic factors. Abdominoperineal resections (APR) were excluded; because low rectal cancers requiring an APR are at higher risk for recurrence, this could have potentially lowered the rates of local failure of the study. Moreover, no perioperative treatment was administered in the form of either chemotherapy or radiation, which significantly deviates from current algorithms. The staging system utilized in this manuscript is now considered obsolete and may have not adequately risk-stratified patients. In this regard, several pathologic features, including tumor budding/deposits and perineural invasion, as well as genetic mutations (MSI-H, KRAS, BRAF) that are nowadays routinely assessed were unknown at the time and thus not investigated. The authors excluded the 3 patients who died postoperatively, which is inappropriate for calculating overall mortality, and their methods of "correcting" the survival rate are not clear, limiting the interpretation of these data. Finally, the oncologic follow-up was limited to physical examination and CEA checks without endoscopy and/or cross-sectional imaging; hence, it is possible that some recurrences were clinically missed.

Relevant Studies   At the time of publication of this study, the local recurrence rates following rectal cancer surgery were approximately 30–40% (2, 3). In order to mitigate the significant high risk of local failure, many centers were routinely employing the use of adjuvant radiation therapy, although no study had demonstrated an improvement in survival (4, 5). In 1986, the year of Heald's seminal paper, Krook et al. completed the accrual for the North Central Cancer Treatment Group study, investigating the role of postoperative radiation alone versus radiation plus fluorouracil after nonstandardized (no TME) proctectomy (6). This was a randomized clinical trial enrolling 204 patients who experienced recurrences in 25% of patients treated with radiation and 13.5% of patients treated with chemoradiotherapy. These findings led to the 1990 National Cancer Institute consensus statement recommending adjuvant chemoradiation for all patients with locally advanced rectal cancer (7). However, as Heald's TME approach alone drastically reduced the local failure to less than 4%, efforts to improve local control became more focused upon optimizing surgical technique rather than providing adjuvant radiation therapy.

Published in 1997, the Swedish Rectal Cancer Trial (SRCT) randomized 1168 adult patients to receive neoadjuvant short-course radiation or to have non-TME surgery alone (8) and reported 5-year local recurrence rates of 11% in the radiation arm and 27% in the surgery only arm ($p < 0.001$). Four years later, the Dutch TME trial demonstrated a persisting benefit in local control at 2 years for patients undergoing preoperative short-course radiotherapy plus TME as compared to TME alone (2.4% vs. 8.2%, $p < 0.001$), thus providing the basis for the current practice of administering neoadjuvant radiotherapy (9). Similarly, the higher incidence of local failure for the radiation plus surgery arm in the Swedish trial (11%) as compared to the Dutch study (2.4%) further highlighted the importance of the TME plane even in the setting of receiving neoadjuvant radiotherapy.

Of note, even though designed as neoadjuvant therapy trials, the net result of the SRCT and the Dutch TME trial were to confirm the primacy of precise surgical technique in the treatment of rectal cancer. This in turn led to worldwide adoption of the TME approach, fostered by an international teaching effort by Prof. Heald and various colleagues. The need for accurate preoperative imaging also led to the development of endoscopic rectal ultrasound and later MRI (10), which are the cornerstones of modern rectal cancer decision making.

REFERENCES

1. Waxman BP. Large bowel anastomoses. II. The circular staplers. The British Journal of Surgery. 1983;70(2):64–7.
2. Hurst PA, Prout WG, Kelly JM, Bannister JJ, Walker RT. Local recurrence after low anterior resection using the staple gun. The British Journal of Surgery. 1982;69(5):275–6.
3. Lasson AL, Ekelund GR, Lindström CG. Recurrence risk after stapled anastomosis for rectal carcinoma. Acta chirurgica Scandinavica. 1984;150(1):85–9.
4. Balslev I, Pedersen M, Teglbjaerg PS, Hanberg-Soerensen F, Bone J, Jacobsen NO, et al. Postoperative radiotherapy in Dukes' B and C carcinoma of the rectum and rectosigmoid. A randomized multicenter study. Cancer. 1986;58(1):22–8.
5. Fisher B, Wolmark N, Rockette H, Redmond C, Deutsch M, Wickerham DL, et al. Postoperative adjuvant chemotherapy or radiation therapy for rectal cancer: results from NSABP protocol R-01. Journal of the National Cancer Institute. 1988;80(1):21–9.
6. Krook JE, Moertel CG, Gunderson LL, Wieand HS, Collins RT, Beart RW, et al. Effective surgical adjuvant therapy for high-risk rectal carcinoma. The New England Journal of Medicine. 1991;324(11):709–15.
7. NIH consensus conference. Adjuvant therapy for patients with colon and rectal cancer. JAMA. 1990;264(11):1444–50.
8. Cedermark B, Dahlberg M, Glimelius B, Påhlman L, Rutqvist LE, Wilking N. Improved survival with preoperative radiotherapy in resectable rectal cancer. The New England Journal of Medicine. 1997;336(14):980–7.
9. Kapiteijn E, Marijnen CA, Nagtegaal ID, Putter H, Steup WH, Wiggers T, et al. Preoperative radiotherapy combined with total mesorectal excision for resectable rectal cancer. The New England Journal of Medicine. 2001;345(9):638–46.
10. Taylor FG, Quirke P, Heald RJ, Moran BJ, Blomqvist L, Swift IR, et al. Preoperative magnetic resonance imaging assessment of circumferential resection margin predicts disease-free survival and local recurrence: 5-year follow-up results of the MERCURY study. Journal of Clinical Oncology: Official Journal of the American Society of Clinical Oncology. 2014;32(1):34–43.

CHAPTER 18

Starting from the Bottom: Endoscopic Surgery in the Rectum

Buess G, Theiss R, Gunther M, Hutterer F, Pichlmaier
H. Leber Magen Darm. 15(6):271-279, 1985

Reviewed by Deborah S. Keller and John H. Marks

Research Question/Objective   The objective of this work was to describe a novel transanal endoscopic operating system and technique that permit microsurgery in the rectal lumen with complete sessile polyp removal and placement of sutures. At the time this study was published, there were no options for endoluminal surgery or minimally invasive surgery. The local excision techniques used for sphincter preservation to this point had high rates of fragmentation, local and distant recurrence, requiring strict patient selection [1]. New options for safe and complete oncologic resection of small carcinomas, villous, and sessile polyps were needed.

Study Design   The study design was a case series performed by a single surgeon at a single institution. The description of the new transanal endoscopic microsurgery platform is analogous to a technical note, with the details of the stereoscopic operating system, the available operating rectoscopes, specially designed endoscopic operating instruments, modified insufflation and suctioning systems to support stable dilation, as well as the system setup, positioning, and step-by-step illustration of the operative technique. The clinical application of the platform for full-thickness excision with lessons learned from performing the cases to facilitate the learning curve corresponds to a prospective observational case series.

Sample Size   The sample size was 12 patients. The intraoperative outcomes were descriptive, and there was no power calculation for a hypothesis-proving sample size. The patient population was 58.3% ($n = 7$) men and 41.7 ($n = 5$) females. The age range was 36–82, with a median age of 63 years. The distal margin ranged from 4 to 15 cm from the anal verge, with sizes ranging from 1 to 33 cm^2. The indications for surgery in the sample were tubulovillous adenoma ($n = 6$), adenocarcinoma ($n = 2$), adenomatosis ($n = 2$), villous adenoma ($n = 1$), and hyperplastic polyp ($n = 1$).

Follow-Up   For this study, there was no follow-up period. All results described the intraoperative setup, procedure, and immediate postoperative outcomes. There was no information on postoperative outcomes after discharge from the hospital or long-term outcomes.

   DOI: 10.1201/9780429285714-18

Inclusion/Exclusion Criteria   No specific inclusion or exclusion criteria were described for this study. The included patients were all adults with extraperitoneal rectal lesions. There were no details on the time frame.

Intervention or Treatment Received   All patients underwent operative intervention, a full-thickness excision with the transanal endoscopic microsurgery platform for a rectal lesion. The technical aspects of the setup were described in detail, including the mechanical dilation of the sphincter complex, exposure by automatic gas insufflation, setup and placement of the stiff oblique angled stereoscopic optical system, selecting the operating rectoscope and surgical instruments, as modifications to the insufflation device for endoscopic operation.

Results   The results show the feasibility of the excision with the novel transanal endoscopic platform. There were no defined metrics, outcomes, or comparative group to report.

Study Limitations   The design was the major limitation, as it was a case series of a single surgeon at a single center. There was also a small sample size of 12 patients. Furthermore, no main outcome measures were cited. Presently, this paper would consist of technical notes or be published along with a checklist for the IDEAL Reporting Guidelines for the surgical evaluation to ensure that the value of the new technology is seen and put into print [2].

Relevant Studies   The challenge of completely excising a low rectal cancer in the narrow confines of the bony pelvis while avoiding a permanent colostomy remains a daunting task for the surgeon. Benign and stage malignant tumors of the lower rectum have traditionally been managed with local excision using the Parks technique. However, this approach has limitations in terms of exposure and visibility of the rectal lumen, as well as higher rates of fragmentation and incomplete excision of the specimen [3]. The technique described in this revolutionary work by Buess established the treatment of choice for early-stage benign and malignant low and mid-rectal tumors, as well as for patients not suitable for radical resection. The stereoscopic view, insufflation, and instrumentation allowed for visualization of both the proximal and distal margins clears with a precise, full-thickness excision to maintain the integrity of the pathology.

While groundbreaking, the technique had its limitations, such as the need for high-cost special instruments and a long learning curve. Atallah and Albert introduced transanal minimally invasive surgery (TAMIS) as an alternate advanced videoscopic transanal platform that addressed some limitations of TEM. The same superior visualization and reach of TEM are realized with TAMIS, but it is performed using standard laparoscopic equipment that reduces the cost and learning curve compared to TEM [4].

The benefits seen from Buess's platform and procedure were widespread. During this same period, Dr. Gerald Marks implemented the first sphincter preservation surgery following high-dose preoperative radiation therapy for very low rectal cancers not amenable to local excision from the bottom up: the transabdominal transanal radical proctosigmoidectomy with coloanal anastomosis, more commonly referred to as the TATA [5]. With the TATA, like the TEM, there is direct visualization of the distal resection margin. By starting the procedure transanal in the intersphincteric plane, the most difficult part of the procedure is completed first with certainty that the distal margin is negative. The procedure was adapted to laparoscopic surgery by Dr. John Marks, maintaining excellent local recurrence, 5-year survival, and functional outcomes without the need for permanent colostomy in patients with cancers in the distal one-third of the rectum [6, 7]. More recently, multiport and single-port robotic platforms have been used for the TATA and transanal excisions, with positive short-term results [8]. The TATA procedure eventually led to the development of the transanal total mesorectal excision (TaTME), which is based on the same principles of closing the rectal lumen, better visualization of the distal rectal resection margin, avoidance of stapling the distal rectum, and less manipulation of the tumor-containing rectum and mesorectum [9]. The evolution of the taTME continues, with an international registry, standardized training courses, and minimally invasive adaptions to the technique [8, 10–12].

The power of this technical description of a new technique nearly 40 years ago continues to have a powerful impact on how rectal cancer is treated today. The surgeon-led surgical innovation was the catalyst for multiple techniques and platforms and will continue to rouse further innovation for the treatment of low rectal cancer.

REFERENCES

1. Hager T, Gall FP, Hermanek P. Local excision of cancer of the rectum. Dis Colon Rectum. 1983;26:149–151.
2. Bilbro NA. New reporting guidelines for IDEAL studies. Br J Surg. 2020;107:1241–1242.
3. Atallah S, Keller D. Why the conventional parks transanal excision for early stage rectal cancer should be abandoned. Dis Colon Rectum. 2015;58:1211–1214.
4. Atallah S, Albert M, Larach S. Transanal minimally invasive surgery: a giant leap forward. Surg Endosc. 2010;24:2200–2205.
5. Marks G, Mohiuddin M, Borenstein BD. Preoperative radiation therapy and sphincter preservation by the combined abdominotranssacral technique for selected rectal cancers. Dis Colon Rectum. 1985;28:565–571.
6. Marks J, Mizrahi B, Dalane S, Nweze I, Marks G. Laparoscopic transanal abdominal transanal resection with sphincter preservation for rectal cancer in the distal 3 cm of the rectum after neoadjuvant therapy. Surg Endosc. 2010;24:2700–2707.
7. Marks JH, Myers EA, Zeger EL, Denittis AS, Gummadi M, Marks GJ. Long-term outcomes by a transanal approach to total mesorectal excision for rectal cancer. Surg Endosc. 2017 Dec;31(12):5248–5257. doi: 10.1007/s00464-017-5597-7. Epub 2017 Jun 22.

8. Marks JH, Perez RE, Salem JF. Robotic transanal surgery for rectal cancer. Clin Colon Rectal Surg. 2021;34:317–324.
9. Sylla P, Rattner DW, Delgado S, Lacy AM. NOTES transanal rectal cancer resection using transanal endoscopic microsurgery and laparoscopic assistance. Surg Endosc. 2010;24:1205–1210.
10. Penna M, Hompes R, Arnold S et al. Transanal total mesorectal excision: international registry results of the first 720 cases. Ann Surg. 2017;266:111–117.
11. Koedam TWA, Veltcamp Helbach M, van de Ven PM et al. Transanal total meso-rectal excision for rectal cancer: evaluation of the learning curve. Tech Coloproctol. 2018;22:279–287.
12. Wynn GR, Austin RCT, Motson RW. Using cadaveric simulation to introduce the concept and skills required to start performing transanal total mesorectal excision. Colorectal Dis. 2018;20:496–501.

CHAPTER 19

Improved Survival with Preoperative Radiotherapy in Resectable Rectal Cancer

Swedish Rectal Cancer Trial: Cedermark B, Dahlberg M, Glimelius B, Påhlman L, Rutqvist LE, Wilking N. N Engl J Med. 336(14):980–987, 1997

Reviewed by Ravi Shridhar

Research Question/Objective   Review Swedish Cancer Rectal Trial.

Study Design   Randomized Phase III

Sample Size   1168 patients

Follow-Up   5-year and 13-year follow-up

Inclusion/Exclusion Criteria

Inclusion

1. Biopsy-proven adenocarcinoma below promontory seen on lateral projection of barium enema
2. Resectable disease
3. Age < 80 years
4. Able to provide informed consent

Exclusion

1. Locally unresectable tumor
2. Tumor amenable to local excision
3. Metastatic disease
4. Prior pelvic radiation therapy
5. Other malignant disease excluding squamous cell carcinoma of skin

Intervention or Treatment Received   Short-course radiotherapy followed by LAR or APR 1 week later versus upfront LAR APR

DOI: 10.1201/9780429285714-19

Results

Outcomes   Between 1987 and 1990, 1168 patients less than 80 years of age with resectable rectal adenocarcinoma were randomized to either undergo upfront LAR or APR or to receive preoperative short-course radiotherapy followed by surgery within 1 week of completion. Total mesorectal excision (TME) was not mandated. The rates of APR vs. LAR were similar between groups. Radiotherapy did not increase post-operative mortality (3% surgery vs. 4% short course, $p = 0.3$). However, in patients treated with a 2-field radiation technique, mortality was considerably higher at 15% (7 out of 48 patients) versus 3% for patients treated with 3–4 field radiation technique ($p < 0.001$) (2, 3). There were more perineal wound infections in patients receiving radiation (20% vs. 10%, $p < 0.001$) (3). After 5 years of follow-up, local recurrence rate was 11% in the radiotherapy group versus 27% in the upfront surgery group ($p < 0.001$). There were significantly more patients with stage I and significantly less stage III patients in the radiated group compared to the surgery alone group ($p = 0.03$, $p = 0.004$), indicating a downstaging effect by the radiation therapy [2, 4]. This translated into a 5-year overall survival benefit in favor of radiated patients (58% vs. 48%, $p = 0.004$).

A long-term follow-up analysis with a 13 year median follow-up showed a persistent local control and overall survival benefit associated with the radiated group [4]. Women in both groups demonstrated a 9–13% increase in overall survival compared to men. Radiated patients displayed a survival rate of 31% compared to 20% in upfront surgery patients ($p = 0.009$). The cumulative local recurrence rate was 9% in the preoperative radiotherapy group and 26% in the surgery group ($p < 0.001$). Local recurrence was reduced in the radiotherapy group regardless of stage (Table 19.1). A lower local recurrence rate was seen at all distances from anal verge but was not statistically significant for tumors >10 cm (Table 19.1). Four of 5 patients with local recurrence after 5 years were in the upfront surgery group, and recurrences were detected up to 12 years after

TABLE 19.1 Swedish Rectal Cancer Trial Local Recurrence			
Local Failure (%)	**RT-Surgery**	**Surgery**	**p**
Tumor Distance from Anal Verge			
<5 cm	10	27	0.003
6–10 cm	9	26	<0.001
>11 cm	8	12	0.3
Stage			
I	4.5	14	<0.001
II	6	22	<0.001
III	23	46	<0.001

surgery. Survival after local recurrence was higher in the upfront surgery group (median 398 days vs. 295 days, $p < 0.001$). One-third of all patients developed metastatic disease, irrespective of the treatment group.

Quality of Life   It has been shown that most of the acute and long-term toxicity from radiation therapy was attributed to early trials utilizing a 2-field radiation technique [3]. Long=term analysis (10 year) from the Uppsala trial utilizing a 3-field technique failed to show any increased in late toxicity [5, 6]. In the Swedish trial, radiated patients had higher rate of hospital admissions within the first 6 months of treatment mainly for gastrointestinal disorders like bowel obstruction [7]. The rates of hospital admissions after 6 months were similar for both groups; however, there were increased admissions for bowel obstruction in radiated patients. Interestingly, risk of inguinal hernia repair was lower in radiated patients. In the follow-up study with the Dutch trial, significant long-term bowel and sexual dysfunction was associated with radiation therapy [8–10].

Study Limitations

Surgical Evaluation   Although it is the only trial to show an overall survival benefit to preoperative radiotherapy, one of the main criticisms of the Swedish trial was that patients did not undergo mandatory TME. The trial demonstrated very high rates of local recurrence in the nonradiated group. It would suggest that the survival benefit associated with radiation was due to inadequate surgical resection. In the follow-up Dutch Trial, TME was mandated and resulted in significantly lower local recurrence rates in the upfront surgical arm. Short-course radiotherapy preoperatively did reduce local recurrency by 50%, but there was no difference in survival in all patients (Table 19.2). A survival benefit was seen in stage III patients with a negative

TABLE 19.2   Short-Course Radiation—Surgery versus Surgery Trials

Trial	N	Preop RT (Gy)	Adjuvant Chemo (C), Chemorads (CRT)	Surgical CRM (%)	LR Total/ LR CRM+	OS (%)	DFS (%)
Uppsala [6]	236	25.5 (5)	None	—	12	40 (6)	—
	235	None	60 Gy (8-week split)	—	21	40 (6)	—
Swedish [2, 4]	553	25 (5)	None	—	9	31 (13)	—
	557	None	None	—	26	20 (13)	—
Dutch [8, 10]	897	25 (5)	None	15.6	5/20	48 (10)	—
	908	None	RT (8%)	16.4	11/24	49 (10)	—
MRC CR07 [12]	674	25 (5)	C (10%)	10	4.4/14	70 (5)	74 (5)
	676	None	CRT-C (12%)	12	11/21	68 (5)	67 (5)

circumferential margin [10]. This was also validated with the MRC C07 trial where intact mesorectum and negative circumferential margin were associated with low rates of local recurrence [11].

Staging   During the era when the Swedish trial was conducted, staging was limited to barium enema CT scans and rigid proctoscopy. This was conducted prior to MRI and endorectal ultrasound staging. Many early-stage patients would have likely been enrolled in that trial where local excision may have been feasible. In addition, lymph node staging was restricted to pathologic analysis unless seen on CT scans.

Radiation Technique   Radiation planning was based on bony landmarks from X-ray films with or without intrarectal contrast. CT-based planning was not utilized. Planning was initially with a 2-field (AP-PA) technique. Borders were based on bony landmarks from the top of L5 to bottom of obturator foramen. This technique was associated with high acute toxicity and higher postoperative mortality. Implementing 3-field (PA and opposed laterals) in the prone position or 4-field (AP-PA and opposed laterals) in the supine or prone position allowed for decreased bowel and bladder toxicity [2, 3].

Currently, patients' radiation treatments are CT planned with full bladder and IV contrast for delineation of draining lymphatics including obturator and iliac vessels up to the bifurcation of the common iliacs, which can have variable positions between L4 and S1. Bowel loops, bowel, genitalia, and hips are contoured, and dose volume histograms are generated to determine cumulative exposure. Female patients who have undergone hysterectomy may have more bowel in the radiation field where advanced techniques like intensity-modulated radiation therapy may have to be employed as bowel-sparing strategies [13].

The understanding of long-term bowel and sexual dysfunction after pelvic radiation has prompted proper patient selection with high-risk disease. In addition to tumor and nodal staging, factors like age, gender, fertility status, menopausal status, and genetic predisposition are taken into consideration for recommending radiation.

Chemotherapy   While chemotherapy was not incorporated into the trial design, chemotherapy during that era was limited to 5-fluorouracil and leucovorin. Capecitabine and oxaliplatin were not available during that era. Molecular testing of molecular satellite instability was just being investigated and wasn't incorporated into treatment decisions to determine benefit immunotherapy, which was also not available during that era.

Total neoadjuvant therapy that incorporates preoperative chemotherapy in addition to radiation has slowly become part of the standard treatment paradigm for stage III rectal cancer. Given the high recurrence rates in stage III patients in the Swedish Trial, a good portion of patients would have benefited from either preoperative or adjuvant chemotherapy.

Sphincter Preservation versus Organ Preservation   Neoadjuvant radiation has shown downstaging and conversion of planned APR to LAR without permanent colostomy. Given the additional effect of chemotherapy in enhancing response and further downstaging, patients with clinical complete response are now being offered active surveillance as part of an organ-preservation strategy. Preoperative radiation has been shown to be associated with decreased bowel function, especially after surgery. Avoiding surgery in patients with complete response will avoid complications from surgery that are enhanced after radiation. Organ-preservation strategies for advanced disease will require total neoadjuvant therapy with chemotherapy. Short-course radiotherapy can be incorporated into neoadjuvant strategies as part of organ preservation but should be incorporated before starting chemotherapy. As an organ-preservation strategy, short-course radiotherapy as the sole modality will likely not be sufficient to obtain clinical complete responses.

Relevant Studies   See "Study Limitations" and Table 19.2.

REFERENCES

1. Benson, A.B., et al., *Rectal Cancer, Version 2.2022, NCCN Clinical Practice Guidelines in Oncology.* J Natl Compr Canc Netw, 2022. **20**(10): pp. 1139–67.
2. Swedish Rectal Cancer Trial, et al., *Improved survival with preoperative radiotherapy in resectable rectal cancer.* N Engl J Med, 1997. **336**(14): pp. 980–7.
3. Swedish Rectal Cancer Trial, *Initial report from a Swedish multicentre study examining the role of preoperative irradiation in the treatment of patients with resectable rectal carcinoma.* Br J Surg, 1993. **80**(10): pp. 1333–6.
4. Folkesson, J., et al., *Swedish Rectal Cancer Trial: long lasting benefits from radiotherapy on survival and local recurrence rate.* J Clin Oncol, 2005. **23**(24): pp. 5644–50.
5. Frykholm, G.J., B. Glimelius, and L. Pahlman, *Preoperative or postoperative irradiation in adenocarcinoma of the rectum: final treatment results of a randomized trial and an evaluation of late secondary effects.* Dis Colon Rectum, 1993. **36**(6): pp. 564–72.
6. Pahlman, L. and B. Glimelius, *Pre- or postoperative radiotherapy in rectal and rectosigmoid carcinoma. Report from a randomized multicenter trial.* Ann Surg, 1990. **211**(2): pp. 187–95.
7. Birgisson, H., et al., *Adverse effects of preoperative radiation therapy for rectal cancer: long-term follow-up of the Swedish Rectal Cancer Trial.* J Clin Oncol, 2005. **23**(34): pp. 8697–705.
8. Kapiteijn, E., et al., *Preoperative radiotherapy combined with total mesorectal excision for resectable rectal cancer.* N Engl J Med, 2001. **345**(9): pp. 638–46.
9. Wiltink, L.M., et al., *Health-related quality of life 14 years after preoperative short-term radiotherapy and total mesorectal excision for rectal cancer: report of a multicenter randomised trial.* Eur J Cancer, 2014. **50**(14): pp. 2390–8.
10. van Gijn, W., et al., *Preoperative radiotherapy combined with total mesorectal excision for resectable rectal cancer: 12-year follow-up of the multicentre, randomised controlled TME trial.* Lancet Oncol, 2011. **12**(6): pp. 575–82.

11. Quirke, P., et al., *Effect of the plane of surgery achieved on local recurrence in patients with operable rectal cancer: a prospective study using data from the MRC CR07 and NCIC-CTG CO16 randomised clinical trial.* Lancet, 2009. **373**(9666): pp. 821–8.
12. Sebag-Montefiore, D., et al., *Preoperative radiotherapy versus selective postoperative chemoradiotherapy in patients with rectal cancer (MRC CR07 and NCIC-CTG C016): a multicentre, randomised trial.* Lancet, 2009. **373**(9666): pp. 811–20.
13. Samuelian, J.M., et al., *Reduced acute bowel toxicity in patients treated with intensity-modulated radiotherapy for rectal cancer.* Int J Radiat Oncol Biol Phys, 2012. **82**(5): pp. 1981–7.

CHAPTER 20

Comparison of Stapled Haemorrhoidopexy with Traditional Excisional Surgery for Haemorrhoidal Disease (eTHos): A Pragmatic, Multicentre, Randomised Controlled Trial

Watson AJ, Hudson J, Wood J, et al. Lancet. 388(10058):2375–2385, 2016

Reviewed by Andrew D. Hawkins and Charles M. Friel

Research Question/Objective   Excisional hemorrhoidectomy either with a closed (Ferguson) or open technique (Milligan–Morgan) is the mainstay procedure for treatment of grade III/IV hemorrhoids. These techniques often result in severe postoperative pain and require local wound care in a sensitive region when open excisional hemorrhoidectomy is performed. Several alternative treatments have been proposed including Doppler-guided hemorrhoidal artery ligation and stapled hemorroidopexy (Longo technique) but have not been previously compared to the gold standard excisional approach. The aim of this study was to compare outcomes for these procedures in patients with hemorrhoids that were refractory to rubber band ligature or hemorrhoidal artery ligation or in patients who were deemed to have hemorrhoids too large for these treatments.

Study Design   This study was a multicenter randomized controlled trial across 32 National Health Service hospitals in England. The primary outcome for this study was the reported quality of life from patient questionnaires up to 24 months after the procedure. The authors used the EQ-5D-3L UK validated questionnaire for quality of life measurement (1). Secondary outcomes were complications including hemorrhage, requirement for blood transfusion, anal stenosis, anal fissure, urinary retention, residual anal skin tags, difficult defecation, wound discharge, pelvic sepsis, and pruritus.

Sample Size   This study screened 1127 patients and randomized 777 patients to receive stapled hemorroidopexy ($n = 389$) or traditional excisional surgery ($n = 388$).

Follow-Up   Study follow-up occurred at five time points between the procedure and 24 months, at which a patient questionnaire was administered. A clinical assessment was performed at a 6-week follow-up appointment

DOI: 10.1201/9780429285714-20

where examination of the anal canal was performed but was not done routinely if patients reported their symptoms had improved.

Inclusion/Exclusion Criteria   Criteria for patient inclusion in this study were adults aged 18 years or older referred to a hospital for surgical treatment of hemorrhoids classified as grades II–IV. Exclusion criteria included previous hemorrhoid surgery, symptomatic incontinence, prior episode of perianal sepsis, inflammatory bowel disease, pregnancy, or prior anal sphincter injury repair. The use of the Ligasure Medtronic and Harmonic Ethicon devices to perform excisional hemorrhoidectomy was excluded.

Intervention   Stapled hemorrhoidopexy involves excision of a ring of tissue above the hemorrhoidal cushions with re-anastomosis of mucosa with staples. A traditional excisional procedure uses electrocautery and intends to excise the hemorrhoidal cushions with either closure of the mucosa with sutures or leaving it open.

Results

Sampling A total of 774 participants were included in the analysis after randomization, 721 participants received surgery, and 570 patients completed the follow-up questionnaire at 24 months. During the 24-month prospective period, 4 patients died in the stapled hemorrhoidopexy group, 37 patients in the stapled hemorroidopexy group received traditional surgery, and 29 in the traditional excisional group received stapled hemorroidopexy based upon patient preference and surgeon assessment.

Cohort Demographics Demographic characteristics between groups were similar with no difference in distribution of disease severity (grade of hemorrhoids and preoperative symptom questionnaires). Consultant (attending) surgeons were more likely to perform stapled hemorrhoidopexy (256 of 358 participants, 78%) than traditional excisional hemorrhoidopexy (225 of 363, 62%). No differences were noted in length of stay, time waiting for surgery, and operative duration. Median follow-up was 731 days for the stapled hemorrhoidopexy group and 731 days for the traditional excisional surgery group.

Quality of Life and Symptom Measures Participants in the stapled hemorrhoidopexy group initially had higher quality of life scores at 1 and 3 weeks, whereas scores were higher in the traditional excisional surgery group at 6 weeks and for the duration of the study (Figure 20.1). The primary outcome was EQ-5D-3L scores at 24 months, which was higher in the traditional excisional surgery group: mean difference -0.070 (95% CI -0.140 to -0.006). Reported incontinence measured using validated tools was higher in the stapled hemorrhoidopexy group (3.8%) versus traditional excisional surgery (3.0%) ($p = 0.0149$). Ninety-four (32%) of 295 participants in the stapled hemorrhoidopexy reported

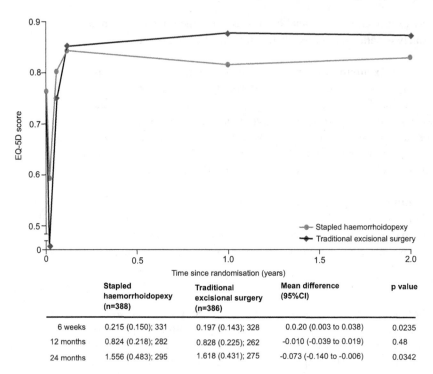

	Stapled haemorrhoidopexy (n=388)	Traditional excisional surgery (n=386)	Mean difference (95%CI)	p value
6 weeks	0.215 (0.150); 331	0.197 (0.143); 328	0.0.20 (0.003 to 0.038)	0.0235
12 months	0.824 (0.218); 282	0.828 (0.225); 262	-0.010 (-0.039 to 0.019)	0.48
24 months	1.556 (0.483); 295	1.618 (0.431); 275	-0.073 (-0.140 to -0.006)	0.0342

Figure 20.1   Validated quality of life questionnaire scores. (*Source:* Adapted from Watson et al.)

symptom recurrence at 12 months compared with 39 (14%) of 287 in the traditional surgery group (OR 2.96, 95% CI 2.02–4.02, $p < 0.0001$). Although not significant, patients in the stapled hemorroidopexy group self-reported more surgical re-interventions. Tenesmus was reported more frequently in the stapled hemorrhoidopexy at 24 months (p =< 0.0001).

Complications and Mortality Of 690 patients enrolled who received treatment with available data, 24 (7%) participants undergoing stapled hemorrhoidopexy and 33 (9%) after receiving excisional surgery had a serious adverse event. These involved hospitalizations for bleeding, urinary retention, and constipation. One patient died in the stapled hemorrhoidopexy group that was unrelated to surgery. Ten participants in the traditional excisional surgery group remained in the hospital or were re-admitted for pain compared to 6 participants in the stapled hemorrhoidopexy group.

Cost Effectiveness Mean cost per patient for excisional hemorrhoidectomy was lower compared to stapled hemorrhoidopexy (£602 vs. £941). The adjusted mean difference in quality-adjusted life years between stapled hemorrhoidopexy versus excisional hemorrhoidectomy was −0.070 (95% CI −0.127 to −0.011).

Study Limitations This study was limited by loss-to-follow-up and lack of participant and surgeon blinding. Given that the primary outcome was a subjective measure, the study design potentially allows for bias due to previously held beliefs regarding the procedure or inaccuracy in patient reporting. Participants were also able to switch groups based on clinician assessment or patient preference due to the open-label and pragmatic study design. However, in a per-protocol analysis including only patients receiving assigned treatment and attending follow-up at least one short-term and long-term follow-up, the difference in reported quality of life between groups was maintained (−0.078, 95% CI −0.153 to 0.002). At the end of the study interval, 22% of participants were lost to follow-up. Clinician assessment and registry data were not uniformly used to assess for hemorrhoid recurrence. A potential means of measuring the incidence of recurrence after these procedures would be to include repeat anorectal examination at study conclusion, but this would be impeded by the sensitivity of performing such an exam in an otherwise unnecessary situation. The study did not include mention of distribution of procedures by surgeon or center, which could introduce additional bias in procedures offered or institutional preference. Surgical technique was not standardized or described in this study.

Relevant Studies The randomized controlled trial by Watson and colleagues had a robust study design with well matched participant groups by demographic characteristics, disease severity, and preoperative symptom scores. Their study included a large number of centers within the National Health Service system in England and patients treated by a variety of provider types including qualified trainees and colorectal specialists. The primary outcome relied on patient-reported quality of life metrics that consistently demonstrated improved scores at 1 year follow-up for patients who underwent excisional hemorrhoidectomy.

Stapled hemorroidopexy or mucoprolapsectomy was introduced in 1998 by Longo and described as removal of 2 cm of mucosa and submucosa between the rectum and anal canal above the dentate line (2). The proposed aim was to avoid postoperative pain by primarily resecting mucosa above the Dentate line and to restore the anatomic position of the hemorrhoidal cushions. The primary criticism of this procedure is a higher recurrence rate compared with traditional techniques (3), 4). It has been theorized that reduced patient satisfaction and resolution of symptoms after stapled hemorrhoidopexy are related misidentifica-tions of residual hemorrhoidal nodules and prolapsed mucosa as hemorrhoid recurrence (5). Ommer and colleagues found in a 6-year retrospective review of stapled hemorroidopexy that a majority of reoperations were for improperly positioned mucosal nodules from the index operation or residual skin tags (6). Several authors have recently proposed modifications, such as the position of the staple line, adequate reduction of mucosal prolapse, or simultaneous excision of perianal skin tags that may result in a reduction in perceived recurrence by patients (7–9).

The trial reviewed here did not find a difference in serious adverse outcomes between stapled and excisional approaches. However, the use of a stapling device presents unique complications including rectal perforation secondary to staple line dehiscence, rectovaginal fistula, and retained staples causing inflammatory polyps that are rarely noted after traditional excisional hemorrhoidectomy (10–12). No major septic complication was reported in a systematic review of 25 randomized controlled trials comparing stapled hemorrhoidopexy with conventional hemorrhoidectomy, but this may represent publishing bias against case reports of rare events (13). McCloud and colleagues calculated a rate of life-threatening sepsis after hemorrhoidopexy as 1.75 per year (over 4 years between 2000 and 2003) versus 0.25 per year for excisional hemorrhoidectomy over a 40-year time period (14). Despite concerns that many of these complications were secondary to an early learning curve with adoption of this procedure, Ravo and colleagues, in a review of 1107 patients from 12 Italian centers, found that most complications occurred after surgeons had performed more than 25 procedures (15). It seems that severe complications are a consequence of technical error with the required purse string sutures being full-thickness rather than in the submucosal plane (16).

The technique of excisional hemorrhoidectomy has been further refined recently with the widespread adoption of vascular sealing devices, improved local anesthetic methods such as pudendal nerve block, and postoperative adjunct medications (17–19). It is possible that with adoption of recommended practices for perioperative pain management recently proposed by the PROSPECT (procedure-specific postoperative pain management) group that initial patient dissatisfaction with excisional techniques can be mitigated (20). Future comparison of these procedures requires standardization of surgical technique, objective assessment of the anal canal at follow-up, and inclusion of recent modifications that have demonstrated improvements to stapled hemorrhoidopexy. The cost-effectiveness of stapled hemorrhoidopexy remains an ongoing concern due to the list price of hemorrhoidal circular staplers used in the procedure (21). In brief, the Watson and colleagues trial suggests that in current everyday practice, excisional hemorrhoidectomy is a more durable option than stapled hemorrhoidectomy.

REFERENCES

[1] EuroQol Group. EuroQol–a new facility for the measurement of health-related quality of life. Health Policy. 1990 Dec 1;16(3):199–208.
[2] Longo A. Treatment of hemorrhoidal disease by reduction of mucosa and hemorrhoidal prolapse with a circular stapler suturing device: a new procedure. In Proceeding of the Sixth World Congress of Endoscopic Surgery, Monduzzi Publishing Co., Rome, 777–784.
[3] Shao WJ, Li GH, Zhang ZH, Yang BL, Sun GD, Chen YQ. Systematic review and meta-analysis of randomized controlled trials comparing stapled haemorrhoidopexy with conventional haemorrhoidectomy. Journal of British Surgery. 2008 Feb;95(2):147–60.
[4] Jayaraman S, Colquhoun PH, Malthaner RA. Stapled hemorrhoidopexy is associated with a higher long-term recurrence rate of internal hemorrhoids compared with conventional excisional hemorrhoid surgery. Diseases of the Colon & Rectum. 2007 Sep;50(9):1297–305.

[5] Tjandra JJ, Chan MK. Systematic review on the procedure for prolapse and hemorrhoids (stapled hemorrhoidopexy). Diseases of the Colon & Rectum. 2007 Jun;50(6):878–92.

[6] Gao XH, Fu CG, Nabieu PF. Residual skin tags following procedure for prolapse and hemorrhoids: differentiation from recurrence. World Journal of Surgery. 2010 Feb;34(2):344–52.

[7] Ommer A, Hinrichs J, Möllenberg H, Marla B, Walz MK. Long-term results after stapled hemorrhoidopexy: a prospective study with a 6-year follow-up. Diseases of the Colon & Rectum. 2011 May 1;54(5):601–8.

[8] Calomino N, Martellucci J, Fontani A, Papi F, Cetta F, Tanzini G. Care with regard to details improves the outcome of Longo mucoprolapsectomy: long term follow up. Updates in surgery. 2011 Sep;63(3):151–4.

[9] Yuan C, Zhou C, Xue R, Jin X, Jin C, Zheng C. Outcomes of modified tissue selection therapy stapler in the treatment of prolapsing hemorrhoids. Frontiers in Surgery. 2022;9.

[10] Chen YY, Cheng YF, Wang QP, Ye B, Huang CJ, Zhou CJ, Cai M, Ye YK, Liu CB. Modified procedure for prolapse and hemorrhoids: lower recurrence, higher satisfaction. World Journal of Clinical Cases. 2021 Jan 1;9(1):36.

[11] Pescatori M, Gagliardi G. Postoperative complications after procedure for prolapsed hemorrhoids (PPH) and stapled transanal rectal resection (STARR) procedures. Techniques in Coloproctology. 2008 Mar;12(1):7–19.

[12] Faucheron JL, Voirin D, Abba J. Rectal perforation with life-threatening peritonitis following stapled haemorrhoidopexy. Journal of British Surgery. 2012 Jun;99(6):746–53.

[13] Fondran JC, Porter JA, Slezak FA. Inflammatory polyps: a cause of late bleeding in stapled hemorrhoidectomy. Diseases of the Colon & Rectum. 2006 Dec;49:1910–3.

[14] Tjandra JJ, Chan MK. Systematic review on the procedure for prolapse and hemorrhoids (stapled hemorrhoidopexy). Diseases of the Colon & Rectum. 2007 Jun;50:878–92.

[15] McCloud JM, Jameson JS, Scott AN. Life-threatening sepsis following treatment for haemorrhoids: a systematic review. Colorectal Disease. 2006 Nov;8(9):748–55.

[16] Ravo B, Amato A, Bianco V, Boccasanta P, Bottini C, Carriero A, Milito G, Dodi G, Mascagni D, Orsini S, Pietroletti R. Complications after stapled hemorrhoidectomy: can they be prevented? Techniques in Coloproctology. 2002 Sep 1;6(2):83.

[17] Calomino N, Martellucci J, Fontani A, Papi F, Cetta F, Tanzini G. Care with regard to details improves the outcome of Longo mucoprolapsectomy: long term follow up. Updates in Surgery. 2011 Sep;63:151–4.

[18] Milito G, Cadeddu F, Muzi MG, Nigro C, Farinon AM. Haemorrhoidectomy with Ligasure™ vs conventional excisional techniques: meta-analysis of randomized controlled trials. Colorectal Disease. 2010 Feb;12(2):85–93.

[19] Xia W, MacFater HS, MacFater WS, Otutaha BF, Barazanchi AW, Sammour T, Hill AG. Local anaesthesia alone versus regional or general anaesthesia in excisional haemorrhoidectomy: a systematic review and meta-analysis. World Journal of Surgery. 2020 Sep;44(9):3119–29.

[20] Lohsiriwat V, Jitmungngan R. Strategies to reduce post-hemorrhoidectomy pain: a systematic review. Medicina. 2022 Mar 12;58(3):418.

[21] Sammour T, Barazanchi AW, Hill AG. Evidence-based management of pain after excisional haemorrhoidectomy surgery: a PROSPECT review update. World Journal of Surgery. 2017 Feb;41(2):603–14.

[22] Kilonzo MM, Brown SR, Bruhn H, Cook JA, Hudson J, Norrie J, Watson AJ, Wood J. Cost effectiveness of stapled haemorrhoidopexy and traditional excisional surgery for the treatment of haemorrhoidal disease. PharmacoEconomics-Open. 2018 Sep;2(3):271–80.

CHAPTER 21

Haemorrhoids—Postulated Pathogenesis and Proposed Prevention

Burkitt DP, Graham-Stewart CW. Postgrad Med J. 51(599):631–636, 1975

Reviewed by Bruce Orkin

Research Question/Objective The objective of this paper is to synthesize the known and hypothesized etiologies of and risk factors for hemorrhoids. The stated hypothesis is that the fundamental cause of hemorrhoids is straining at viscid stools, which are the result of fiber-depleted diets.

Study Design The authors discuss the nature of hemorrhoids utilizing epidemiological, clinical, and very limited experimental evidence. A hypothesis of the underlying pathogenesis developed by one of the authors and salient observations by the other inform the discussion. Using this information, the authors conclusions are described as reasoned deductions rather than as any specific experimental results.

Although not specifically stated, this paper focuses entirely upon internal hemorrhoids, and external hemorrhoids were not considered at all.

Sample Size Not applicable.

Follow-up Not applicable.

Inclusion/Exclusion Criteria Not applicable.

Intervention or Treatment Received Not applicable.

Results This article repeats the etiologic hypotheses of Graham-Stewart (1962) and relies heavily on the limited and inconclusive experimental evidence contained therein.

Their first assumption is that venous dilatation in hemorrhoids is confined to the superior/internal hemorrhoidal plexus. This dilation is due to straining at stool against a tight anal sphincter which results in retrograde flow in these vessels. This is described as a "vascular pump and tube-valve mechanism" (Graham-Stewart 1963). Despite the authors' convictions, this mechanism has never been proven or even suggested by actual experimental evidence.

DOI: 10.1201/9780429285714-21

Their second assumption is that there is a distinction between two types of internal hemorrhoids, vascular and mucosal. There is no actual evidence that these are distinct entities, and nowhere else in the literature is this categorization used. Indeed, most clinicians recognize that internal hemorrhoids represent variable combinations of these two findings, and it is well recognized that vascular dilation and prolapsing mucosa and submucosa are variable components of all internal hemorrhoids.

A number of possible factors influencing the development of hemorrhoids were examined. Those that did not seem to be directly related include heredity, predisposing anatomic features, nutrition aside from fiber, occupation, climate, psychiatric issues, senility/aging, endocrine abnormalities, gastrointestinal "irritation," infections, and pregnancy. Although none of these is definitively ruled out, they seem to have little to no effect. Pregnancy in general was not felt to be causative; however, it is well-known that pregnant patients often develop hemorrhoidal problems, especially thrombosed external hemorrhoids.

Factors that were deemed most likely to be related include constipation with straining at stool and a low fiber diet leading to small hard stools and prolonged intestinal transit times. These are felt to be closely related to one another.

The authors do point out that it was difficult to come to clear conclusions based on the literature available in 1975 because of a lack of a clear, accepted definition of hemorrhoids, the lack of population studies, and the fact that the majority of the literature is from Western countries and so may not be generalizable. In addition, the limited experimental data are very poor and generally inconclusive.

However, they go on to state that the direct cause of hemorrhoids is raised intra-abdominal pressure with straining to evacuate hard stools.

This is a summary article discussing the pathogenesis of internal hemorrhoids reflecting the opinions of the authors based on their hypotheses, observations, deductions, and some experimental evidence. They conclude that there is no evidence that any other etiological factor is as significant as low fiber intake and resultant constipation and straining.

Study Limitations   There is very little actual relevant experimental evidence regarding the etiology of hemorrhoids contained in this study or the rest of the medical literature. Indeed, the studies that have been attempted are all inconclusive. Therefore, the authors conclusions are based on subjective observations and opinions and so are biased and not supported by objective data.

Relevant Studies

Definition   The actual definition of hemorrhoids is difficult since hemorrhoidal vessels and cushions are part of the normal anatomy of the anal canal, and there is a broad spectrum of hemorrhoidal disease including internal and external hemorrhoids, vascular dilation, mucosal laxity, prolapse, thrombosis, and gangrene.

Incidence   Even the incidence of hemorrhoidal disease is very difficult to ascertain since most data are highly suspect and subjective. In most parts of the world, virtually any anorectal complaint is often attributed to hemorrhoidal disease. Self-reporting and physician identification of hemorrhoids are unreliable, and population studies are even less accurate (Loder et al. 1994).

Pathogenesis   The pathophysiology of hemorrhoidal development is poorly understood. None of the proposed theories of the pathogenesis of hemorrhoids from antiquity to today have been proven (Loder et al. 1994). Even to this day, surprisingly little research on the etiology of hemorrhoids has been performed (Loder et al. 1994, Brisinda 2000, Lohsiriwat 2012, Sandler 2018, Pata et al. 2021, Pigot et al. 2005). In spite of this lack of evidence, it is generally believed that constipation leads to chronic straining and hard stools resulting in degeneration of the supportive tissue in the anal canal and distal displacement of the anal cushions (Johanson and Sonnenberg 1990, Loder et al. 1994, Sandler and Peery 2019).

A large number of histologic changes in the anal vasculature and suspensory tissues and in local mediators and enzymes have been described. However, it is not known whether these are causative or resultant or if they are even related to hemorrhoidal disease (Lohsiriwat 2012).

Review of the medical literature shows that most papers focus on treatment methods and outcomes (Brisinda 2000).

The Authors   Denis Parsons Burkitt, MD (1911–1993), was an Irish-born surgeon. He made two major contributions to medical science related to his experiences in Africa. He identified the childhood lymphoma now known as Burkitt's lymphoma and the role of dietary fiber in bowel function and disease. He came to believe that a diet lacking in fiber contributed to the development of many disorders that are more common in industrialized countries such as constipation, hemorrhoids, and colorectal cancer.

Burkitt's seminal paper, the "Effect of dietary fiber on stools and transit times, and its role in the causation of disease" (Burkitt et al. 1972), is of primary importance in any discussion of hemorrhoids and constipation. Herein, he reported his observations of bowel habits and stools as well as the results of over 1000 transit time studies performed in various populations in different locations. He found that high-fiber diets resulted in large, soft stools and in rapid intestinal transit, while low-fiber diets produce small, firm stool that traverses the gut slowly. This work and others show that this phenomenon does not depend on ethnicity and that changes in diet will rapidly result in altered bowel habits (Burkitt 1979, Johanson and Sonnenberg 1990, Sandler and Peery 2019).

Colin Woodward Graham-Stewart (unknown—2000) was a general surgeon who competed his surgical training at St. Thomas's Hospital in London. He was subsequently appointed consultant surgeon to Harrogate District Hospitals. He wrote his MBBM thesis in 1962 for the University of London on the etiology of hemorrhoids (Graham-Stewart 1962). Much of the paper discussed here is based on that work. In his thesis, he described a set of experiments that were attempted to try and validate his hypotheses. He tried to measure vascular pressure changes within the hemorrhoidal vessels in a very small number of male and female patients, pregnant women, older patients, and controls. However, because of the crude techniques and small numbers of subjects, these studies did not show any clear patterns and so were inconclusive (Graham-Stewart 1963, 1975).

Loder, et al.'s comprehensive discussion of this subject concludes that virtually all data regarding the incidence and etiology of hemorrhoidal disease are suspect (Loder et al. 1994). Even constipation as a factor has been called into question (Johanson and Sonnenberg 1994).

The authors of this paper are well-informed, thoughtful, and experienced. Their thoughts on this problem are interesting and well-reasoned; however, their conclusions can only be accepted as being speculative (Sandler and Peery 2019).

Conclusion   Although the detailed hypotheses of the etiology of internal hemorrhoids promoted in this article are interesting, none have borne the test of time. This returns us to the generally accepted conclusion, based on expert opinion rather than research data, that constipation and straining are important in the development of hemorrhoids and that this is often related to fiber intake. That, then, is the primary lasting message of this paper.

REFERENCES

Brisinda G. How to treat haemorrhoids. Prevention is best; haemorrhoidectomy needs skilled operators. BMJ. 2000 Sep 9;321(7261):582–3. doi: 10.1136/bmj.321.7261.582. PMID: 10977817; PMCID: PMC1118483.

Burkitt D. Don't forget fibre in your diet: to help avoid many of our commonest diseases. London: Martin Dunitz, 1979.

Burkitt DP, Graham-Stewart CW. Haemorrhoids–postulated pathogenesis and proposed prevention. Postgrad Med J. 1975 Sep;51(599):631–6. doi: 10.1136/pgmj.51.599.631. PMID: 1105503; PMCID: PMC2496194.

Burkitt DP, Walker ARP, Painter NS. Effect of dietary fibre on stools and transit times, and its role in the causation of disease. Lancet. 1972 Dec 30;2(7792):1408–12. doi: 10.1016/s0140-6736(72)92974-1.

Graham-Stewart CW. The Aetiology of Haemorrhoids. Section 1, M.S. Thesis, University of London, 1962.

Graham-Stewart CW. What causes hemorrhoids? A new theory of etiology. Dis Colon Rectum. 1963 Sep–Oct;6:333–44. doi: 10.1007/BF02618390. PMID: 14063156.

Graham-Stewart CW. Letter: nature of piles. Lancet. 1975 Oct 4;2(7936):665. doi: 10.1016/s0140-6736(75)90153-1. PMID: 52040. doi: 10.1016/s0140-6736(75)90153-1

Johanson JF, Sonnenberg A. The prevalence of hemorrhoids and chronic constipation. An epidemiologic study. Gastroenterology. 1990 Feb;98(2):380–6. doi: 10.1016/0016-5085(90)90828-o. PMID: 2295392.

Johanson JF, Sonnenberg A. Constipation is not a risk factor for hemorrhoids: a case-control study of potential etiological agents. Am J Gastroenterol. 1994 Nov;89(11):1981–6. PMID: 7942722.

Loder PB, Kamm MA, Nicholls RJ, Phillips RK. Haemorrhoids: pathology, pathophysiology and aetiology. Br J Surg. 1994 Jul;81(7):946–54. doi: 10.1002/bjs.1800810707. PMID: 7922085

Lohsiriwat V. Hemorrhoids: from basic pathophysiology to clinical management. World J Gastroenterol. 2012;18(17):2009–17. PMID: 22563187. doi: 10.3748/wjg.v18.i17.2009.

Pata F, Sgró A, Ferrara F, Vigorita V, Gallo G, Pellino G. Anatomy, physiology and pathophysiology of haemorrhoids. Rev Recent Clin Trials. 2021;16(1):75–80. doi: 10.2174/15748871156 66200406115150. PMID: 32250229.

Pigot F, Siproudhis L, Allaert FA. Risk factors associated with hemorrhoidal symptoms in specialized consultation. Gastroenterol Clin Biol. 2005; 29: 1270–4. PMID: 16518286. doi: 10.1016/s0399-8320(05)82220-1.

Sandler RS, Peery AF. Rethinking what we know about hemorrhoids. Clin Gastroenterol Hepatol. 2019 Jan;17(1):8–15. doi: 10.1016/j.cgh.2018.03.020. PMID: 29601902; PMCID: PMC7075634.

CHAPTER 22

Laparoscopic Peritoneal Lavage or Sigmoidectomy for Perforated Diverticulitis with Purulent Peritonitis: A Multicenter, Parallel-Group, Randomized, Open-Label Trial

Vernix S, Musters GD, et al. The Lancet. 386:1269–1277, 2015

Reviewed by Norbert Garcia-Henriquez

Research Question/Objective   In recent years, laparoscopic lavage has been proposed as an alternative to surgery, specifically sigmoidectomy in patients with complicated diverticulitis. The authors aimed to assess the superiority of laparoscopic lavage compared to surgery in patients with purulent peritonitis as it pertains to overall long-term morbidity and mortality.

Study Design   The Ladies (DIVA and LOLA) trial is a multicenter, parallel-group, randomized, open-label superiority trial carried out in 34 teaching and 8 academic hospitals throughout Belgium, Italy, and the Netherlands. Specifically, it was designed to compare laparoscopic lavage and sigmoidectomy for complicated diverticulitis as defined by purulent peritonitis in the LOLA group and to compare Hartmann's procedure versus sigmoid colectomy with primary anastomosis in both purulent and feculent peritonitis in the DIVA group. In this particular trial, the LOLA group was assessed.

The primary outcome of the study consisted of major morbidity and mortality within 12 months. Secondary outcomes included operative times, length of hospital stay, days alive and outside of the hospital, short-term morbidity and mortality, incisional hernia rates, reinterventions within 12 months, and health-related quality of life. Major morbidity was defined as a surgical intervention, abdominal wall dehiscence, abscess requiring percutaneous drainage, urosepsis, myocardial infarction, renal failure, and respiratory insufficiency within 30 days after operation or in hospital.

A post hoc analysis was performed in order to determine the incidence of recurrent diverticulitis as well as the incidence of underlying perforated cancer diagnosed during follow-up.

DOI: 10.1201/9780429285714-22

Sample Size   In an effort to obtain an appropriate number of patients for the data analysis, the authors concluded a sample size of 264 patients was required to detect a 15% difference in the composite end point with an expected rate of 25% in the sigmoidectomy group and 10% in the lavage group at 12 months. Included were a two-sided likelihood ratio test and a power of 90%. The assumption of 10% major morbidity and mortality is based on the reported morbidity and mortality by Toorenvliet et al. [1], whereas the 25% was based on adjusted data from the scientific literature as the authors exclusively included patients with a Hinchey III classification [2].

Follow-Up   Total follow-up time for the study period was 12 months. Upon convalescence from the index operation, patients were followed up at least once in the outpatient setting and after sigmoidoscopy and stoma reversal per institutional protocol. If patients were not in active follow-up with the surgeon within 12 months, the patients were contacted and follow-up verified.

Inclusion/Exclusion criteria   All patients with signs of peritonitis and suspected perforated diverticulitis were eligible for inclusion. CT scan evaluation had to demonstrate diffuse free intraperitoneal air or fluid in order to be classified as perforated diverticulitis. Those patients with dementia, previous sigmoidectomy, pelvic radiation, chronic high-dose steroid treatment (>20 mg daily), <18 or >85 years of age, preoperative shock requiring inotropic support, or Hinchey classification I or II were excluded from the final analysis. Of note, those with Hinchey IV or overt perforation could only be allocated to the DIVA group of the study.

Intervention   Laparoscopic lavage was performed by irrigating the abdominal cavity with up to 6 L of warm saline and placing an abdominal drain through a designated port site. Sigmoidectomy with primary anastomosis was performed based on American Society of Colon and Rectal Surgeons. A protective ileostomy was created at the discretion of the surgeon.

Results   From July 1, 2010, to the early termination of the trial date of February 22, 2013, the authors randomized 90 patients to the LOLA group of the study: 47 to laparoscopic lavage and 43 to sigmoidectomy. Patients in the trial were included from 30 hospitals (28 from the Netherlands, 1 Belgian, and 1 Italian). The baseline characteristics of the included patients did not differ. The mean age in the analyzed patients was 63 years, 58% of which were men (Table 22.1). The proportion of patients with ASA grade III or IV was lower in the lavage group. Within the surgery group, 20 patients were allocated to a Hartmann's procedure and 22 to sigmoidectomy with primary anastomosis, where 1 was converted to a Hartmann's procedure and 1 crossed to the lavage group as the patient could not be placed in stirrups because of recent knee surgery. A total of 14 patients were diverted with an ileostomy. One patient in the lavage group was converted to an open Hartmann's procedure due to feculent peritonitis. Seven sigmoidectomies were performed and completed by the laparoscopic platform, where the remainder were converted to open upon randomization.

TABLE 22.1   Baseline Characteristics in Randomly Assigned Patients with Perforated Diverticulitis

	Laparoscopic Lavage (n = 46)	Sigmoidectomy (n = 42)
Age (years)	62.3 (12.7)	64.0 (12.3)
Sex		
Men	26 (57%)	25 (60%)
Women	20 (43%)	17 (40%)
Body-mass index (kg/m²)*	27.6 (6.2)	27.0 (4.4)
ASA		
I	10 (22%)	8 (19%)
II	21 (46%)	13 (31%)
III	5 (11%)	13 (31%)
IV	3 (7%)	2 (5%)
Missing	7 (15%)	6 (14%)
Previous diverticulitis†	12 (32%)	10 (26%)
Previous laparotomy‡	4 (9%)	3 (7%)
Disease severity preoperative		
APACHE II	7.3 (4.2)	9.0 (4.8)
POSSUM PS	20.8 (6.2)	22.8 (6.2)
POSSUM OS	17.1 (0.5)	20.0 (2.2)
Interval from ER to Surgery (h)	13 (8–32)	13 (6–42)
Number of patients operated on by a gastrointestinal surgeon	37 (80%)	36 (86%)

Source: Data are mean (SD), n (%), or median (IQR) ASA = American Society of Anesthesiologists classification. APACHE II = acute physiology and chronic health evaluation II. POSSUM-PS = physiology and operative severity score for the enumeration of mortality and morbidity—physiology score. POSSUM-OS = POSSUM operative score. ER = moment of presentation at the emergency department. *n = 40 in the laparoscopic lavage group, n = 39 in the sigmoidectomy group. †n = 38 in the laparoscopic lavage group; n = 38 in the sigmoidectomy group. ‡n = 45 in the laparoscopic lavage group; n = 41 in the sigmoidectomy group

The LOLA group of the Ladies trial was terminated early for safety reasons where the DSMB (data and safety monitoring board) evaluated the final data on 46 lavage and 40 sigmoidectomy patients. Upon their third analysis of the data, the major morbidity and mortality was 35% and 18% in the lavage and sigmoidectomy groups, respectively. The majority of these adverse events were in the form of surgical reintervention; 18 in the lavage group and 2 in the sigmoidectomy group (in-hospital interventions) ($p = 0.0011$). Overall surgical reinterventions were 28 in the lavage group and 11 in the sigmoidectomy group ($p = 0.0219$).

During the 12-month follow-up, no differences were noted in the incidence of the composite primary end point (30 lavage group vs. 25 in the sigmoidectomy group; OR 1.28, 95% CI 0.54–3.03, $p = 0.5804$). The mean operative time was shorter for the lavage group (60 minutes) compared to the sigmoidectomy group (120 minutes), and the lengths of hospital stay did not differ between the two groups.

The combined major morbidity and mortality rates within 30 days after surgery or in hospital were higher in the lavage group, 39% compared to 19% in the sigmoidectomy group: OR 2.74, 95% CI 1.03–7.27, $p = 0.0427$). The majority of the former is attributed to the higher rate of reinterventions (Table 22.2).

Nine patients in the lavage group required reintervention due to persistent sepsis (feculent peritonitis or overt perforation). One patient was diagnosed with an underlying cancer on final pathology. Seven patients had a Hartmann's procedure, 1 a primary anastomosis with ileostomy, and 1 patient had 4 relaparotomies after lavage followed by delayed elective sigmoidectomy. Two other patients died from multiorgan failure. Three patients in the sigmoidectomy group required reintervention for an acute fascial dehiscence, an unconfirmed anastomotic leak, and a negative second look laparotomy in a patient with an open abdomen. One patient died from an arterial embolism, and another 2 died shortly after an extended hospital stay because of renal or respiratory failure. On final pathology, 2 patients were discovered to have colon cancer, both of which were treated with adjuvant chemotherapy.

With regard to stomal reversal surgery, 5 of 11 patients underwent surgery in the lavage group, whereas 24 of 35 patients underwent surgery in the sigmoidectomy group. With regard to quality of life, no differences were noted in the main scores of the SF-36, GIQLI, and EQ5D questionnaire.

Lastly, in a *post hoc* subgroup analysis for patients aged younger or above 60 years of age, the primary end point did not differ between the two treatment groups. *Post hoc* stratified analysis for patients with a low ASA grade (I or II) or high ASA (III or IV) did not demonstrate a significant between-group difference in the primary outcome (OR 1.36 95% CI 0.51–3.62, $p = 0.5337$).

Study Limitations   In this study, which was terminated early, laparoscopic lavage for purulent perforated diverticulitis did not result in a reduction in the composite end point of major morbidity and mortality compared to sigmoidectomy at 12 months. Although laparoscopic lavage did result in a higher acute reintervention rate, 76% of patients were discharged without

TABLE 22.2   Serious Adverse Events, Defined as Major Morbidity

	Laparoscopic Lavage (n = 46)		Sigmoidectomy (n = 42)		p-Value
	Patients	**Events**	**Patients**	**Events**	
Short-term serious adverse events	18 (39%)	39	8 (19%)	14	0.0427
Death	2 (4%)	2	1 (2%)	1	0.6237
Surgical reintervention	9 (20%)	15	3 (7%)	3	0.1230
Abscess with drainage	9 (20%)	12	0	0	0.0027
Fascial dehiscence	0	0	3 (7%)	3	0.1046
Myocardial infarction	0	0	1 (2%)	1	0.4775
Respiratory failure	6 (13%)	6	2 (5%)	2	0.1955
Renal failure	2 (4%)	2	2 (5%)	2	0.9207
Long-term serious adverse events	17 (37%)	30	17 (40%)	20	0.1156
Death	2 (4%)	2	5 (12%)	5	0.1875
Surgical reintervention	13 (28%)	16	5 (12%)	6	0.1156
Abscess with drainage	2 (4%)	4	2 (5%)	2	0.9207
Fascial dehiscence	5 (11%)	5	5 (12%)	5	0.4359
Sigmoid carcinoma	5 (11%)	5	2 (5%)	2	0.3047
Recurrent diverticulitis	9 (20%)	9	1 (2%)	1	0.0315
Composite primary outcome (major morbidity or mortality at 12 months)	30 (67%)		25 (60%)		0.5804

Source: Data are *n* (%), unless otherwise stated. Short term is defined as within 30 days or in hospital; long term is defined as after 30 days or discharge and within 12 months

requiring any further surgery. This said, the higher morbidity rates did not result in excess mortality, which suggests that patients that fail laparoscopic lavage can be rescued if reintervention is performed in a timely manner.

Although this is indeed a well written and informative study, one of its most critical limitations is that it was underpowered and thus obviated the study's inability to conclude on noninferiority. That said, as the authors have mentioned, a noninferiority type of study with mortality as the primary end point would require a very large sample size. With the proper number of patients and longer follow-up, perhaps noninferiority would easily come to light.

In the meantime, although laparoscopic lavage seems like a viable option for patients with Hinchey Class III, it is associated with higher reintervention rates, which can be mitigated with definitive resection. Along those lines, this study allows us to properly inform our patients. However, even though surgery is a better option, the technical challenges and potential surgical complications, especially at the time of end colostomy reversal, cannot be understated.

REFERENCES

1. Toorenvliet BR, Swank H, Schoones JW, Hamming JF, Bemelman WA. Laparoscopic peritoneal lavage for perforated colonic diverticulitis: a systematic review. *Colorectal Dis* 2010; 12:862–867.
2. Abbas S. Resection and primary anastomosis in acute complicated diverticulitis: a systematic review of the literature. *Int J Colorectal Dis* 2007; 22: 351–357.

CHAPTER 23

Surgery versus Conservative Management for Recurrent and Ongoing Left-Sided Diverticulitis (Direct Trial): An Open-Label, Multicentre, Randomised Controlled Trial

van de Wall BJM, Stam MAW, Draaisma WA, Stellato R, Bemelman WA, Boermeester MA, Broeders IAMJ, Belgers EJ, Toorenvliet BR, Prins HA, Consten ECJ: DIRECT trial collaborators. The Lancet. 2(1):P13–22, 2017

Reviewed by Tyler McKechnie, Cagla Eskicioglu, and Jason F. Hall

Research Question/Objective   Both non-operative management and elective anterior resection are acceptable approaches to managing persistent and recurrent uncomplicated left-sided diverticulitis (1). Prior to completion of this study, no high-quality study had compared nonoperative and operative management for this patient population. Moreover, no study had taken into consideration quality of life (QoL) and postoperative complications. This randomized controlled trial was designed to compare nonoperative management to elective anterior resection in patients with persistent or recurrent symptoms after an episode of left-sided diverticulitis. The primary aim was to determine which approach afforded better QoL.

Study Design   This was an open-label, randomized controlled trial conducted across 26 centers in the Netherlands that compared nonoperative management to elective anterior resection in patients with persistent or recurrent symptoms after an episode of left-sided diverticulitis. The index episode had to be confirmed on computed tomography (CT), ultrasonography, and/or endoscopy. Recurrent diverticulitis was defined as 3 or more presentations with signs and symptoms in keeping with acute diverticulitis within a 2-year period and with at least 3 months between each presentation. Ongoing complaints were defined as persistent left-sided abdominal pain or change in bowel habits for at least 3 months following the index episode, accompanied by signs of inflammation on CT or endoscopy. The primary outcome was health-related quality of life as measured by the Gastrointestinal Quality of Life Index (GIQLI) at 6 months following study enrollment/surgery. The secondary outcomes included other quality of life scores [i.e., EuroQol five dimensions questionnaire (EQ-5D), Visual Analogue Score for pain (VAS-pain), 36-item Short Form health survey (SF-36)], and postoperative morbidity and mortality. Data were analyzed with independent t-tests and according to the intention-to-treat principle.

DOI: 10.1201/9780429285714-23

Sample Size   Assuming the minimum clinically important difference (MID) of the GIQLI score was 10, sample size calculations with a *p*-value of 0.05 and power of 90% supposed that 97 patients per group were required to adequately power this study. Throughout the study period of July 1, 2010, to April 1, 2014, 431 patients were assessed for eligibility. Of these, 109 patients met the inclusion criteria. Randomization allocated 56 patients to the nonoperative management group, and 53 patients to the elective surgery group. The study was terminated early due to failure to recruit.

Follow-Up   Patients completed QoL questionnaires at inclusion and at 3- and 6-months following inclusion or surgery. Postoperative morbidity and mortality were recorded at 30 days and 6 months.

Inclusion/Exclusion Criteria   This study included patients between 18 and 75 years of age presenting to one of the 26 centers involved in this study with either ongoing abdominal complaints or recurrent diverticulitis following an index episode of left-sided diverticulitis. Patients who were greater than American Society of Anesthesiologists (ASA) Class III, had absolute indications for operations (i.e., peritonitis, stricture, fistula), had a high suspicion of underlying colorectal malignancy, and had undergone previous anterior resection for diverticular disease were excluded.

Intervention or Treatment Received   Patients assigned to the nonoperative management group were treated with a combination of the following measures in keeping with practice patterns in the Netherlands at the time of the study: (1) lifestyle measures, (2) supplementary dietary fibre, (3) laxatives as needed, (4) analgesics as needed. Antibiotics and mesalamine were not routinely used in this group. Patients assigned to the surgery group underwent elective anterior resection within 3 months of randomization. The preferred operative approach was a laparoscopic anterior resection with primary anastomosis without diverting loop ileostomy.

Results   Fifty-six patients (median age 56.5 years, 57% female, mean body mass index (BMI) 27.8 kg/m^2) were randomized to nonoperative management, 43 of which ultimately received it (76.8%); 53 patients (median age 54.1 years, 72% female, mean BMI 28.7 kg/m^2) were randomized to operative management, 47 of which ultimately received it (88.7%). Most patients were included for persistent symptoms as opposed to recurrent disease ($n = 69$, 63.3%). In patients with persistent symptoms, the median duration of symptoms prior to inclusion was 31 weeks (IQR 16–81). In patients with recurrent disease, the mean number of episodes prior to inclusion was 4. The majority of index episodes of left-sided diverticulitis were diagnosed on CT and colonoscopy. The surgery group had worse index episodes as per Hinchey classification, with 19% of patients having Hinchey II disease compared to 11% in the nonoperative group. There were also 2 patients in the surgery group with Hinchey III/IV disease. Mean GIQLI (nonoperative: 92.2 +/–21.3; surgery: 92.6 +/–22.8) and VAS-pain (nonoperative: 69.3 SD 13.6; surgery: 63.3 SD 21.7) scores were similar at baseline between groups.

On intention-to-treat analysis, mean GIQLI score at 6 months was significantly higher in the surgery group compared to the nonoperative group (114.4 SD 22.3 vs. 100.4 SD 22.7, MD 14.2, 95%C% 7.2–21.1, $p < 0.0001$). The GIQLI improved by more than 10 points (MID) in 70% of patients in the surgery group and in 34% of patients in the nonoperative group. There was no difference in outcomes between patients with persistent disease and patients with recurrent disease. The per-protocol analysis yielded similar results to the intention-to-treat analysis. There were also significant improvements in the secondary quality of life measures at 6 months in the surgery group compared to the nonoperative group (EQ-5D: 0.84 SD 0.20 vs. 0.73 SD 0.19, $p = 0.0013$; VAS-pain score: 23.9 SD 23.4 vs. 48.3 SD 22.9, $p < 0.0001$; SF-36 physical score: 43.5 SD 8.8 vs. 39.5 SD 7.0, $p = 0.016$).

Of the patients in the surgery group, 98% of patients had laparoscopic surgery, conversion rate to open was 6.5%, and the incidence of temporary loop ileostomy formation was 21%. All but one of the patients had their stoma reversed within 6 months of its formation. Minor perioperative complications (Clavien-Dindo I/II) occurred in 38% of patients, major postoperative complications (Clavien-Dindo III-V) occurred in 28% of patients, and the incidence of anastomotic leak was 15%.

In the nonoperative management group, 7 (13%) patients developed recurrent diverticulitis in the 6-month follow-up period. All recurrences were managed nonoperatively. Thirteen patients (23%) in the nonoperative group had persistent abdominal complaints for which they ultimately underwent elective anterior resection.

Study Limitations   The study was closed prematurely due to inability to recruit to the targeted sample size. It is possible that early closure of the study could have resulted in overestimation of the treatment effect (2). There were important differences in baseline characteristics of both groups. Patients in the surgery group were more likely to have greater Hinchey scores at the time of their index episode of diverticulitis. As such, it is possible that they reported greater improvements in postoperative quality of life measures as a result of the worse baseline disease. Additionally, there was a lack of standardization in the nonoperative management group. Patients in this group likely received a range of lifestyle and medical recommendations. For example, mesalamine use was not ubiquitous amongst patients in this group (3). Since this was not a placebo-controlled trial, it is possible that part of the improvement in the surgical group was explained by the placebo effect that accompanies interventions (4).

Relevant Studies   Prior to this randomized controlled trial, most data comparing nonoperative and operative management for persistent and/or recurrent left-sided diverticulitis were derived from low-quality observational studies. A systematic review and meta-analysis of 21 studies in 2016 by

Andeweg et al. suggested that elective laparoscopic anterior resection for recurrent uncomplicated diverticulitis improved quality of life according to the SF-36 score and decreased incidences of chronic abdominal complaints compared to nonoperative management (5). They concluded that while there may be improved outcomes following elective surgery for these patients, high-quality prospective data would be required to confirm these findings.

The DIRECT trial, as discussed, followed and confirmed these findings. The long-term data from this trial have also since been published in 2019 (6). At 5-year follow-up, the mean GIQLI score was significantly greater in the surgery group compared to the nonoperative group (118.2 SD 21.0 vs. 108.5 SD 20.0, MD 9.7, 95% CI 1.7–17.7, p = 0.018). Secondary quality of life measures were also significantly improved in the surgery group compared to the nonoperative group at 5 years, including the EQ-5D score (p = 0.016), SF-36 physical score (p = 0.03), SF-36 mental score (p = 0.01), and VAS-pain score (p = 0.011). Twenty-six patients from the nonoperative group (46%) had undergone elective anterior resection at 5 years follow-up. Overall, the long-term data suggest that patients with persistent and/or recurrent left-sided diverticulitis benefit from elective anterior resection.

The LASER trial, published in 2021 in *JAMA Surgery*, is the only other randomized, controlled trial addressing this clinical question (7). This was a multicenter, prospective, open-label randomized controlled trial that randomized 128 patients with persistent, recurrent, or complicated left-sided diverticulitis to either nonoperative management or elective laparoscopic anterior resection. Patients were eligible if they had 3 or more episodes of uncomplicated left-sided diverticulitis within 2 consecutive years, 1 or more episode(s) of complicated left-sided diverticulitis, or if they had persistent pain or change in bowel habits for more than 3 consecutive months after an index episode of CT-proven left-sided diverticulitis. Their findings were similar to the DIRECT trial; specifically, the difference between GIQLI scores at randomization and 6 months follow-up was a mean of 11.96 points higher in the surgery group than in the nonoperative group (11.76 SD 15.89 vs. −0.2 SD 19.07, MD 11.96, 95% CI 3.72–20.19, p = 0.005). The rate of major perioperative morbidity in the patients undergoing elective laparoscopic anterior resection was lower than in the DIRECT trial (10%).

In conclusion, the available data comparing nonoperative and operative management for persistent and recurrent left-sided diverticulitis suggest operative management by way of elective laparoscopic anterior resection offers improved QoL and decreased risk of recurrence for these patients. Further studies with less stringent inclusion criteria and within the North American context are required to increase the generalizability of these findings.

REFERENCES

1. Al Harakeh H, Paily AJ, Doughan S, Shaikh I. Recurrent Acute Diverticulitis: When to Operate? Inflamm Intest Dis. 2018;3(2):91–9.
2. Bassler D, Briel M, Montori VM, Lane M, Glasziou P, Zhou Q, et al. Stopping Randomized Trials Early for Benefit and Estimation of Treatment Effects: Systematic Review and Meta-Regression Analysis. JAMA. 2010;303(12):1180–7.
3. Stollman N, Magowan S, Shanahan F, Quigley EMM. A Randomized Controlled Study of Mesalamine After Acute Diverticulitis: Results of the DIVA Trial. J Clin Gastroenterol. 2013;47(7):621–9.
4. Jonas WB, Crawford C, Colloca L, Kaptchuk TJ, Moseley B, Miller FG, et al. To What Extent Are Surgery and Invasive Procedures Effective Beyond a Placebo Response? A Systematic Review with Meta-Analysis of Randomised, Sham Controlled Trials. BMJ Open. 2015;5(12):e009655.
5. Andeweg CS, Berg R, Staal JB, ten Broek RPG, van Goor H. Patient-reported Outcomes After Conservative or Surgical Management of Recurrent and Chronic Complaints of Diverticulitis: Systematic Review and Meta-Analysis. Clin Gastroenterol Hepatol. 2016;14(2):183–90.
6. Bolkenstein H, Consten E, van der Palen J, van de Wall B, Broeders I, Bemelman W, et al. Long-Term Outcome of Surgery versus Conservative Management for Recurrent and Ongoing Complaints After an Episode of Diverticulitis: 5-Year Follow-Up Results of a Multicenter Randomized Controlled Trial (DIRECT-Trial). Ann Surg. 2019;269(4):612–20.
7. Santos A, Mentula P, Pinta T, Ismail S, Rautio T, Juusela R, et al. Comparing Laparoscopic Elective Sigmoid Resection With Conservative Treatment in Improving Quality of Life of Patients with Diverticulitis: The Laparoscopic Elective Sigmoid Resection Following Diverticulitis (LASER) Randomized Clinical Trial. JAMA Surg. 2021;156(2):129–36.

Randomized Clinical Trial of Antibiotics in Acute Uncomplicated Diverticulitis

Chabok A, Pahlman L, Hjern F, et al.: AVOD Study Group. Br J Surg. 99(4):532–539, 2012

Reviewed by Richard Garfinkle and Marylise Boutros

Research Question/Objective   Recent evidence has challenged the routine use of antibiotics in the management of uncomplicated diverticulitis. The objective of this study was to evaluate the effect of antibiotic omission on the development of complications in the management of left-sided acute uncomplicated colonic diverticulitis.

Study Design   This was an open-label, multicenter randomized controlled trial (RCT) that recruited patients from 2003–2010 from 10 hospitals in Sweden and 1 hospital in Iceland. Block randomization, stratified by participating center, was performed. The primary outcome was in-hospital complications, defined as bowel perforation with free air, abscess or fistula. Secondary outcomes included hospital length of stay, the need for antibiotics (among those randomized to nonantibiotic treatment), as well as recurrent diverticulitis, sigmoid resection, and abdominal pain/bowel habits at 1 year.

Sample Size   Assuming a baseline incidence of complications *with* antibiotics of 1.5%, the investigators estimated requiring 240 patients in each group to detect a 5% absolute increase in the incidence of complications *without* antibiotics. Among 669 patients randomized, 623 patients were included in the primary analysis: 314 in the antibiotics group and 309 in the nonantibiotics group. Forty-one patients were lost to follow-up, leaving 582 patients available for analysis at 1-year follow-up.

Follow-Up   The primary outcome (complications) was assessed in-hospital within 30 days of treatment initiation for the index presentation of uncomplicated diverticulitis. Long-term secondary outcomes, including recurrent diverticulitis, sigmoid resection, and abdominal pain/bowel habits, were assessed at 1-year follow-up.

Inclusion/Exclusion Criteria   Adult (>18 years old) patients with CT-confirmed acute uncomplicated left-sided colonic diverticulitis were eligible for the study. Exclusion criteria included sepsis on presentation, presence of diverticulitis complications on CT scan (abscess, fistula, or free air), immunosuppression, pregnancy, or ongoing antibiotic therapy for another condition.

DOI: 10.1201/9780429285714-24

Intervention or Treatment Received   The control arm of the trial received intravenous fluid with broad-spectrum antibiotics (intravenous followed by transition to oral). The experimental arm received intravenous fluids alone without antibiotics. All patients were admitted to hospital, and in-patient management, including discharge criteria, was otherwise similar in both groups.

Results

CONSORT Diagram   Among 669 randomized patients, 46 (21 in the antibiotics arm and 25 in the nonantibiotics arm) were excluded from the primary analysis, most commonly for not meeting proper inclusion criteria. Five patients were found to have complicated diverticulitis on the final CT report, resulting in their exclusion as well. In total, 314 patients were included in the antibiotics group and 309 patients in the nonantibiotics group.

Clinical Characteristics   The median age of included patients was 58 years (range: 23–88), and the majority of patients were female (64.4%). Less than one-half (39.6%) of patients had a previous history of diverticulitis, and this was more common in the nonantibiotics arm (44.8% vs. 35.6%, $p = 0.020$). Mean white blood cell counts (WBC) (antibiotics arm: 12.6 ±3.1 vs. nonantibiotics arm: 12.3 ±3.3, $p = 0.276$) and C-reactive protein (CRP) levels (100 ±62 vs. 91 ±61, $p = 0.070$) were similar in both groups, as were abdominal pain, body temperature, and abdominal tenderness.

Primary Outcomes   In total, 9 patients developed diverticulitis complications while in hospital: 6 with sigmoid perforation and 3 with abscess formation. In the antibiotics arm, 3 patients developed sigmoid perforations and underwent emergency surgery. In the nonantibiotics arm, 3 patients developed sigmoid perforation (with 1 requiring emergency surgery), and 3 patients developed an abscess. The incidence of complications was similar in both groups (1.0% vs. 1.9%, $p = 0.302$).

Secondary Outcomes   Hospital length of stay was similar in both groups at approximately 3 days (2.9 ±1.9 vs. 2.9 ±1.6, $p = 0.717$). Ten patients (3.2%) allocated to the nonantibiotics arm were ultimately started on antibiotics because of increasing CRP level, fever, or abdominal pain. No diverticulitis complications occurred in these patients. Conversely, 3 patients (1.0%) in the antibiotics arm discontinued treatment because of allergic side effects. During the 1-year follow-up period, 41 patients were lost to follow-up. Only 8 patients (0.6% vs. 1.9%, $p = 0.148$) underwent sigmoid resection, either for symptomatic diverticular disease or diverticulitis complications. Recurrent diverticulitis was also similar in both groups (15.8% vs. 16.2%, $p = 0.881$). On regression analysis, the only factor significantly associated with recurrent diverticulitis was a history of previous diverticulitis episodes prior to the index presentation (adjusted OR: 2.78, 95% CI 1.76–4.41). Symptoms of abdominal pain and changes in bowel habits were also no different on long-term follow-up.

Subgroup Analyses   In the per-protocol analysis, there remained no association between antibiotic omission and the development of diverticulitis complications. Furthermore, in subgroup analyses of patients with more severe symptoms (abdominal pain score >8 or abdominal tenderness score >3) and higher inflammatory parameters (CRP level >150 mg/L, WBC count >15 × 10^9 cells/L, fever >38.5° C), the incidence of diverticulitis complications, and recurrent diverticulitis remained similar in both groups.

Study Limitations   One criticism of this study was the failure of each participating site to register all eligible patients that were approached for study inclusion. Eligible patients who refused to participate in the study may have been systematically different from those who gave consent, which could have resulted in selection bias. The study also recruited patients over an 8-year period, during which time other changes in the management of uncomplicated diverticulitis may have occurred.

Diverticulitis complications were also a difficult outcome to study in this patient population. While it is a good measure of safety when considering antibiotic omission, it is very rare for patients with uncomplicated diverticulitis to progress to a complicated state after treatment; it is therefore not the most relevant outcome in this clinical scenario. Despite a twofold increase in the incidence of complications in the nonantibiotics arm (1.9% vs. 1.0%), the absolute increase was very small, and the findings were not significant. Patient-reported outcomes, persistent disease, time to recovery, as well as healthcare utilization (e.g., emergency room visits, treatment for ongoing symptoms) may have been more suitable end points to which the study could have been powered.

Finally, while antibiotic omission is more likely to impact short-term outcomes rather than long-term outcomes, the follow-up period of 1 year was likely too short to reliably measure recurrent diverticulitis. Most recurrences occur within 2 years of a patient's index presentation, but a significant proportion will occur thereafter.[1] Furthermore, there was a very low rate of elective surgery in the study cohort, which the authors attributed to the country's general policy to not operate on patients with a history of uncomplicated disease.

Relevant Studies   This RCT, often referred to as the AVOD trial, was the first trial to assess nonantibiotic therapy in diverticulitis. Prior to its publication, only one large observational series (from the same authors) reported on the outcomes of nonantibiotic therapy in the management of acute uncomplicated diverticulitis.[2] Among 311 patients hospitalized for diverticulitis, Hjern et al. compared 193 (62%) patients who did not receive antibiotic therapy to 118 (38%) who did. During follow-up, only 7 (4%) patients went on to require antibiotics for worsening symptoms, and the need for surgery as well as recurrent diverticulitis were similar between groups. Several additional observational series were ultimately published, with no study reporting worse outcomes with nonantibiotic treatment.[3–5]

TABLE 24.1 RCTs Comparing Antibiotic to Nonantibiotic Therapy in the Management of Acute Uncomplicated Diverticulitis

Author	Study Years	Country	Number of Patients	Primary Outcome	Results
Chabok et al.[6]	2003–2010	Sweden and Iceland	623	Diverticulitis complications	Antibiotics: 1.0 vs. nonantibiotics: 1.9%, $p = 0.302$
Daniels et al.[7]	2010–2012	Netherlands	528	Time to full recovery	Antibiotics: 12 days vs. nonantibiotics: 14 days, HR 0.91(95% CI 0.78-X)
Jaung et al.[8]	2015–2019	New Zealand and Australia	178	Length of hospital stay	Antibiotics: 40.0 hours (95% CI 24.4–57.6) vs. nonantibiotics: 45.8 hours (95% CI 26.5 to 60.2), $p = 0.20$
Mora-Lopez et al.[9]	2016–2020	Spain	488	Hospital admission	Antibiotics: 5.8% vs. nonantibiotics: 3.3%; mean difference 2.6% (95% CI 6.32 to −1.17)

More importantly, three additional RCTs were published in 2017, 2020, and 2021, respectively (Table 24.1).[6–9] Despite slightly different inclusion criteria, data analysis plans, and primary outcomes, the conclusions of all three RCTs were concordant with that of the AVOD trial: nonantibiotic therapy was safe and provided equivalent outcomes to treatment with antibiotics. Furthermore, follow-up studies of the AVOD and DIABOLO (Daniels et al.) trials reported no differences in long-term rates of recurrent diverticulitis or need for surgery.[10,11] Of note, the most recent RCT out of Spain is the only one to evaluate nonantibiotic therapy in the outpatient setting[9]; the three other trials required hospitalization for all patients.

Despite the evidence that continues to support nonantibiotic therapy for acute uncomplicated diverticulitis, there has been reluctance, particularly within North America, for surgeons and other physicians to abandon antibiotics in the routine management of these patients.[12] Several concerns have been expressed, including the lack of a North American trial (all of the data are currently from Europe or Australia), patient expectations to receive antibiotics, and the potential for medicolegal ramifications.[13] In their 2020 revised clinical practice parameters, the American Society of Colon and Rectal Surgeons endorsed non-antibiotic therapy in appropriate patients with uncomplicated diverticulitis[14]; it will be interesting to survey the adoption of this practice in the years to come.

REFERENCES

1. Garfinkle R, Almalki T, Pelsser V, et al. Conditional risk of diverticulitis after non-operative management. Br J Surg. 2020;107(13):1838–1845.
2. Hjern F, Josephson T, Altman D, et al. Conservative treatment of acute colonic diverticulitis: are antibiotics always mandatory? Scand J Gastroenterol. 2007;42(1):41–47.
3. de Korte N, Kuyvenhoven JP, van der Peet DL, et al. Mild colonic diverticulitis can be treated without antibiotics. A case-control study. Colorectal Dis. 2012;14(3):325–330.
4. Isacson D, Andreasson K, Nikberg M, Smedh K, Chabok A. No antibiotics in acute uncomplicated diverticulitis: does it work? Scand J Gastroenterol. 2014;49(12):1441–1446.
5. Brochmann ND, Schultz JK, Jacobsen GS, Øresland T. Management of acute uncomplicated diverticulitis without antibiotics: a single-center cohort study. Colorectal Dis. 2016;18(11):1101–1107.
6. Chabok A, Pahlman L, Hjern F, Haapaniemi S, Smedh K; AVOD Study Group. Randomized clinical trial of antibiotics in acute uncomplicated diverticulitis. Br J Surg. 2012;99(4):532–539.
7. Daniels L, Unlu C, de Korte A, et al. Dutch Diverticular Disease (3D) Collaborative Study Group. Randomized clinical trial of observational versus antibiotic treatment for a first episode of CT-proven uncomplicated acute diverticulitis. Br J Surg. 2017;104(1):52–61.
8. Jaung R, Nisbet S, Gosselink MP, et al. Antibiotics do not reduce length of hospital stay for uncomplicated diverticulitis in a pragmatic double-blind randomized trial. Clin Gastroenterol Hepatol. 2021;19(3):503–510.
9. Mora-Lopez L, Ruiz-Edo N, Estrada-Ferrer O, et al. Efficacy and safety of non-antibiotic outpatient treatment in mild acute diverticulitis (DINAMO-study): a multicentre, randomised, open-label, noninferiority trial. Ann Surg. 2021;274(5):e435–e442.
10. Isacson D, Smedh K, Nikberg M, Chabok A. Long-term follow-up of the AVOD randomized trial of antibiotic avoidance in uncomplicated diverticulitis. Br J Surg. 2019;106(11):1542–1548.
11. van Dijk ST, Daniels L, Unlu C, et al. Long-term effects of omitting antibiotics in uncomplicated acute diverticulitis. Am J Gastroenterol. 2018;113(7):1045–1052.
12. Francis NK, Sylla P, Abou-Khalil M, et al. EAES and SAGES 2018 consensus conference on acute diverticulitis management: evidence-based recommendations for clinical practice. Surg Endosc. 2018;33(9):2726–2741.
13. Garfinkle R, Sabboobeh S, Demian M, et al. Patient and physician preferences for antibiotics in acute uncomplicated diverticulitis: a Delphi consensus process to generate noninferiority margins. Dis Colon Rectum. 2021;64(1):119–127.
14. Hall J, Hardiman K, Lee S, et al. The American Society of Colon and Rectal Surgeons clinical practice guidelines for the treatment of left-sided colonic diverticulitis. Dis Colon Rectum. 2020;63(6):728–747.

CHAPTER 25

Laparoscopic Ileocaecal Resection versus Infliximab for Terminal Ileitis in Crohn's Disease: A Randomized Controlled, Open-Label, Multicentre Trial

Ponsioen CY, de Groof EJ, Eshuis EJ, Gardenbroek TJ, Bossuyt PMM, Hart A, Warusavitarne J, Buskens CJ, van Bodegraven AA, Brink MA, Consten ECJ, van Wagensveld BA, Rijk MCM, Crolla RMPH, Noomen CG, Houdijk APJ, Mallant RC, Boom M, Marsman WA, Stockmann HB, Mol B, de Groof AJ, Stokkers PC, D'Haens GR, Bemelman WA: LIR!C study group (1). Lancet Gastroenterol Hepatol. 2(11):785–792, 2017

Reviewed by Allison M. Ammann, Ian M. Paquette, and Carla F. Justiniano

Research Question/Objective The initial management of mild to moderately active ileocecal Crohn's disease often begins with steroids and immunomodulators. For those who fail conservative management or who have severely active disease, a biologic (e.g., infliximab) is typically employed. However, maintenance medical treatment can negatively affect quality of life. Surgical resection has generally been reserved for those who fail conservative management. This study aimed to compare health-related quality of life and treatment outcomes among patients with Crohn's disease who failed initial treatment and were then randomized to ileocecal resection or infliximab.

Study Design This was a randomized controlled, open-label, parallel group trial that examined patients with active Crohn's of the terminal ileum who failed ≥3 months of conventional therapy with glucocorticoids, thiopurines, or methotrexate. Twenty-nine hospitals in the United Kingdom and Netherlands were involved. Patients were randomized in a 1:1 fashion to the infliximab or ileocecal resection arms. The primary outcome was disease-specific quality of life assessed by the Inflammatory Bowel Disease Questionnaire (IBDQ). Secondary outcomes were general quality of life measured with the Short Form-36 (SF-36) health survey, days unable to participate in social life, days on sick leave, morbidity, and body image and cosmesis.

Sample Size A total of 143 patients, the target sample size per the power calculation, were randomly assigned to infliximab (70) or laparoscopic ileocecal resection (73) and included in the intention-to-treat analysis.

DOI: 10.1201/9780429285714-25

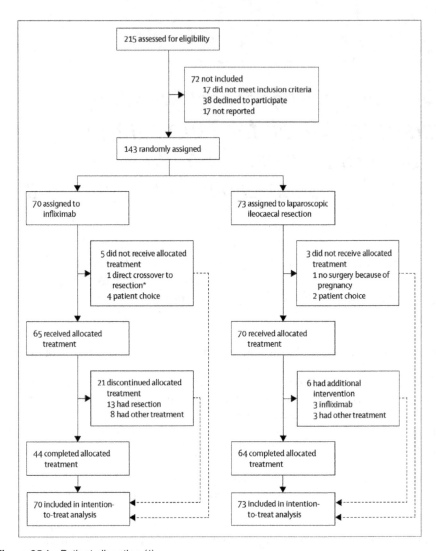

Figure 25.1 Patient allocation (1).

However, only 44 patients received the allocated infliximab treatment, while only 64 received the allocated laparoscopic ileocecal resection (Figure 25.1). Median age was 27 (IQU 22–40). Baseline characteristics were similar, except for smoking status, which was higher in the resection group.

Follow-Up Patients were evaluated by a surgeon or gastroenterologist in clinic at 2 and 6 weeks and at 3, 6, 9, and 12 months after the start of treatment. Patients underwent colonoscopy at 1-year to evaluate for inflammation using the Crohn's Disease Endoscopic Index of Severity (CDEIS) or the modified Rutgeerts score in the resection group. Indicators of remission were a CDEIS score of less than 6 and a Rutgeerts score of less than 2b. Chart review was performed at the 1-year follow-up for additional steroid courses, Crohn's-related surgery, perianal fistula, use of biological agents, concurrent use of immunomodulators, and follow-up colonoscopies.

Inclusion/Exclusion Criteria   Patients were 18–80 years old with active terminal ileal Crohn's unsuccessfully treated with ≥3 months of conventional therapy (glucocorticoids, thiopurines, or methotrexate). Exclusion criteria were previous ileocecectomy, obstructive ileal Crohn's that would likely require surgery (as indicated by prestenotic dilatation or absence of inflammation on screening imaging), diseased small bowel segment >40 cm, or abdominal abscess. Patients with an American Society of Anesthesiologist scores of III–IV were excluded.

Intervention or Treatment Received   Infliximab versus laparoscopic ileocecal resection were the two treatment arms. The infliximab arm received three infusions of 5 mg/kg at weeks 0, 2, and 6 weeks and maintenance infusions every 8 weeks. Variation existed in further treatment with dose escalation to every 6 weeks and/or dose increase to 10 mg/kg allowed with insufficient response as well as combination therapy with azathioprine or mercaptopurine, although combination was not mandatory. The surgery arm patients were allowed a 4-week steroid taper course while awaiting surgery. Ileocecal resection was performed laparoscopically.

Results   At 2 weeks, resection patients reported significantly worse quality of life than those in the infliximab group (mean difference −20.7 [95% CI −30.0 to −11.3]). This became nonsignificant at 6 weeks. The mean IBDQ scores at 12 months were similar between the infliximab [172.0 (95% CI 164.3–179.7)] and the resection groups [178.1 (95% CI 171.1–185.0)] with a mean difference of 6.1 points (95% CI −4.2 to 16.4, $p = 0.25$). The mean SF-36 total score was significantly lower in the infliximab group than in the resection group at 6 months [105.6 (95% CI 101.5–109.8) vs. 112.7 (95% CI 108.7–116.7)]. At 12 months, there was no difference in the mean SF-36 total score in the infliximab [106.5 (95% CI 102.1–110.9)] and the resection groups [112.1 (95% CI 108.0–116.2)]; mean difference of 5.6 (95% CI −0.4 to 11.6). Patients in the laparoscopic ileocecal resection group reported more days on sick leave [3.4 days (SD 7.1)] than those in the infliximab group [1.4 days (4.7), $p < 0.0001$]. The mean number of days patients were unable to participate in social life were similar [1.1 (SD 4.5) in the infliximab group vs. 1.8 (6.3) in the resection group ($p = 20$)]. An additional 20% of patients in the infliximab group underwent ileocecal resection in the first year after enrollment due to treatment failure. Of the patients in the surgical group, 9% required medical treatment following resection. There were notable surgical complications in 6% of the operations performed.

Study Limitations   Pertinent limitations were acknowledged by the authors. First, blinding was inherently not possible. At enrollment, endoscopic disease severity was not required to be reported. Not all patients underwent follow-up endoscopy at 12 months. Initiation or maintenance of immunomodulators after primary therapy was at the discretion of treating physicians. Therapeutic drug levels were not regularly monitored. Finally, the study population was primarily young and healthy adult patients, albeit this largely reflects the population impacted by Crohn's.

The authors concluded that laparoscopic resection in patients with limited, nonstructuring, ileocecal Crohn's disease is a reasonable alternative to infliximab therapy as quantified by short-term quality of life and disease recurrence. Although in the context of a randomized controlled trial, the data do provide real-world variability in the medical management of Crohn's disease across the 29 centers included.

Relevant Studies   Previously, management of Crohn's disease relied on a "step-up" approach aimed at symptomatic improvement starting with steroids, aminosalicylates, or thiopurines followed by medical escalation only after symptomatic failure. This resulted in high rates of medical treatment failure and surgical intervention. More recently, therapy has evolved toward preventing early disease progression with disease-modifying medications (i.e., biologics) and aggressive monitoring of remission though both clinical (e.g., improved abdominal pain and bowel habits) and endoscopic (e.g., resolution of inflammation or ulceration) measures, also called a treat-to-target approach (2). This involves a multidisciplinary team discussion and personalized treatment approach focused on the optimization of both medical and surgical interventions (3, 4).

The presented study was the first to examine medical versus surgical management of Crohn's disease with limited, predominantly inflammatory terminal ileitis for whom conventional treatment was unsuccessful. Long-term follow-up of this study published recently examined data for 94% of the patients included in the original trial and showed that laparoscopic ileocecal resection remained appropriate at 5 years. A total of 74% of patients who initially had an ileocecal resection did not need additional biological treatment, 42% did not need additional treatment for disease flares, and no patients required a different Crohn's-related resection. Meanwhile, 48% of patients who received infliximab treatment required a Crohn's disease-related resection (5). Long-term quality of life was not reported. The 1-year cost analysis of the same cohort showed that surgical management was associated with lower direct healthcare costs and high quality-adjusted life-years (6). Thus, while surgical treatment was and is still often considered a complication of Crohn's treatment, in this specific cohort of patients it may be utilized as primary treatment rather than merely a rescue.

This concept is further supported by a recent meta-analysis examining relapse in Crohn's disease after surgical, medical, and combined (surgery and biologic) therapeutic approaches. Recurrence rates were lower after ileocecal resection as compared to medical therapy for both clinical [OR 2.5 (95% CI 1.53–4.08), $p <$ 0.0001] and surgical [OR 3.60 (95% CI 1.06–12.3, $p = 0.041$)] recurrences. Clinical recurrence was defined as symptoms plus the need for new medications while surgical recurrence was the need for reoperation.

The sequelae of surgery with its inherent risks and long-term complications like adhesions and obstruction warrants mention. Yet, the presented study and others have now shown that with the deployment of a minimally invasive approach, the morbidity of an ileocecal resection is overall low (7). Thus, early minimally invasive surgery at the time of limited disease allows the patient to profit from the aforementioned benefits of lower cost and decreased recurrence while minimizing the disadvantages of having experienced surgery once if the patient were to need repeat surgery (8, 9).

Although the presented study does not indicate a definitive answer as to which treatment is superior, and long-term quality of life data for this cohort is not available, it does beg the consideration of surgical resection in patients with limited, nonstricturing, and immunomodulatory-refractory ileocecal Crohn's. This has been reflected in the recent American Society of Colon and Rectal Surgeons Clinical Practice Guidelines for the Management of Crohn's Disease and by the European Crohn's and Colitis Organization Guidelines on surgical management of Crohn's disease (10, 11).

REFERENCES

1. Ponsioen CY, de Groof EJ, Eshuis EJ, Gardenbroek TJ, Bossuyt PMM, Hart A, et al. Laparoscopic ileocaecal resection versus infliximab for terminal ileitis in Crohn's disease: a randomised controlled, open-label, multicentre trial. Lancet Gastroenterol Hepatol. 2017;2(11):785–92.
2. Torres J, Mehandru S, Colombel JF, Peyrin-Biroulet L. Crohn's disease. Lancet. 2017;389(10080):1741–55.
3. Linda Ferrari AF. Operative indications and options in intestinal Crohn's disease. Semin Colon Rectal Surg. 2022;33(1).
4. Eula Plana Tetangco ACS. Medical treatment of intestinal Crohn's disease. Semin Colon Rectal Surg. 2022;33(1).
5. Stevens TW, Haasnoot ML, D'Haens GR, Buskens CJ, de Groof EJ, Eshuis EJ, et al. Laparoscopic ileocaecal resection versus infliximab for terminal ileitis in Crohn's disease: retrospective long-term follow-up of the LIR!C trial. Lancet Gastroenterol Hepatol. 2020;5(10):900–7.
6. de Groof EJ, Stevens TW, Eshuis EJ, Gardenbroek TJ, Bosmans JE, van Dongen JM, et al. Cost-effectiveness of laparoscopic ileocaecal resection versus infliximab treatment of terminal ileitis in Crohn's disease: the LIR!C Trial. Gut. 2019;68(10):1774–80.
7. Lee Y, Fleming FJ, Deeb AP, Gunzler D, Messing S, Monson JR. A laparoscopic approach reduces short-term complications and length of stay following ileocolic resection in Crohn's disease: an analysis of outcomes from the NSQIP database. Colorectal Dis. 2012;14(5):572–7.
8. Holubar SD, Dozois EJ, Privitera A, Cima RR, Pemberton JH, Young-Fadok T, et al. Laparoscopic surgery for recurrent ileocolic Crohn's disease. Inflamm Bowel Dis. 2010;16(8):1382–6.

9. Carvello M, Danese S, Spinelli A. Surgery versus medical therapy in luminal ileocecal Crohn's disease. Clin Colon Rectal Surg. 2022;35(1):72–7.

10. Lightner AL, Vogel JD, Carmichael JC, Keller DS, Shah SA, Mahadevan U, et al. The American Society of Colon and rectal surgeons clinical practice guidelines for the surgical management of Crohn's disease. Dis Colon Rectum. 2020;63(8):1028–52.

11. Adamina M, Bonovas S, Raine T, Spinelli A, Warusavitarne J, Armuzzi A, et al. ECCO guidelines on therapeutics in Crohn's disease: surgical treatment. J Crohns Colitis. 2020;14(2):155–68.

CHAPTER 26

Crohn's Disease Management after Intestinal Resection: A Randomised Trial

De Cruz P, Kamm MA, Hamilton AL, Ritchie KJ, Krejany EO, Gorelik A, Liew D, Prideaux L, Lawrance IC, Andrews JM, Bampton PA, Gibson PR, Sparrow M, Leong RW, Florin TH, Gearry RB, Radford-Smith G, Macrae FA, Debinski H, Selby W, Kronborg I, Johnston MJ, Woods R, Elliot RPt, Bell SJ, Brown SJ, Connell WR, Desmond PV. Lancet. 385(9976):1406–1417, 2015

Reviewed by Alessandro Fichera

Research Question Objective   Recurrence in Crohn's disease (CD) remains a common problem with significant impact on quality of life. Endoscopic recurrence at the anastomosis occurs in up to 90% of CD patients at 1 year. Medical therapy has made significant improvement in this field, but the indications and algorithms for surveillance and targeted postoperative medical prophylaxis of disease recurrence have not been standardized. This study was designed to identify the optimal medical management and surveillance strategy to prevent postoperative disease recurrence.

Study Design   This is a randomized prospective trial of consecutive patients undergoing intestinal resection of all macroscopic CD with an endoscopically accessible anastomosis from 17 centers in Australia and New Zealand. Patients were assigned in a 2:1 ratio to colonoscopy at 6 months (active care) or no colonoscopy (standard of care). Initial therapy was based on risk of recurrence. High risk was defined as having one or more of the following factors: smoking, perforating disease, or previous resection. The primary study end point was the presence and severity of endoscopic recurrence at 18 months after surgery using the Rutgeerts score. Endoscopic recurrence was defined as Rutgeerts score >i2. Secondary end point included clinical recurrence, based on Crohn's Disease Activity Index (CDAI), need for further surgery, C-reactive protein elevation, and drug efficacy in prevention of mucosal recurrence. Colonoscopy were performed at 6 months in the active group and at 18 months on all comers. The most distal anastomosis was scored. Endoscopic recurrence was defined according to the records scored by the endoscopist, and photographs were reviewed centrally by two investigators. Three secondary measure of endoscopic disease activity were also reported: the Crohn's Disease Endoscopic Index of Severity (CDEIS), the Simple Endoscopic Score for Crohn's disease (SES-CD), and a count of the number of ulcers at the anastomosis.

DOI: 10.1201/9780429285714-26

Sample Size   The power calculation was based on expected endoscopic disease recurrence at 18 months of 60% for standard care and 35% for active care based on previous studies. To allow for a 31% dropout, a total of 170 patients were needed.

Follow-Up   Patients were assessed clinically 2 weeks before surgery, at surgery, 1 month after surgery, every 2 months for the first year, at 15 and 18 months. CDAI was assessed preoperatively and at 6, 12, and 18 months. Colonoscopy was performed at 6 months for the active group and at 18 months for all comers.

Inclusion/Exclusion Criteria   Patients undergoing intestinal resection of all macroscopic CD with an endoscopically accessible anastomosis were included. Patents were excluded if they had an end stoma, the anastomosis was not endoscopically accessible, there was persistent macroscopic disease after surgical resection, or there was a perforation of the gastrointestinal tract or pregnancy.

Intervention or Treatment Received   All patients received metronidazole 400 mg twice daily for 3 months postoperatively. If metronidazole was not well tolerated, they received 200 mg twice daily, once daily, or ceased taking the drug. Patients at a high risk of disease recurrence also received azathioprine 2 mg/kg per day or 6-mercaptopurine 1.5 mg/kg per day for 18 months postoperatively. Patients intolerant to a thiopurine received adalimumab for 18 months until study conclusion. Patients receiving prednisolone had this drug tapered to zero within 12 weeks of surgery. When endoscopic recurrence was detected in the active care group at 6 months, low-risk patients stepped up to thiopurine, patients at high risk receiving a thiopurine stepped up to adalimumab induction followed by 40 mg every 2 weeks, and those receiving 40 mg adalimumab every 2 weeks stepped up to 40 mg adalimumab weekly.

Results   A total of 174 (83% high-risk) CD patients were enrolled and received at least one dose of the study drug. In the active care group, 39% of patients received stepped-up treatment. At 18 months, endoscopic recurrence occurred in 49% of patients in the active care group and 67% in the standard care group (modified intention to treat, $p = 0.03$), and when further adjusted for treatment step-up, the OR for endoscopic recurrence was 0.33 ($p = 0.01$). Smoking ($p = 0.02$) and the presence of 2 or more clinical risk factors including smoking ($p = 0.05$) increased the risk of endoscopic recurrence. Complete mucosal normality was maintained in 22% of patients in the active care versus 8% in the standard care group ($p = 0.03$). In the active care group, of those with 6 months recurrence who stepped up treatment, 38% of patients were in remission 12 months later; conversely, of those in remission at 6 months who did not change therapy, recurrence occurred in 41% of patients 12 months later. The incidence and type of adverse and severe adverse events did not differ significantly between groups. There was no correlation between clinical recurrence defined as CDAI > 200 ($p = 0.08$) or CDAI > 150 ($p = 0.30$) and endoscopic recurrence.

Study Limitations Recurrence was defined as a Rutgeerts score >i2. The Rutgeerts score combines endoscopic changes in the neoterminal ileum and at the anastomosis. The question remains whether anastomotic lesions are related to ischemic changes instead of the progression of disease, and alternative scoring systems have been developed. Furthermore, the authors questioned whether the noted endoscopic recurrence would be clinically meaningful as the study did not have long enough follow-up to look for progression of disease. Lastly drug optimization based on serum levels and metabolite testing was not performed.

Relevant Studies In 2017 the American Gastroenterological Association published guidelines for management of CD in surgical remission, recommending endoscopic monitoring at 6–12 months after surgery irrespective of postoperative medical therapy (1). Based on the findings of this trial (2), the AGA issued a strong recommendation because of the high likelihood of benefit from detection of endoscopic recurrence by colonoscopy, the risk of which is as high as 90% within 1 year of surgery especially in those patients not receiving any prophylaxis. This monitoring may prompt the initiation of medical therapy if endoscopic recurrence is detected. They also concluded that there is insufficient clinical evidence to inform how often endoscopic monitoring should be performed following the initial postoperative colonoscopy (1).

The POCER study has really changed the way we approach surgical remission in CD. While it has opened new avenues for a treat-to-target approach, it has generated debate and controversy around the timing of first evaluation and frequency thereafter, the clinical relevance of the current endoscopic scoring, alternative and less invasive diagnostic modalities to colonoscopy, correlation between clinical and endoscopic disease activity and treatment strategies for recurrence in patients that have failed biologic treatment, to mention a few.

In a recent study from China, CD patients underwent postoperative colonoscopy within 30 days. Changes were noted at the anastomosis and in the neoterminal ileum early in the postoperative course (3). Anastomotic ulcerations were associated with postoperative recurrence ($p = 0.046$), and elevated fecal calprotectin at 14 days could predict the presence of anastomotic ulcers ($p = 0.027$). Given the evidence in the POCER study that, despite aggressive surveillance and medical therapy, some patients show progression of disease, perhaps the first colonoscopy should be performed sooner especially in high-risk patients and fecal calprotectin could be an valuable adjunct (4).

The Rutgeerts score has been traditionally used to grade the severity of endoscopic lesions in the neo-terminal ileum and ileocolonic anastomosis (5). However, recent studies have proposed separating aphthous lesions in the neoterminal ileum from those confined to the anastomosis, as questions remain whether anastomotic lesions are related to postsurgical ischemic changes instead of progression of disease. A recently published prospective multicenter study developed two separate endoscopic grading systems (REMIND score) for anastomotic and ileal lesions after surgery for ileal or ileocolonic CD (6). Among 193 patients with a median follow-up of 3.82 years, clinical recurrence-free survival after surgery was significantly shorter in patients with ileal lesions compared to those without, and patients with exclusively ileal lesions had poorer clinical long-term outcomes than patients with exclusively anastomotic lesions. These data suggest that patients with ileal lesions could benefit from escalation of treatment.

Previous studies have looked at postoperative use of biologics to modify the natural course of the disease with excellent results (7–9). Biologic therapy is not without morbidity and added cost and therefore should be individualized. This study introduced for the first time the concept of early endoscopic risk stratification and a treat-to-target approach based on the risk of the current and endoscopic findings. In order to determine whether preoperative treatment with anti-TNFα therapy influenced postoperative response, a large multicenter retrospective analysis of CD patients who underwent intestinal resection before and after anti-TNFα therapy was introduced in Japan and was recently published (10). After stratifying patients by anti-TNFα exposure prior to surgery, the postoperative administration of anti-TNFα was found to be effective in the biologic-naïve group with lower reoperation rates but not in the group that failed biologic therapy before operation. Therefore, determining optimal postoperative prophylaxis strategy for biologic-experienced patients requires further exploration.

REFERENCES

1. Nguyen, G.C., et al., *American Gastroenterological Association Institute Guideline on the Management of Crohn's disease after surgical resection.* Gastroenterology, 2017. **152**(1): pp. 271–5.
2. De Cruz, P. and M.A. Kamm, *Letter: management of post-operative Crohn's disease—thiopurines vs adalimumab-authors' reply.* Aliment Pharmacol Ther, 2016. **43**(1): pp. 170–1.
3. Guo, Z., et al., *Endoscopic evaluation at 1 month after ileocolic resection for Crohn's disease predicts future postoperative recurrence and is safe.* Dis Colon Rectum, 2022. **65**(3): pp. 382–9.
4. Qiu, Y., et al., *Fecal calprotectin for evaluating postoperative recurrence of Crohn's disease: a meta-analysis of prospective studies.* Inflamm Bowel Dis, 2015. **21**(2): pp. 315–22.
5. Rutgeerts, P., et al., *Predictability of the postoperative course of Crohn's disease.* Gastroenterology, 1990. **99**(4): pp. 956–63.
6. Hammoudi, N., et al., *Postoperative endoscopic recurrence on the neoterminal ileum but not on the anastomosis is mainly driving long-term outcomes in Crohn's disease.* Am J Gastroenterol, 2020. **115**(7): pp. 1084–93.
7. Regueiro, M., et al., *Infliximab reduces endoscopic, but not clinical, recurrence of Crohn's disease after ileocolonic resection.* Gastroenterology, 2016. **150**(7): pp. 1568–78.
8. Regueiro, M., et al., *Infliximab prevents Crohn's disease recurrence after ileal resection.* Gastroenterology, 2009. **136**(2): pp. 441–50 e1; quiz 716.

9. Savarino, E., et al., *Adalimumab is more effective than azathioprine and mesalamine at preventing postoperative recurrence of Crohn's disease: a randomized controlled trial.* Am J Gastroenterol, 2013. **108**(11): pp. 1731–42.

10. Shinagawa, T., et al., *Rate of reoperation decreased significantly after year 2002 in patients with Crohn's disease.* Clin Gastroenterol Hepatol, 2020. **18**(4): pp. 898–907 e5.

CHAPTER 27

Recurrence of Crohn's Disease after Ileocolic Resection Is Not Affected by Anastomotic Type: Results of a Multicenter, Randomized, Controlled Trial

McLeod RS, Wolff BG, Ross S, Parkes P, McKenzie M: CAST Trial. Dis Colon Rectum. 52(5):919–927, 2009

Reviewed by Jacopo Crippa and Antonino Spinelli

Research Question/Objective   The trial by McLeod et al. (1), also known as the CAST Trial, was designed to evaluate the difference in the recurrence rate of Crohn's disease (CD) at the anastomotic site after ileocolic resection with two different types of anastomoses: mechanical side-to side (STSA) or manual end-to-end (ETEA). Recurrence after resection for CD occurs frequently after primary surgery (app. 40%), and the great majority are located at the anastomotic site (app. 90%). The pathological features behind recurrence are still unknown. This remains a highly debated topic even today, years after the publication of the CAST Trial, as ECCO (European Crohn's and Colitis Organization) was created as a specific working group aimed to shed light on this matter by collecting cutting-edge evidence (2). One hypothetical factor that may increase the chances for recurrence is the effect induced by fecal statis, given, for example, by a narrow anastomotic lumen, that might induce the disease relapse. Microbiome alteration and bacteria translocation consequent to a slow transit may in fact play a role in the development of recurrence (3). To reduce the risk of fecal stasis, a wider anastomosis is advisable to limit the resistance given by the narrowing of the bowel lumen.

For its technical peculiarity, STSA is wider than ETEA, with the diameter of the latter depending more on the bowel lumen and wall thickness. STSA may then reduce CD recurrence, based on the rationale of reduced fecal stasis through a wider anastomosis.

Study Design   This study is a single-blind randomized controlled trial involving multiple centers from 3 countries: 10 Canadian hospitals, 6 Americans, and 1 British. Randomization was performed intraoperatively after assessing the feasibility and safety of both anastomotic techniques and excluding other sites of disease.

DOI: 10.1201/9780429285714-27

Sample Size A 20% absolute risk rate decrease in anastomotic recurrence based on an estimated 40% recurrence rate after ileocolic anastomosis was utilized as the primary outcome to calculate the sample size, for a total of 200 patients to be recruited (180 plus 10% loss to follow-up). The accrual was too slow and stopped at 170 patients giving the study a 70% power instead of 80% to depict a 20% difference in recurrence rate or 80% power to depict a 23% difference.

Follow-Up Crohn's Disease Activity Index (CDAI) and Inflammatory Bowel Disease Questionnaire (IBDQ) were completed, and blood work including C-reactive protein was performed at 12 months after surgery and compared to baseline. In addition, a colonoscopy was utilized to assess the presence of recurrence using a modified Rutgeert's score (4). When signs of recurrence occurred before 12 months, the colonoscopy was performed in advance.

Inclusion/Exclusion Criteria To be included, patients with CD located only to the distal ileum and right colon had to be scheduled for elective ileocolic resection. Patients were excluded if they previously received another gastrointestinal resection for CD, if they required a defunctioning ileostomy, or if medications used to treat CD could not be discontinued postoperatively.

Intervention or Treatment Received Once they met the inclusion criteria, patients were randomized intraoperatively to mechanical side-to side (STSA) or manual end-to-end (ETEA) anastomosis. Peculiarities of the surgical techniques were decided in advance and provided to the operating surgeons.

Results A total of 171 patients were included in the study in a 42-month span. One patient was excluded because he did not receive an ileocolic resection. The remaining 170 patients successfully received the treatment (84 STSA/86 ETEA). Operative time was shorter in the STSA group (113 vs. 138 minutes, $P = 0.0009$) along with the time to perform the anastomosis (15 vs. 31 minutes, $P < 0.0001$). Postoperative outcomes were similar, included anastomotic leak rate and reoperation rate (7% for leak and reintervention in both groups, not statistically significant). All reoperations occurred because of leak/intra-abdominal abscess. Median postoperative stay was 6 days in both groups.

Thirty-one patients (18.1%) were lost to follow-up. Of them, 20 refused to undergo a colonoscopy at 12 months. A total of 56 patients (40.3%) developed a recurrence at the anastomotic site, with no significant difference between the groups (37.9% STSA vs. 42.5% ETEA groups, $p = 0.55$). Almost half of the patients that recurred had a symptomatic disease, and no difference between the groups was found (22.7% vs. 21.9%, $p = 0.92$).

A secondary analysis was performed between patients who developed recurrence versus those who did not (56/83). Length of time since diagnosis, number of previous resections, smoking status, fistula or abscess present at surgery, type of procedure (laparoscopic or open), length of small bowel affected by CD, postoperative azathioprine (AZA) maintenance therapy, compliance with postoperative AZA maintenance therapy, and CDAI at 6 weeks were analyzed as factors potentially related to recurrent disease. After multivariate analysis, previous resection was the only risk factor for recurrence (endoscopic [1.78; 95% CI 1.06 to 2.90, $P = 0.028$] and symptomatic recurrence [2.00; 95% CI 1.14 to 3.60, $P = 0.0016$]). Compliance to therapy with AZA was associated with a statistically significant reduced risk of symptomatic recurrence but not of overall recurrence.

Study Limitations   The sample size and patients' follow-up are two important points of debate and may have weakened the trial results in a relevant way. Accrual did not reach the expected number of 200 patients. The reason of this flaw must be found in the perioperative therapy for CD. AZA, a mainstay for CD therapy, was not even planned as a postoperative treatment within the trial. Two years after the beginning of the trial, AZA as postoperatory therapy was allowed in order to expand the inclusion criteria and therefore the potential eligible patients for the trial. Nevertheless, physicians were less prone to enroll patients given the protocol's strict indications on perioperative therapy, and consequently, due to a slow accrual, the trial was close in advance. Maintenance therapy in CD may certainly affect relapse, thus reducing the magnitude of the anastomosis impact on the main outcome of the study, as confirmed by the secondary analysis. The introduction of AZA as possible postoperative therapy during the enrollment phase might present a confounding factor in the present study.

Another potential limitation is the 18% of loss to follow-up. This loss is relevant and may have underpowered the study, which never even reached the estimated target accrual of 200 patients.

Relevant Studies   A certain number of previous studies have suggested a role of the anastomosis type in CD relapse at this site (5), providing small and inconclusive evidence. The trial by McLeod et al. (1) truly set a milestone on this topic for both its objective and randomized nature. Much has changed since the trial, including the advent of biologic therapy, which generated a paradigm shift in CD therapy (6). The introduction of targeted therapies had an unprecedent impact, enough to consider trials performed before their debut as potentially outdated.

Another remarkable impact resulted from the introduction of a novel anastomotic technique described by Kono et al. (7), called KONO-S anastomosis. "S," as in supporting, reflects a key in its design, which allows for the fixed orientation of the anastomotic bowel, thus maintaining a large lumen diameter. A retrospective trial suggested its potential in reducing CD relapse irrespective of postoperative treatment (Infliximab) (7).

New randomized trials have been designed to compare standard side-to-side anastomosis and KONO-S anastomosis such as NCT03256240 (8). Results are awaited, as these might set a new standard in CD surgery. Along with these notable findings, the type of anastomosis might not be the only modifiable surgical factor to affect relapse in CD. Recent evidence suggests that the mesentery might play a role as described by Coffey et al. (9) A significant reduction in CD recurrence at the anastomotic site was seen in patients who underwent mesentery excision during ileocecal resection (10). The SPICY trial aims to demonstrate a difference in recurrence rate after mesentery excision compared to standard surgery (11). As new trials are proposed, nowadays the recurrence rates after primary CD surgery do not differ greatly since the publication of the CAST trial, and the research community has failed to fill this gap, although this may change in the near future as the results from ongoing trials are released.

REFERENCES

1. McLeod RS, Wolff BG, Ross S, Parkes R, McKenzie M, Investigators of the CT. Recurrence of Crohn's disease after ileocolic resection is not affected by anastomotic type: results of a multicenter, randomized, controlled trial. Dis Colon Rectum. 2009;52(5):919–27.
2. Riviere P, Bislenghi G, Hammoudi N, Verstockt B, Brown S, Oliveira-Cunha M, et al. Results of the Eighth Scientific Workshop of ECCO: pathophysiology and risk factors of postoperative Crohn's disease recurrence after an ileocolic resection. J Crohns Colitis. 2023.
3. Wright EK, Kamm MA, Wagner J, Teo SM, Cruz P, Hamilton AL, et al. Microbial factors associated with postoperative Crohn's disease recurrence. J Crohns Colitis. 2017;11(2):191–203.
4. Rutgeerts P, Geboes K, Vantrappen G, Kerremans R, Coenegrachts JL, Coremans G. Natural history of recurrent Crohn's disease at the ileocolonic anastomosis after curative surgery. Gut. 1984;25(6):665–72.
5. Scarpa M, Angriman I, Barollo M, Polese L, Ruffolo C, Bertin M, et al. Role of stapled and hand-sewn anastomoses in recurrence of Crohn's disease. Hepatogastroenterology. 2004;51(58):1053–7.
6. Cosnes J, Nion-Larmurier I, Beaugerie L, Afchain P, Tiret E, Gendre JP. Impact of the increasing use of immunosuppressants in Crohn's disease on the need for intestinal surgery. Gut. 2005;54(2):237–41.
7. Kono T, Ashida T, Ebisawa Y, Chisato N, Okamoto K, Katsuno H, et al. A new antimesenteric functional end-to-end handsewn anastomosis: surgical prevention of anastomotic recurrence in Crohn's disease. Dis Colon Rectum. 2011;54(5):586–92.
8. https://beta.clinicaltrials.gov/study/NCT03256240 (accessed June 5, 2023).
9. Coffey CJ, Kiernan MG, Sahebally SM, Jarrar A, Burke JP, Kiely PA, et al. Inclusion of the mesentery in ileocolic resection for Crohn's disease is associated with reduced surgical recurrence. J Crohns Colitis. 2018;12(10):1139–50.
10. Turri G, Carvello M, Ben David N, Spinelli A. Intriguing role of the mesentery in ileocolic Crohn's disease. Clin Colon Rectal Surg. 2022;35(4):321–7.
11. van der Does de Willebois EML, SPICY Study Group. Mesenteric SParIng versus extensive mesentereCtomY in primary ileocolic resection for ileocaecal Crohn's disease (SPICY): study protocol for randomized controlled trial. BJS Open. 2022;6(1).

CHAPTER 28

Are Random Biopsies Still Useful for the Detection of Neoplasia in Patients with IBD Undergoing Surveillance Colonoscopy with Chromoendoscopy?

Moussata D, Allez M, Cazals-Hatem D, et al. Gut. 67:616–624, 2018

Reviewed by Totadri Dhimal and Zhaomin Xu

Research Question   Until recently, the standard practice for colorectal cancer surveillance in patients with inflammatory bowel disease (IBD) was to obtain large samples of nontargeted (random) biopsies in 2–4 quadrants, every 10 cm of colonic segments. However, this practice has been challenged by evidence that new endoscopic technologies, such as high-definition (HD) colonoscopy and chromoendoscopy (CE), can significantly improve the detection of dysplasia in patients with IBD. As a result, targeted biopsies may be sufficient for the surveillance of neoplasia in IBD patients, compared to the standard practice of random biopsies.

Authors of the study compared the detection of dysplasia in surveillance colonoscopies using random biopsies versus targeted biopsies in patients with IBD who underwent HD colonoscopy with CE. They also aimed to assess patient risk factors that increased the likelihood of neoplasia and to identify patients who may still require random biopsies.

Study Design   This was a large prospective cohort study performed across 14 French academic departments of gastroenterology by the Groupe d'Études et de Thérapeutiques des Affections Inflammatoires du tube Digestif (GETAID). All patients underwent HD colonoscopy with CE and targeted biopsy of visible lesion and random quadrant biopsies every 10 cm. Biopsy samples were analyzed by local GI pathologist, and all samples with a diagnosis of dysplasia were sent to be reviewed by a panel of five expert GI pathologists. Data were analyzed using the Mann–Whitney U test, chi-square for quantitative and qualitative data, and multivariable logistic regression was used to detect risk factors for neoplasia.

Sample Size   This study screened 1058 patients with inflammatory bowel disease (IBD). Of these, 1000 met the inclusion and exclusion criteria and were enrolled in the study. Of the 1000 enrolled patients, 495 had ulcerative colitis, and 505 had Crohn's disease.

DOI: 10.1201/9780429285714-28

Inclusion/Exclusion Criteria   The inclusion criteria for this cohort study were: (1) patients with ulcerative colitis (UC) with extensive colitis (proximal to the splenic flexure) and colonic Crohn's (involving at least one-third of the colon) for >8 years; (2) patients with left-sided UC for >15 years; (3) patients with concomitant primary sclerosing cholangitis (PSC); and (4) other indications for surveillance colonoscopy in patients with IBD. Patients with poor bowel prep or incomplete colonoscopy were excluded from the study. Of 1058 patients recruited, 1000 met the inclusion criteria, 57 were excluded because of poor bowel prep, and 1 patient had an incomplete colonoscopy due to an anesthetic problem.

Intervention or Treatment Received   All patients underwent HD colonoscopy with CE with targeted biopsy of all visible lesions plus nontargeted random biopsies every 10 cm.

Results   The median age of patients was 45 with UC patients being slightly older (median age 48) than Crohn's patients (43). About 57% of UC patients were male compared to 37% of Crohn's patients. Most patients were in remission with 97% of UC patients with a Clinical Activity Index of <3 and 93% of Crohn's patients with a Harvey-Bradshaw index of <3. About 68% of UC patients were taking mesalamine, and 13% were on immunosuppressants compared to 54% and 36% for Crohn's patients.

A total of 35,630 biopsies were performed during the 1000 surveillance colonoscopies, with an average of 35.6 biopsies performed per colonoscopy. Of those, 1044 suspicious lesions were identified, and 3801 targeted specimens were obtained from these lesions and surrounding mucosa. In total, 112 neoplastic lesions were identified, and 94 of them were treated endoscopically. Sixteen patients had 18 neoplastic lesions, which included 5 macroscopic cancers and 13 dysplastic lesions, all of which were not amenable to endoscopic treatment and were referred for surgical resection.

The remaining 31,865 biopsies were obtained by random sampling, which detected 68 dysplastic biopsies at 28 sites (0.21%), and 24 of these sites had low-grade dysplasia (LGD) and 4 sites had high-grade dysplasia (HGD). In total, 94 patients had 140 neoplastic sites on their surveillance biopsy, 75 patients (80%) had 112 neoplastic lesions identified on targeted biopsies, and 19 patients (20%) had 28 neoplastic sites on at least one random biopsy sample. Overall dysplasia yields of random biopsies were 0.2% (68/31,865). Cancer was detected in 5 patients by targeted biopsy but never on random biopsies alone.

There was increased likelihood of finding neoplasia on random and targeted biopsy when patients had the following risk factors: age >45 years, a personal history of neoplasia, concomitant PSC, and strictly normal colon. Multivariable analysis showed the likelihood of finding neoplasia was 2.8% in 358 patients with

0 risk factors, 7.8% in 410 patients with 1 risk factor, 19.2% in 182 patients with 2 risk factors, and 34.0% in 50 patients with 3–4 risk factors.

Increased likelihood of detecting neoplasia with random biopsy alone was associated with a personal history of neoplasia, concomitant PSC, and a tubular colon. Multivariable analysis showed the likelihood of finding neoplasia was 0.5% in 782 patients with 0 risk factors, 5.1% in 197 patients with 1 risk factor, and 23.8% in 21 patients with 2–3 risk factors.

Follow-Up   A follow-up was done for patients with dysplasia in random biopsies to assess its impact on further management. Of 7 patients with dysplasia in random biopsy, 1 patient was lost to follow-up. Six underwent surgical resection with 3 having multifocal (MF) LGD, 2 having MF LGD and HGD, and 1 having MF LGD, HDG, and CRC on surgical specimen. There were 12 patients with dysplasia on random biopsies only, of which 3 underwent colectomy. Out of these 3, 1 had MF LGD and the rest MF LGD & HGD. The remaining 9 patients underwent endoscopic surveillance. Of those 9 who underwent surveillance, 1 was lost to follow-up, 4 had no dysplasia on subsequent colonoscopy, 3 had LGD, and 1 patient had subsequent rectal cancer, who was referred for surgical resection with specimen revealing MG LGD, HGD, and CRC.

Study Limitations   Overall, this is a well designed prospective cohort study that demonstrated the low yield for random biopsies in IBD patients with no risk factors. Since it is not a randomized control trial, the long-term outcomes data between the targeted versus random biopsies group are not explored. Further evaluation needs to be done to better understand whether the small number of patients with missed dysplasia on targeted biopsies have any worse outcome compared to patients undergoing random biopsies. As targeted biopsies with HD colonoscopy and CE become more common, it is important to study the following factors: incidence of CRC in IBD patients undergoing targeted biopsies, rate of dysplasia on subsequent surveillance colonoscopy, timing of surveillance colonoscopies, as well as mortality and morbidity associated with surgical resection in patients with dysplasia.

Relevant Studies   Patients with chronic inflammatory bowel disease are at increased risk of developing colorectal cancer. Surveillance colonoscopy to detect dysplasia has been shown to improve cancer-related mortality (1). Rubin et al. showed in their mathematical model that the probability of detecting dysplasia was 90% with 33 biopsies (2). In addition, Bernstein et al. described a 19% and 42% likelihood of detecting CRC concomitantly in patients with endoscopic LGD and HGD, respectively (3). Thus the standard of care in patients with IBD surveillance has been to perform random biopsies in 2–4 quadrants every 10 cm segment of colon to maximize the rate of dysplasia detection. The downside to such random biopsies is that they are costly and time-consuming. Multiple studies have shown that targeted biopsies detect dysplasia at a higher rate than random biopsies with the use of high-definition colonoscopy and chromoendoscopy (4–7), while others have shown no improvement in dysplasia detection versus conventional colonoscopy with random biopsies (8). Watanabe et al. found in their study that targeted biopsies were as good as random biopsies while also noting the cost-effectiveness of the targeted approach (9). However, consensus was not reached at the 2015 SCENIC International Convention on whether to recommend targeted biopsies over standard practice of random sampling given the lack of robust evidence at the time. This current study by Moussata et al. added to the growing body of literature that indicate targeted biopsies are sufficient for the detection of dysplasia in patients with IBD with low-risk characteristic (10, 11). Since the 2015 SCENIC guidelines, the American Gastroenterological Association (AGA) has endorsed new guidelines based on this current study and on others that random biopsies are not required when HD colonoscopy and CE are implemented (12). However, there is still a role for random biopsies in patients with risk factors such as PSC and personal history of neoplasm or tubular colon since the likelihood of identifying dysplasia on random biopsies is high (10, 11). Therefore, thanks to the work of Moussatta et al. and others, the widespread recommendation for nontargeted biopsies has decreased, leading to cost and time savings, but whether they can be eliminated completely remains up for debate.

REFERENCES

1. Choi CH, Rutter MD, Askari A, Lee GH, Warusavitarne J, Moorghen M, et al. Forty-Year Analysis of Colonoscopic Surveillance Program for Neoplasia in Ulcerative Colitis: An Updated Overview. Am J Gastroenterol. 2015;110(7):1022–34.
2. Rubin CE, Haggitt RC, Burmer GC, Brentnall TA, Stevens AC, Levine DS, et al. DNA Aneuploidy in Colonic Biopsies Predicts Future Development of Dysplasia in Ulcerative Colitis. Gastroenterology. 1992;103(5):1611–20.
3. Bernstein CN, Shanahan F, Weinstein WM. Are We Telling Patients the Truth About Surveillance Colonoscopy in Ulcerative Colitis? Lancet. 1994;343(8889):71–4.
4. Soetikno R, Subramanian V, Kaltenbach T, Rouse RV, Sanduleanu S, Suzuki N, et al. The Detection of Nonpolypoid (Flat and Depressed) Colorectal Neoplasms in Patients With Inflammatory Bowel Disease. Gastroenterology. 2013;144(7):1349–52, 52e1–6.
5. Subramanian V, Ramappa V, Telakis E, Mannath J, Jawhari AU, Hawkey CJ, et al. Comparison of High Definition With Standard White Light Endoscopy for Detection of Dysplastic Lesions During Surveillance Colonoscopy in Patients With Colonic Inflammatory Bowel Disease. Inflamm Bowel Dis. 2013;19(2):350–5.
6. Marion JF, Waye JD, Israel Y, Present DH, Suprun M, Bodian C, et al. Chromoendoscopy Is More Effective Than Standard Colonoscopy in Detecting Dysplasia During Long-term Surveillance of Patients With Colitis. Clin Gastroenterol Hepatol. 2016;14(5):713–9.
7. Har-Noy O, Katz L, Avni T, Battat R, Bessissow T, Yung DE, et al. Chromoendoscopy, Narrow-Band Imaging or White Light Endoscopy for Neoplasia Detection in Inflammatory Bowel Diseases. Dig Dis Sci. 2017;62(11):2982–90.
8. Mooiweer E, van der Meulen-de Jong AE, Ponsioen CY, Fidder HH, Siersema PD, Dekker E, et al. Chromoendoscopy for Surveillance in Inflammatory Bowel Disease Does Not Increase Neoplasia Detection Compared With Conventional Colonoscopy With Random Biopsies: Results From a Large Retrospective Study. Am J Gastroenterol. 2015;110(7):1014–21.

9. Watanabe T, Ajioka Y, Mitsuyama K, Watanabe K, Hanai H, Nakase H, et al. Comparison of Targeted vs Random Biopsies for Surveillance of Ulcerative Colitis-Associated Colorectal Cancer. Gastroenterology. 2016;151(6):1122–30.

10. Moussata D, Allez M, Cazals-Hatem D, Treton X, Laharie D, Reimund JM, et al. Are Random Biopsies Still Useful for the Detection of Neoplasia in Patients With IBD Undergoing Surveillance Colonoscopy With Chromoendoscopy? Gut. 2018;67(4):616–24.

11. Hu AB, Burke KE, Kochar B, Ananthakrishnan AN. Yield of Random Biopsies During Colonoscopies in Inflammatory Bowel Disease Patients Undergoing Dysplasia Surveillance. Inflamm Bowel Dis. 2021;27(6):779–86.

12. Murthy SK, Feuerstein JD, Nguyen GC, Velayos FS. AGA Clinical Practice Update on Endoscopic Surveillance and Management of Colorectal Dysplasia in Inflammatory Bowel Diseases: Expert Review. Gastroenterology. 2021;161(3):1043–51e4.

CHAPTER 29

Long-Term Results of the Side-to-Side Isoperistaltic Strictureplasty in Crohn's Disease: 25-Year Follow-Up and Outcomes

Michelassi F, Mege D, Rubin M, Hurst RD. Ann Surg. 272(1):130–137, 2020

Reviewed by Erin B. Fennern and David W. Dietz

Research Question/Objective   The management of diffuse jejunoileitis in fibrotic Crohn's disease (CD) poses specific challenges for the surgeon. The side-to-side isoperistaltic strictureplasty (SSIS), first described by Michelassi in 1996,[1] is a bowel-sparing procedure suitable for the management of long and/or multiple segments of fibrostenotic jejunoileal disease. The aim of this study was to review the long-term outcomes of SSIS with respect to safety, rates of recurrence or failure, and the risk of missed small bowel cancer.

Study Design   This study was a cohort study of patients who underwent SSIS for the management of CD by Dr. Michelassi and Dr. Hurst between 1992 and 2016. A prospective database of patients operated on for abdominal CD included data on demographics, surgical history, medical treatments for CD, use of total parenteral nutrition (TPN), intraoperative data (length and location of diseased bowel, associated procedures), and outcomes. Data on outcomes included length of stay and 30-day complications following SSIS, as well as subsequent endoscopic or radiographic diagnosis of recurrence either at and/or away from the site of SSIS; subsequent surgical interventions for recurrence (specified as requiring a revision or complete resection of the SSIS; failure of SSIS was defined as need for resection); and additional long-term outcomes (anemia, subsequent steroid/ medication/TPN use, development of small bowel adenocarcinoma, etc.).

Sample Size   Out of 2101 patients operated on for abdominal CD, 60 underwent an SSIS for the treatment of diffuse jejunoileitis (2.9% of the overall CD cohort).

Follow-Up   One patient died on postoperative day 8 of a pulmonary embolism and was therefore unable to be followed long-term. Of the 59 remaining SSIS patients, the median follow-up was 11 years, with a range between 1 month and 25 years. There was complete follow-up to within 12 months of the study for 47 patients.

Inclusion/Exclusion Criteria   The indications for the performance of SSIS were either an area of affected small bowel greater than 10% of the entire small

DOI: 10.1201/9780429285714-29

bowel length and/or extensive disease affecting a segment longer than 2 feet. Patients were not considered for an SSIS if the strictures could be handled by simpler techniques (such as the Heineke–Mikulicz or Finney procedure), if the strictures were associated with an inflammatory or dysplastic mass, or if they had underlying severely thickened and friable mesentery (making the transection and manipulation needed to form an SSIS too challenging).

Treatment Received   The SSIS technique involves division of the small bowel and underlying mesentery at the midpoint of the segment with fibrostenotic disease. The proximal end is brought over the distal one in a side-to-side fashion, and a longitudinal layer of interrupted seromuscular stitches is formed using nonabsorbable suture. A longitudinal full-thickness enterotomy is then created on both loops, approximately 5 mm out from the seromuscular layer. The ends of the bowel are spatulated to avoid blind stumps. A running, full-thickness stitch is formed with absorbable suture to create the inner layer of the back wall of the entero-enterostomy. This inner layer is then continued anteriorly as a running full-thickness Connell suture, which is then reinforced with an outer layer of interrupted seromuscular stitches of nonabsorbable suture.

Results

Cohort Demographics and Index Procedures   All 60 patients underwent SSIS, with 1 patient undergoing a synchronous second SSIS at the time of index procedure. The average age was 36 (range of 12–69 years). Around half of patients ($n = 29$, 48%) were treated with steroids within the 3 months prior to the index procedure, and the majority ($n = 35$, 58%) had previously undergone abdominal surgery for CD. Thirteen patients (22%) were maintained on TPN preoperatively. In 33 patients (55%), a portion of the affected loop required resection prior to performance of the SSIS (median length of resected bowel was 20 cm, and median length of spared bowel was 53 cm).

Safety   Postoperative morbidity was observed in 7 patients (12%), with 2 patients requiring procedural intervention (return to OR and percutaneous drainage). One patient died of a pulmonary embolism on postoperative day 8. TPN was discontinued in all 13 patients prior to discharge. At discharge, all 59 surviving patients experienced resolution of their preoperative symptoms of obstruction. There were no suture line leaks in this cohort.

Recurrence and Failure   Thirty-six patients (61% of the 59 patients with follow-up data) developed recurrence, which was defined by the presence of endoscopic or radiographic confirmatory findings in the setting of clinical symptoms of disease. The median time to a first episode of recurrence was 4.5 years, with a range of 1–20 years.

Among the 36 patients with one or more episodes of recurrence, a total of 22 patients required surgical treatment for the first episode (37% of the overall cohort), 11 of whom experienced recurrence at the SSIS site. To treat those 11 cases, 5 required resection, and 6 required a revision of their SSIS. (An additional 4 patients developed recurrence at the SSIS site but did not require surgical intervention for their first episode of recurrence.)

While 22 patients required surgical intervention for a first episode of recurrence, 12 out of those 22 patients subsequently required additional surgical treatment for later episodes of recurrence. Of those 12, only 5 occurred at the original SSIS, and 7 occurred at another site.

With failure of SSIS defined as a need for removal of the SSIS, the overall rate of failure in this cohort was 8 out of 59 (14%). Of these 8 failures, 5 occurred at the time of the patient's first episode of recurrence, and an additional 3 occurred at subsequent episodes of recurrence.

Incidence of Adenocarcinoma   No cases were reported in this cohort during the period of follow-up.

Study Limitations   Within this cohort study, the largest potential sources of bias stem from differential follow-up and loss to follow-up, as well as the absence of data on potential confounding factors. Specifically, these are the patients of only two surgeons, both of whom practiced at tertiary referral centers in major metropolitan centers in the United States. We don't have any data on socioeconomic status or insurers, but it's likely that these patients don't represent a generalizable subset of abdominal CD patients with respect to personal resources and supports or access to healthcare. Moreover, this cohort may not be generalizable to GI surgeons without extensive experience in the management of complex abdominal CD.

Moreover, without an appropriate comparison group, the data do not allow for causative inferences about the potential impact of SSIS on recurrence, relative to other operative procedures for the treatment of diffuse jejunoileitis in CD.

Relevant Studies

Safety   With a 12% overall complication rate and a 5% major complication rate at 30 days, this cohort's outcomes support the existing data that show the SSIS procedure to be safe. Postoperative complication rates after standard resection and anastomosis[2-4] and in other strictureplasty procedures[5] for abdominal CD are estimated to be similar. Another prospective cohort of SSIS procedures performed at 6 different centers found a complication rate ranging from 5.7% to 20.8%,[6] demonstrating the reproducibility of these findings.

Small bowel adenocarcinoma is extremely rare, and there is consensus that the risk is increased in patients with abdominal CD.[7] However, no cases of small bowel adenocarcinoma at the site of SSIS was observed in this cohort, and, thus far, no cases of adenocarcinoma have been described in any other SSIS cohort.

Risk of Recurrence   Recurrence in this study was reported to occur in 61% of patients at a median time of 4.5 years from index operation. Overall, 37% of the cohort required at least one additional operative intervention for recurrence, with 19% requiring operative intervention at the site of the index SSIS during the first episode of recurrence. Overall, 14% of patients required removal of their index SSIS over the time they were followed.

Put another way, however, the data demonstrated that 86% of patients were able to keep a median of length of 53 cm of small bowel that would have been lost at the index operation, had a standard resection technique been utilized. These findings reflect an improvement in the rate of recurrence relative to standard resection. About a quarter of patients who undergo ileocolic resections with anastomoses subsequently require additional resections within 5 years,[8] and the rate of reoperation is estimated to be even higher among patients with diffuse jejunoileitis for whom the SSIS procedure was developed.[9] Moreover, in a meta-analysis of studies of patients who underwent any strictureplasty procedure (of whom only 5% underwent SSIS), recurrence was observed in 39% of patients (with 30% requiring surgical treatment).[10] This suggests a potential protective effect of SSIS on disease progression and recurrence, relative to both standard resection and other strictureplasty techniques.

REFERENCES

1. Michelassi F. Side-to-side isoperistaltic strictureplasty for multiple Crohn's strictures. *Dis Colon Rectum*. 1996;39(3):345–349. doi:10.1007/BF02049480
2. Alves A, Panis Y, Bouhnik Y, Pocard M, Vicaut E, Valleur P. Risk factors for intra-abdominal septic complications after a first ileocecal resection for Crohn's disease: a multivariate analysis in 161 consecutive patients. *Dis Colon Rectum*. 2007;50(3):331–336. doi:10.1007/s10350-006-0782-0
3. Yamamoto T, Allan RN, Keighley MR. Risk factors for intra-abdominal sepsis after surgery in Crohn's disease. *Dis Colon Rectum*. 2000;43(8):1141–1145. doi:10.1007/BF02236563
4. Kanazawa A, Yamana T, Okamoto K, Sahara R. Risk factors for postoperative intra-abdominal septic complications after bowel resection in patients with Crohn's disease. *Dis Colon Rectum*. 2012;55(9):957–962. doi:10.1097/DCR.0b013e3182617716
5. Dietz DW, Fazio VW, Laureti S, et al. Strictureplasty in diffuse Crohn's jejunoileitis: safe and durable. *Dis Colon Rectum*. 2002;45(6):764–770. doi:10.1007/s10350-004-6294-x
6. Michelassi F, Taschieri A, Tonelli F, et al. An international, multicenter, prospective, observational study of the side-to-side isoperistaltic strictureplasty in Crohn's disease. *Dis Colon Rectum*. 2007;50(3):277–284. doi:10.1007/s10350-006-0804-y
7. von Roon AC, Reese G, Teare J, Constantinides V, Darzi AW, Tekkis PP. The risk of cancer in patients with Crohn's disease. *Dis Colon Rectum*. 2007;50(6):839–855. doi:10.1007/s10350-006-0848-z
8. Fichera A, Michelassi F. Surgical treatment of Crohn's disease. *J Gastrointest Surg*. 2007;11(6):791–803. doi:10.1007/s11605-006-0068-9
9. Watanabe K, Sasaki I, Fukushima K, et al. Long-term incidence and characteristics of intestinal failure in Crohn's disease: a multicenter study. *J Gastroenterol*. 2014;49(2):231–238. doi:10.1007/s00535-013-0797-y
10. Yamamoto T, Fazio VW, Tekkis PP. Safety and efficacy of strictureplasty for Crohn's disease: a systematic review and meta-analysis. *Dis Colon Rectum*. 2007;50(11):1968–1986. doi:10.1007/s10350-007-0279-5

CHAPTER 30

Regional Ileitis: A Pathologic and Clinical Entity

Crohn BB, Ginzburg L, Oppenheimer GD. JAMA. 99(16): 1323–1329, 1932

Reviewed by Ada Graham and Neil Hyman

Research Question/Objective While reviewing cases of surgical excision for inflammatory masses of either the large or small intestine performed by Dr. A.A. Berg at Mount Sinai Hospital, the authors identified a subset of 14 patients noted to have inflammation isolated to the terminal ileum that did not encroach beyond the ileocecal valve. Furthermore, these cases did not appear to be related to other benign intestinal processes such as tuberculosis, typhoid, or appendicitis. When comparing the clinical presentation and pathologic findings of the resected segments, these patients appeared to share a common clinical entity, termed "regional ileitis" by the authors. The purpose of this study was to define the clinical presentations, pathologic findings, and management of this newly recognized disease.

Study Design A detailed retrospective review was performed of patients who presented with a similar constellation of symptoms and pathologic findings. The aim of the study was to describe the pathologic and clinical details of this disease mainly affecting young adults and characterized by "a subacute or chronic necrotizing and cicatrizing inflammation." Gross findings, histologic sections, physical findings, clinical course of the disease, radiologic findings, differential diagnosis and treatment were all reviewed/discussed.

Sample Size A total of 14 patients typically presenting with fever, diarrhea, and "emaciation," eventually leading to obstruction and with an associated right lower quadrant mass requiring surgery, comprise the study cohort.

Follow-Up The course after surgery was observed to be "benign," and all patients who survived the operation were noted to be alive and well. One patient developed recurrent disease proximal to the anastomosis; the length of follow-up is not specified.

Inclusion/Exclusion Criteria Inclusion criteria consisted of patients with the symptoms just described who at surgery were found to have exclusively terminal ileal (TI) disease extending to the ileocecal (IC) valve. The disease was described as beginning "abruptly" in the ileum and increasing in intensity as it approached the IC. The valve-fistulas to the colon or abdominal wall were "familiar." All patients had been ill for at least a year. Exclusion criteria included

DOI: 10.1201/9780429285714-30

patients with any previously recognized granulomatous or inflammatory condition such as tuberculosis, foreign body perforations, or Hodgkin's disease.

Intervention or Treatment Received   Patients either underwent ileocolic resection or ileocolic bypass to the transverse colon.

Results   A remarkably timeless description of the findings, both gross and microscopic, is provided. The authors observe how the disease tends to become milder as one approaches the normal proximal margin of resection. They acknowledge that more acute disease mimics acute appendicitis and that the TI is noted to be thickened, edematous, and "soggy." Indeed, half of the patients already had already undergone a previous right lower quadrant exploration for presumed appendicitis.

In the study cohort, the average age is 32 years old, with a 2:1 male predominance. The most common physical findings are a palpable mass in the right iliac region, evidence of fistulae, emaciation/anemia, scar from a previous appendectomy, and evidence of intestinal obstruction.

Intraoperative and pathologic findings are succinctly described. The TI mesentery was "greatly thickened" and contained numerous "hyperplastic glands." They also describe isolated lesions separate from the "main mass" (skip lesions). They hypothesized that lesions ("oval mucosal ulcerations") occurring on the mesenteric border of the small bowel were the early/primary lesions (what we would now call "aphthous ulcers"). Furthermore, they explicitly described the linear ulcers and cobblestoning of the mucosa so characteristic of the disease. They described strictures, bowel wall thickening, and proximal dilatation. They also note that in the "older phases" of disease, the acute inflammatory reaction is replaced by a "fibrostenotic process."

They note that free perforation was not observed and that the "chronic" perforation leads to a walling off process by neighboring viscera that often leads to fistulas (they specifically describe ileosigmoid fistulas). They observe that simply draining the associated abscess leads to an enterocutaneous fistula and that simple suture is ineffective. The authors describe distinct clinic courses including an inflammatory, obstructive (most common), and fistulizing phenotype. They report that the one recurrence occurred just proximal to the ileocolic anastomosis.

Study Limitations   The small sample size and inability to perform endoscopic evaluation prior to surgery likely limited the author's ability to describe early findings, as well as to describe extra-ileal manifestations which are now known to occur with Crohn's disease. For example, they believe that the disease is restricted to the TI (hence the name "regional ileitis") and that perirectal abscesses/fistulas are not seen. But they note that the "most important differentiation" is from ulcerative colitis and that when the proximal colon alone is involved, this leads to "confusion." It is noted that cases with perianal disease are associated with colitis, although they distinguish this from regional enteritis.

Relevant Studies   After the publication of this paper, several case series were presented, both from Mount Sinai and elsewhere, confirming and extending the findings of this paper. Subsequent studies expanded on the nature of Crohn's disease to include perianal manifestations,[1] concomitant colonic involvement,[2] and Crohn's colitis,[3] among other clinical features. Intestinal bypass with exclusion was soon felt to be the safest surgical option,[4] but the danger of cancer in the bypassed segment ultimately established resection as the procedure of choice.[5] A related historical footnote relates to the controversial choice of bypass rather than resection for President Dwight Eisenhower in 1956 when he required laparotomy for a bowel obstruction related to structuring disease of the TI.[6]

REFERENCES

1. Penner A, Crohn BB. Perianal fistulae as a complication of regional ileitis. Annals of Surgery. 1938;108(5):867–73.
2. Colp R. A case of nonspecific granuloma of the terminal ileum and cecum. Surgical Clinics of North America. 1934;14:443–9.
3. Lockhart-Mummery HE, Morson BC. Crohn's disease (regional enteritis) of the large intestine and its distinction from ulcerative colitis. Gut. 1960;1:87–105.
4. Ginzburg L, Garlock JH. Regional- ileitis. Annals of Surgery. 1942;116(6):906–12.
5. Greenstein AJ, Janowitz HD. Cancer in Crohn's disease. The danger of a by-passed loop. American Journal of Gastroenterology. 1975;64(2):122–4.
6. Heaton LD, et al. President Eisenhower's operation or regional enteritis: a footnote to history. Annals of Surgery. 1964;159:661–6.
7. Bornstein J, Steinhagen R. History of Crohn's disease. In Fichera A, Krane M (eds). *Crohn's Disease: Basic Principles*. 2015, Springer, pp. 1–13.
8. Ginzburg, L. The road to regional enteritis. Mt. Sinai Journal of Medicine. 1974;41(2):272–5.
9. Kovalicik PJ. Early history of regional enteritis. Current Surgery. 1982;39(6):395–400.

HISTORICAL NOTE

The lifelong drama and markedly disparate accounts of the origins of this paper are legendary and have been beautifully outlined by Bornstein and Steinhagen.[7] According to Dr. Ginzburg,[8] his interest in inflammatory masses of the intestine dated back to when he was house staff on Dr. Berg's service. He recruited Dr. Oppenheimer, who was working in pathology as a research assistant, to collaborate on analyzing 53 such cases. In this group, he found 12 cases with inflammation restricted to the terminal ileum (Crohn added two cases), who comprise the study cohort for the 1932 landmark paper.

Suffice it to say that Dr. Ginzburg believed that Dr. Crohn had "no role whatsoever" in the research represented in this manuscript, clearly a major source of angst to him as regional ileitis quickly became known as Crohn's disease. In direct contradistinction, Dr. Crohn believed the manuscript represented his collaborative effort with Dr. Berg, who had suggested adding the two "younger men" as coauthors.[9]

Irrespective, both Dr. Ginzburg and Dr. Crohn highlight the central role of Dr. Berg, who "with unnecessary modesty" declined to be a coauthor. This is of particular interest since the editorial policy of *JAMA* at that time was to list authors alphabetically; it seems likely we would now call this "Berg's disease" had he accepted.

CHAPTER 31

Proctocolectomy with Ileal Reservoir and Anal Anastomosis

Parks AG, Nicholls RJ, Belliveau P. Br J Surg. 67(8):533–538, 1980

Reviewed by Arman Erkan

Research Question/Objective Preserving the function while treating the disease is the classic surgical dilemma. Diseases like ulcerative colitis and polyposis coli pose a typical challenge, where complete excision of colonic and rectal mucosa may achieve cure; however, patients' quality of life may be significantly impacted by a permanent ileostomy. The objective of this article was to describe a novel surgical technique that strives for gastrointestinal continuity while eliminating diseased/at risk mucosa. This is achieved by combining two major preceding advances: an ileal reservoir described by Kock (1) and endoanal anastomosis described by the same author (Parks) (2).

Study Design This study was a case series from a single colorectal surgery unit in the UK. A novel operation was performed on patients with ulcerative colitis and polyposis coli who expressed a strong aversion to living with a permanent ileostomy. Postoperative complications and long-term functional outcomes including the number of evacuations per day, need for self-catheterization, and daytime and nighttime continence were evaluated. Furthermore, although not in the form of a calculated index, quality of life measures were assessed.

Sample Size This study included a total of 21 patients. Of these, 17 had ulcerative colitis and 4 had polyposis coli. Among patients with ulcerative colitis, 16 had medically refractory disease and 1 had malignancy. Similarly, 1 patient with polyposis coli had carcinoma.

Follow-Up The mean follow-up period for 20 patients was 13.5 months (2–34 months). In addition to pouch function, overall health, social and work life, and sexual and urinary function were assessed over time. All but 1 patient were satisfied with the outcomes and preferred the quality of life after this new operation over permanent ileostomy.

Inclusion/Exclusion Criteria The operation was performed on patients with ulcerative colitis and polyposis coli aged 14–47. Patients with ulcerative colitis either had medically refractory disease or malignancy. Of patients with polyposis coli, 1 had malignancy, and 1 was not a candidate for ileorectal

DOI: 10.1201/9780429285714-31

anastomosis due to possible inadequate follow-up. A strong motivation
to avoid a permanent ileostomy was necessary on the patients' end.

Treatment   The surgery consists of abdominal and perineal components. First, the
entire colon is removed. Dissection is carried out close to the rectal wall below the
rectosigmoid junction to avoid neural injury. The rectum is transected just below the
peritoneal reflection leaving a stump of 6–8 cm. Then an ileal pouch 15 cm in length
is constructed from the last 50 cm of ileum. This segment is folded twice to obtain an
S-shape, where proximal two limbs are 15 cm and the distal limb is 20 cm (an extra
5 cm of exit conduit). Ileum is opened on its antimesenteric border. The inner edges of
the adjacent loops are sutured together to form the posterior wall. The two outer edges
are then folded and sutured together to form the anterior wall and complete the pouch.

On the perineal portion, the rectal mucosa is elevated by injecting adrenaline-
containing normal saline. Mucosectomy is performed beginning from the
dentate line to the cut edge of the rectum. Finally, the exit conduit of the pouch
is passed through the rectal stump and anastomosed to the anal canal. Stool is
diverted with a temporary loop ileostomy, which is closed in 4–6 weeks.

Following ileostomy closure, patients are instructed to catheterize the pouch 4
times a day. About half of the patients will gain the ability to evacuate the pouch
spontaneously.

Results

Patients   In total, 21 patients with ages ranging from 14 to 47 years (mean 30.7)
underwent the new operation. There were 17 patients with ulcerative colitis and 4 with
polyposis coli. Eight patients with ulcerative colitis had previous subtotal colectomy
(3-stage procedure); in 9 patients proctocolectomy and pouch were performed at the
same time (2-stage procedure). One patient with polyposis coli had a previous ileorectal anastomosis; this was converted to a pouch for the likelihood of inadequate
surveillance.

General Outcome   All patients were in good health at the time of follow-up.
Patients with ulcerative colitis were within normal weight range. Women who
suffered amenorrhea started to have menstruation. All previously employed
patients returned to work except for 1. One patient had pouchitis. Most importantly, all patients but 1 were satisfied with the outcomes and preferred the quality of life with pouch over that after ileostomy. One patient had found pouch
catheterization unacceptable and had undergone pouch excision.

Complications   There was no mortality. Nine patients had postoperative
complications (43%), 3 pelvic abscess, 3 small bowel obstruction, and 1 each of
the remaining 3 pouch hemorrhage, chest infection, and deep vein thrombosis. Two of the pelvic abscesses discharged through the anastomosis, and the

pouch hemorrhage was controlled endoscopically. The complication rate was decreased in the second half of the series, possibly due to experience with the procedure. No urinary or sexual complications occurred.

Pouch Function   Ten patients gained the ability to evacuate spontaneously. Average number of evacuations was 3.8/day (1–6/day). The frequency diminished 6 months after ileostomy closure. All patients were continent of stool during the day, and there was 1 patient with night-time incontinence. Two patients needed to use pad during the day for mucus discharge, and 3 at night.

Study Limitations   This was a single-center case series, subject to selection bias. The authors acknowledged that this procedure was still under trial and was only offered to patients who were not candidates for ileorectal anastomosis. Although the outcomes were outstanding, especially in terms of function and quality of life, there was no comparison with a different group like permanent ileostomy or ileorectal anastomosis. The variation in follow-up times was high.

Relevant Studies   This is a seminal article in the field of pouch surgery, validating the utilization of ileal pouch in the surgical treatment of ulcerative colitis and polyposis coli, also acting as a bridge between prior attempts to avoid an ileostomy and contemporary practice.

The ileoanal anastomosis evolved naturally to restore alimentary continuity after the elimination of colorectal mucosa. The history of ileoanal anastomosis starts with Nissen in 1933, when he reported the case of a 10-year-old patient with polyposis (3). There were further reports by Best (4), Ravitch (a leading pediatric surgeon and a pioneer of mechanical stapling devices in the United States) (5), and Goligher (6) in the following years. However, the function was far from satisfactory as the number of bowel movements, rates of urgency, and incontinence were high, resulting in poor quality of life.

In the meantime, animal experiments were carried out by Valiente and Bacon (7). Their work marks the beginning of the pouch concept. In the late 1960s, Kock developed a valve mechanism within an ileal pouch that provided continence with ileostomy (1). In this way, patients did not need to wear an external appliance and were able to empty the pouch intermittently by catheterizing rather than living with a continuous uncontrolled flow of intestinal content into the bag. This, however, still included an ostomy and required multiple reoperations due to complications related to the valve mechanism. Kock had moved the pouch out of the pelvis into the abdominal cavity but showed that it was applicable in humans.

Parks and Nicholls converged these two approaches by anastomosing an S-shaped ileal reservoir to the anal canal. After an initial report with a smaller group of 5 patients (8), they published the current article where they gave a detailed description of the technique, postoperative complications, and long-term functional outcomes. Between the two reports, they started to construct a larger pouch using the last 50 cm of ileum rather than the 30 cm as described in the initial report. There was no mortality, but morbidity was 42%, reflecting the similarly high rates today. As they did not carry out a dissection in the lower pelvis, no sexual or urinary complications occurred, but the price for leaving a long rectal cuff and a long exit conduit was the need for catheterization to evacuate in half of the cohort. The rates of incontinence were also low due to the same mechanism; however, some patients still experienced mucus discharge.

Other important concepts described in their article were staged approach (what is known today as 2-stage and 3-stage procedures), pouchitis, pouch failure and subsequent pouch excision, and quality of life.

The pouch procedure continued to evolve in time. Utsunomiya described a simpler pouch configuration in J-shape by using staplers (9). This design resulted in more frequent defecation; however, it eliminated the need for intubation. Nicholls later reported a 4-limbed W-shaped pouch that did not require intubation and still had low frequency similar to the S-pouch (10). Although its outcomes were promising, the W-pouch never gained popularity due to its complex and time-consuming construction. Among these pouch types, J-pouch withstood the test of time and became the most commonly performed pouch type as it is easier to construct and eliminates the need for catheterization due to the lack of an efferent limb (11). On the other hand, surgeons who perform pouch procedures should also be familiar with S-pouch as it is still occasionally performed to gain an extra 2–3 cm in cases where a J-pouch won't reach the pelvic floor even after mesenteric lengthening maneuvers. The efferent limb should be kept as short as possible to allow spontaneous evacuation (12).

In the late 1980s, with further advancement of surgical staplers, a double stapled technique became possible, leading to easier transanal anastomosis without the need for mucosectomy. Fazio's review of 1005 patients became a milestone by showing lower complication rates and better sphincter function after double stapled anastomosis (13).

Similar to the morbidity, pouch failure rates have remained high between 3% and 15%. Permanent diversion with or without pouch excision was recommended after pouch failure. But dissatisfaction of patients urged surgeons to look for alternatives. This led to revisional pouch surgery. Remzi reported a success rate of 85% with abdominopelvic salvage surgery for initially failed pouches (14).

Pouch surgery remains a complex operation with high morbidity. Subspecialization and centralization are key for achieving better outcomes. Therefore, more institutions are establishing dedicated IBD centers.

REFERENCES

1. Kock NG. Intra-abdominal "reservoir" in patients with permanent ileostomy. Preliminary observations on a procedure resulting in fecal "continence" in five ileostomy patients. Arch Surg. 1969;99(2):223–31.
2. Parks AG. Transanal technique in low rectal anastomosis. Proc R Soc Med. 1972;65(11):975–6.
3. Nissen R. Demonstrationen aus der operativen Chirurgie, no 39. Berlin Surgical Society. Zentralbl Chir. 1933;15:888.
4. Best RR. Anastomosis of the ileum to the lower part of the rectum and anus; a report on experiences with ileorectostomy and ileoproctostomy, with special reference to polyposis. Arch Surg (1920). 1948;57(2):276–85.
5. Ravitch MM, Sabiston DC, Jr. Anal ileostomy with preservation of the sphincter; a proposed operation in patients requiring total colectomy for benign lesions. Surg Gynecol Obstet. 1947;84(6):1095–9.
6. Goligher JC. The functional results after sphincter-saving resections of the rectum. Ann R Coll Surg Engl. 1951;8(6):421–38.
7. Valiente MA, Bacon HE. Construction of pouch using pantaloon technic for pull-through of ileum following total colectomy; report of experimental work and results. Am J Surg. 1955;90(5):742–50.
8. Parks AG, Nicholls RJ. Proctocolectomy without ileostomy for ulcerative colitis. Br Med J. 1978;2(6130):85–8.
9. Utsunomiya J, Iwama T, Imajo M, Matsuo S, Sawai S, Yaegashi K, et al. Total colectomy, mucosal proctectomy, and ileoanal anastomosis. Dis Colon Rectum. 1980;23(7):459–66.
10. Nicholls RJ, Pezim ME. Restorative proctocolectomy with ileal reservoir for ulcerative colitis and familial adenomatous polyposis: a comparison of three reservoir designs. Br J Surg. 1985;72(6):470–4.
11. Lovegrove RE, Heriot AG, Constantinides V, Tilney HS, Darzi AW, Fazio VW, et al. Meta-analysis of short-term and long-term outcomes of J, W and S ileal reservoirs for restorative proctocolectomy. Colorectal Dis. 2007;9(4):310–20.
12. Pescatori M. A modified three-loop ileoanal reservoir. Dis Colon Rectum. 1988;31(10):823–4.
13. Fazio VW, Ziv Y, Church JM, Oakley JR, Lavery IC, Milsom JW, et al. Ileal pouch-anal anastomoses complications and function in 1005 patients. Ann Surg. 1995;222(2):120–7.
14. Remzi FH, Fazio VW, Kirat HT, Wu JS, Lavery IC, Kiran RP. Repeat pouch surgery by the abdominal approach safely salvages failed ileal pelvic pouch. Dis Colon Rectum. 2009;52(2):198–204.

CHAPTER 32

Oxaliplatin, Flurouracil, and Leucovorin as Adjuvant Treatment for Colon Cancer

Andre T, Boni C, Mouneji-Boudiaf L, Navarro M, Tabernero J, Hickish T, Topham C, Zaninelli M, Clingan P, Bridgewater J, Tabah-Fisch I, deGramont A. N Engl J Med. 350:2343–2351, 2004

Reviewed by Larissa Temple

Research Question/Objective To compare the efficacy of 6 months of adjuvant fluoruracil, leucovorin (FL) with and without oxaliplatin after surgical resection for stages II and III colon cancer.

Study Design Multicentered randomized controlled clinical trial.

Sample Size 2246 patients.

Follow-Up Median follow-up 37.9 months.

Inclusion/Exclusion Criteria INCLUSION: Ability to consent, stage II–III colon cancer (>15 cm from anal margin, above anterior reflection), initiated chemotherapy <7 weeks postoperative, 18–75 years of age, KPS >60, CEA >10 ng/ml. EXCLUSION: Prior chemotherapy, immunotherapy, or radiotherapy, adequate blood counts, liver and kidney function.

Results The majority of patients received a median of 12 cycles of chemotherapy [74% FL oxaliplatin (FOLFOX) vs. 86.5% in FL alone]. Most patients received the planned dose (84% FOLFOX vs. 97.7% FL). There was a statistically and clinically significant difference in recurrence rates (26.1% vs. 21.1%, $p = 0.002$) and disease-free survival (78.2% vs. 72.9%, $p = 0.002$) in patients who received FOLFOX compared to patients who were treated with FL alone. Patients treated with FOLFOX had more toxicities including febrile neutropenia (1.8%) and sensory neuropathy (12.4% that reduced to 1% at 12 months), but there was no difference in deaths during treatment (6 patients/group).

Study Limitations Reported disease-free survival rather than overall survival and short follow-up for overall survival. Samples too small to really evaluate the role of oxaliplatin for patients with stage II colon cancer. No surgical QA.

DOI: 10.1201/9780429285714-32

Relevant Studies While earlier studies had demonstrated the improved oncologic outcomes with FOLFOX in patients with metastatic disease, there were no data for adjuvant treatment, and patients continued to be treated with 5FU and leucovorin. As such, this trial was pivotal in advancing therapeutic options for patients with stage II–III colon cancer. These data, showing acceptable toxicity and improved 3-year disease-free survival, changed the approach to adjuvant chemotherapy.

This adjuvant trial was practice changing and also interesting because of its utilization of a 3-year end point. Historically, 5-year overall survival was considered gold standard, but given the time to obtain the data and potential confounding of newer treatments in patients with recurrence over the study period, there was a real interest in a 3-year end point. Pooled data from large randomized adjuvant colon cancer trials demonstrated that a 3-year overall disease-free survival end point was highly correlated with 5-year overall survival (Sargent et al., 2005; Sargent, 2007).

While the 3-year end point changed clinical practice, in 2015, the authors reported their 6-year overall survival data as well as some meaningful subgroup analyses (Andre et al., 2015). With a median follow-up of 9.5 years, the 10-year overall survival of 71.7% versus 67.1% for FOLFOX versus FL remained significantly different 25% ($p = 0.043$). In addition, the authors reported OS survival in patients with stage II (78.4% vs. 79.5, $p = 0.98$) and stage III (67.1% vs. 59.0%, = 0.016) treated with FOLFOX versus FL. Among the 2246 patients, a subset were dMMR (95) or BRAF mutant (94), and dMMR was found to be prognostic (HR 2.02 1.15–3.55, $p = 0.014$). Overall, the data at 10 years support the use of FOLFOX in stage III disease and in patients with dMMR and BRAF. There were no long-term data regarding neurotoxicity. These longer-term outcomes confirmed the initial findings and also provided more information regarding the impact of the treatment in subgroups.

Over the last decade, there have been important nuances to treating with FOLFOX. In a recent paper reporting data on a cohort of 6501 stage III colon cancer patients in RCTs who were treated between 1998–2003 and 2004–2009 (Salem et al., 2020), there were significant differences in oncologic outcomes including time to recurrence (73% vs. 76%), 3-year disease-free survival (74.7% vs. 72.3%), survival after recurrence (27% vs. 17 months), and overall 5-year survival (80.9% vs. 75.7%). While there may be several explanations, it does seem that advances in therapeutic options for metastatic disease are a contributing factor. The potential utilization of FOLFOX for high-risk stage II pMMR tumors based on molecular profiling will require further study. The role of FOLFOX in the era of newer agents for dMMR tumors remains to be determined.

While the oncologic benefit of oxaliplatin in the adjuvant setting is clear, it has known toxicity. In fact, in the initial study, 1 year after treatment almost 30% of patients had persistent neuropathy although the majority was grade 1 (83%) (Andre et al., 2004). In an effort to decrease the toxicity of treatment, there has been interest in decreasing the duration of treatment. The International Duration Evaluation of Adjuvant (IDEA) Therapy collaborative (Andre et al., 2020) reported on pooled data from 6 RCTs evaluating 3 versus 6 months of FOLFOX/CAPOX in patients with stage III colon cancer with disease-free survival being the primary end point with other secondary end points reported. The authors also demonstrated a significant difference in toxicity while on treatment when comparing 3 versus 6 months of chemotherapy (FOLFOX [37.6% vs. 56%] and CAPOX [25% vs. 36%]) (Grothey et al., 2018). Among the 12,835 patients in the 6 trials, with a median of 72-month follow-up, the data did not demonstrate noninferiority in disease-free survival patients treated with 3 months (82.4%) versus 6 months (82.8%), but the authors questioned the clinical significance of 0.4% absolute difference. Interestingly, given the differences in 3 versus 6 months in patients treated with FOLFOX versus CAPOX as well as T4 and N2 tumors, they concluded that 3 months of adjuvant CAPOX was appropriate for most patients with stage III colon cancer. In addition to RCTs comparing 3 versus 6 months of adjuvant therapy, others have evaluated the role of a 6-month chemotherapy schedule with only 3 months of oxaliplatin (Kim et al., 2022). In this recently published RCT, 1788 patients were randomized to 6 months versus 3 months of fluorouracil (FU) with 3 months of oxaliplatin. In patients treated with fluoropyrimidine for 3 versus 6 months and 3 months of oxaliplatin, the 3-year survival rates met noninferiority (84.7% vs. 83.7%) criteria, although this was more evident with capecitabine when compared to FU. Thus the authors recommended 3 months of capecitabine and oxaliplatin and 3 months of oxaliplatin rather than 6 months of FU therapy.

In summary, Andre's FOLFOX-versus-5FULV randomized trial, significantly changed adjuvant treatment paradigms for patients with colon cancer. Regardless of initially reporting surrogate end points, the oncologic benefits were shown durable over extended follow-up. Longer-term data support the benefit of FOLFOX in stage III versus stage II, and its impact is still evident with dMMR tumors. Subsequent studies have attempted to decrease the toxicity of treatment by comparing 3 versus 6 months of FOLFOX as well as 3 versus 6 months of oxaliplatin with 6 months of FU. Interestingly, data suggest that capecitabine may result in better outcomes in patients receiving 3 months of oxaliplatin compared to FU. The majority of patients can be treated with capecitabine and oxaliplatin, although high-risk tumors appear to still benefit from 6 months of FOLFOX. Further work is required to better identify high-risk stage II tumors who may benefit from more than FU, the role of immunotherapy in the adjuvant setting for dMMR tumors and the role of ctDNA in making treatment decisions.

REFERENCES

Andre T, Boni C, Mouneji-Boudiaf L, Navarro M, Tabernero J, Hickish T, Topham C, Zaninelli M, Clingan P, Bridgewater J, Tabah-Fisch I, deGramont A. Oxaliplatin, flurouracil, and leucovorin as adjuvant treatment for colon cancer. N Engl J Med, 2004; 350: 2343–51.

Andre T, deGramont A, Vernery D, Chibaudel B, Bonnetain F, Tijeras-Raballand A, Scriva A, Hickish T, Tabernero J, VanLaethem JL, Banzi M, Maartense E, Shmueli E, Carlsson GU, Scheithauer W, Papamichael D, Moehler M, Landolfi S, Demetter P, Colote S, Tournigand C, Louvet C, Duval A, Flejou JF, deGramont A. Adjuvant fluorouracil, leucovorin and oxaliplatin in stage II to III colon cancer: updated 10 year survival and outcomes according to BFAF Mutation and Mismatch repair status of the MOSAIC Study. J Clin Oncol, 2015; 33: 4176–87.

Andre T, Meyerhardt J, Iveson T, Sobrero A, Yoshino T, Souglakos I, Grothey A, Niedzwiecki D, Saunders M, Labianca R, Tamanaka T, Boukovinas I, Vernerey D, Meyers J, Harkin A, Torri V, Oki E, Georgoulias V, Taieb J, Shields A, Shi Q. Effect of duration of adjuvant chemotherapy for patients with stage II colon cancer (IDEA collaboration): final results of a prospective pooled analysis of six randomized phase 3 trials. Lancet, 2020; 21: 1621–29.

Grothey A, Sobrero A, Shields A, Yoshino T, Paul J, Tajeb J, Souglakos J, Shi Q, Kerr R, Labianca R, Meyerhardt J, Vernerey D, et al. Duration of adjuvant chemotherapy for stage III colon cancer. N Engl J Med, 2018; 378: 1177–88.

Kim ST, Kim SY, Lee J, Hyeon Yun S, Kim HC, Lee WY, Kim TW, Hong YS, Lim SB, Baek JY, Oh JH, Ahn JB, Shin SJ, Han SW, Kim SG, Kang SY, Sym SJ, Zang DY, Kim YH, Choi IS, Kan JH, Kim MJ, Park YS. Oxaliplatin (3 month v 6 months) with 6 months fluoropyrimidine as adjuvant therapy in patients with stage II/II colon cancer: KCSG C009-07. J Clin Onco, 2022; 40: 3868–77.

Salem ME, Yin J, Goldberg RM, Pederson LD, Wolmark N, Alberts SR, Taieb SR, Marshal JL, Lonardi S, Yoshino T, Kerr RS, Yothers G, Grothey A, Andre T, DeGramont A, Shi Q. Evaluation of the change of outcomes over a 10 year period in patients with stage III colon cancer: pooled analysis of 6501 patients treated with fluorouracil, leucovorin and oxaliplatin in ACCENT database. Ann Onc, 2020; 31: 480–86.

Sargent DJ, Wiend HS, Haller DG, et al. Disease free survival vs overall survival as a primary end point for adjuvant colon cancer studies: individual patient data from 20898 patients on 18 randomized trials. J Clin Oncol, 2005; 23: 8664–70.

CHAPTER 33

Duration of Adjuvant Chemotherapy for Stage III Colon Cancer

Grothey A, Sobrero AF, Shields T, et al. N Engl J Med. 378(13):1177–1188, 2018

Reviewed by Mohamedtaki A. Tejani

Research Question/Objective   Although it was well established that adjuvant FOLFOX improved disease-free (DFS) and overall survival (OS) in patients with resected stage III colon cancer (1, 2), the ideal duration of therapy was unknown. Six months was the adopted historical standard based on studies with fluorouracil (3), but the risk of oxaliplatin-related sensory neuropathy goes up significantly depending on the cumulatively administered dose. Oxaliplatin-related neuropathy can be severe and persistent with the potential to significantly impact quality of life. The central aim of this International Duration Evaluation of Adjuvant Therapy (IDEA) collaboration of six clinical trials of adjuvant therapy was to evaluate the hypothesis that 3 months of FOLFOX or CAPOX chemotherapy would be noninferior to 6 months of therapy in the rate of DFS at 3 years.

Study Design   IDEA was a collaboration of six randomized, phase 3 clinical trials enrolling patients with resected stage III colon cancer in 12 countries. Patients were randomly assigned to receive 3 months or 6 months of chemotherapy. The primary end point of the six trials was DFS, which is defined as the time from the date of randomization to date of first relapse, diagnosis of a secondary colorectal cancer, or death from any cause, whichever occurred first. Preplanned analyses included assessments of noninferiority of 3 months versus 6 months of therapy within subgroups that were defined according to the T/N stage and chemotherapy regimen.

Sample Size   A total of 13,025 patients with resected stage III colon cancer were enrolled in the IDEA trials. Of these patients, 12,834 met the criteria for the modified intention-to-treat analysis. Noninferiority of 3 months versus 6 months of therapy would be claimed if the upper limit of the two-sided 95% confidence interval of the hazard ratio did not exceed 1.12. This margin was chosen on the basis of clinical acceptability, since it corresponded to a worsening of 2.7 percentage points in the 3-year DFS from 72% to 69.3% as determined by consensus among the IDEA researchers.

Follow-Up   Study follow-up occurred at a median of 41.8 months. At the time of database lock, 3263 events of disease recurrence or death (96.3% of the estimated events) had occurred.

 DOI: 10.1201/9780429285714-33

Inclusion/Exclusion Criteria   Criteria for patient inclusion in these six studies were outlined as adults with resected stage III colon cancer. All T and N stages including T4 and N2 were included.

Intervention   Patients were randomly assigned in a 1:1 manner to receive 3 months or 6 months of therapy. Five of the six trials allowed the use of either FOLFOX or CAPOX, which are known to be pharmacologically similar (4, 5). This nonrandomized choice of regimen was made by the treating physicians.

Results

Sampling   Although most of the characteristics of the patients and their tumors were similar across trials, there were some notable differences. The percentage of patients with T4 tumors varied from 12.1% to 29.5%. The percentage of patients with N2 tumors varied from 25.2% to 32.5%. Overall, 40% of patients received CAPOX and 60% FOLFOX.

Treatment Adherence   For fluorouracil/capecitabine, the mean percentage of doses that were delivered was 92.4% and 91.2%, respectively, in the 3-month group as compared with 81.6% and 78% in the 6-month group. For oxaliplatin, the mean percentage of FOLFOX and CAPOX doses were 91.4% and 89.8% respectively, in the 3-month group as compared with 72.8% and 69.3% in the 6-month group.

Primary End Point   Noninferiority of 3 months of therapy versus 6 months was not confirmed in the modified intention-to-treat population (hazard ratio 1.07, 95% confidence interval 1.00 to 1.15). The 3-year rates of disease-free survival were 74.6% (95% CI 73.5–75.7) in the 3-month therapy group as compared to 75.5% (95% CI 74.4–76.7) in the 6-month therapy group.

Adverse Events   A shorter duration of adjuvant therapy was associated with significantly lower rates of adverse events than a longer duration. Neuropathy of grade 2 or higher was substantially lower in the 3-month group (16.5% with FOLFOX and 14.2% with CAPOX) when compared to the 6-month group (47.7% with FOLFOX and 44.9% with CAPOX).

Subgroup Analysis According to Treatment   Among patients who received FOLFOX, 6 months of adjuvant therapy was superior to 3 months (HR 1.16, 95% CI 1.06–1.26) with a difference in 3-year DFS rate of 2.4 percentage points (73.6% vs. 76.0%). However, among the patients who received CAPOX, the hazard ratio for DFS was 0.95, which met the prespecified margin for noninferiority. The 3-year DFS rates were 75.9% and 74.8% for 3 months and 6 months of CAPOX, respectively.

Subgroup Analysis According to Tumor and Nodal Stage   In an exploratory analysis of the combined regimens, among patients with T1, T2, or T3 and N1 cancer (low risk), 3 months of therapy was noninferior to 6 months with a 3-year DFS rate of 83.1% and 83.3%, respectively (HR 1.01, 95% CI 0.9–1.12). Among patients with cancer that were classified as T4, N2, or both (high risk), the DFS rate for a 6-month duration of therapy was superior to that for a 3-month duration (64.4% vs. 62.7%) for the combined treatments (HR 1.12, 95% CI 1.03–1.23).

Study Limitations   IDEA had a few limitations. The six trials were conducted in varied settings that led to intertrial differences. The study did not test the discontinuation of oxaliplatin at 3 months while continuing a fluoropyrimidine, a common clinical practice. Subgroup analyses were performed without adjustment for multiplicity. The study design did not have a randomization for CAPOX or FOLFOX. Also, there were no standardized follow-up procedures, including imaging and lab assessment intervals.

Relevant Studies   Prior to this study, the historical standard for adjuvant chemotherapy for resected stage III colon cancer was 6 months of chemotherapy. IDEA did not confirm noninferiority for 3 months of therapy in the overall cohort, but the difference in 3-year DFS rate was 0.9 percentage points, which is a difference of limited clinical relevance. In patients treated with CAPOX, 3 months of therapy was as effective as 6 months, particularly in the low-risk subgroup.

The IDEA results provide a strong framework for individual discussions between oncologists and patients regarding choice of treatment regimen and duration of therapy balanced against individual risk of recurrence and toxicity, especially persistent neuropathy.

REFERENCES

1. Andre T, Boni C, Mounedji-Boudiaf L, et al. Oxaliplatin, fluorouracil, and leucovorin as adjuvant treatment for colon cancer. N Engl J Med 2004; 350: 2343–51.
2. Andre T, Boni C, Navarro M, et al. Improved overall survival with oxaliplatin, fluorouracil and leurovorin as adjuvant treatment in stage II or III colon cancer in the MOSAIC trial. J Clin Oncol 2009; 27: 3109–16.
3. Haller DG, Catalano PJ, Macdonald JS, et al. Phase III study of fluorouracil, leucovorin and levamisole in high-risk stage II and III colon cancer: final report of Intergroup 0089. J Clin Oncol 2005; 23: 8671–8.
4. Haller DG, Tabernero J, Maroun J, et al. Capecitabine plus oxaliplatin compared with fluorouracil and folinic acid as adjuvant treatment for stage III colon cancer. J Clin Oncol 2011; 29: 1465–71.
5. Twelves C, Wong A, Nowacki MP, et al. Capecitabine as adjuvant treatment for stage III colon cancer. N Engl J Med 2005; 352: 2696–704.

CHAPTER 34

Standardized Surgery for Colonic Cancer: Complete Mesocolic Excision and Central Ligation—Technical Notes and Outcomes

Hohenberger W, Weber K, Matzel K, Papadopoulos T, Merkel S.
Colorectal Dis. 11(4):354–364, discussion 364–365, 2009

Reviewed by Matthew R. Albert

Research Question/Objective Total mesorectal excision (TME), as initially described by Heald over 30 years ago, has become the standard surgical technique for the management of rectal cancer. Similarly, the mesocolic planes are found to be well-defined throughout the abdomen, leading many to hypothesize that perhaps the same surgical principles for the management of rectal cancer could be applied to the surgical resection of colon cancer with similar improvement in oncologic outcomes.

Study Design Prospectively obtained data from 1329 consecutive patients of a single gastrointestinal surgical department in Erlangen, Germany, with R0-resection of colon cancer between 1978 and 2002 were analyzed. The primary end point was cancer-related survival. Secondary end points included locoregional recurrence, lymph node yield, as well as postoperative morbidity and mortality. Patient data of three subdivided time periods were compared (1978–1984, 1985–1994, and 1995–2002) corresponding with stepwise changes in the surgical technique and the introduction of a standardized surgical approach.

Sample Size A total of 1329 patients were included in the final analysis, after exclusion of 109 patients (7.6%).

Follow-Up Median follow-up time was 103 months (range 1–335). Patients were followed for minimum of 5 years, quarterly for the first 2 years and semiannually thereafter.

Inclusion/Exclusion Criteria Only patients with a solitary adenocarcinoma of the colon above 16 cm were analyzed. Patients were excluded preoperatively from analysis if they had a prior history of colon cancer or synchronous lesion, or if they had a malignancy in the setting of FAP, or if they had chronic ulcerative colitis. Another 109 patients were excluded from evaluation postoperatively for incomplete resection (not R0 resection), surgical mortality (42 patients, 2.9%), or if they had unknown locoregional or metastatic disease at the final time of analysis (2006).

Intervention or Treatment Received   Over the treatment period, the surgeons implemented, during two different time periods, changes to their standardized approach to segmental colon resection of right and left colon cancers with complete mesocolic excision (CME).

Results   The concept of TME was applied to the analogous mesocolic planes that continue to the pelvis and are termed complete mesocolic excision (CME). Central to the technique of CME is sharp separation of the parietal and visceral fascia to expose the entire mesocolon with intact visceral fascia, adequately exposing the colon and intact mesocolon with its lymphovascular supply, thus allowing central ligation of the supplying arteries within 10 cm on either side of tumor. The technique emphasizes two important oncologic principles: (1) that of a preserved intact mesocolon, theoretically preventing microscopic tumor spillage, and (2) maximal lymph node harvesting through true central vascular ligation.

While the overall 5-year local recurrence rate was 4.9%, recurrence rates in colon cancer decreased from 6.5% in the period from 1978 to 1984 and again to 3.6% in 1995–2002 following application of complete mesocolic excision. Locoregional recurrence increased with increasing depth of invasion (pT) and increased number of metastatic lymph nodes (pN). (See Tables 34.1–34.3.)

TABLE 34.1   Cancer-Related Survival M0 R0 1978–2002 (5-year rates, n = 1329)

	n	Univariate Analysis			Multivariate Analysis		
		5-Year Survival	95% CI	p	Relative Risk	95% CI	p
All	1329	85.0	83.0–87.0				
pT1	118	98.0	95.3–100	<0.001	1.0		
pT2	186	99.5	98.5–100		1.2	0.3–4.9	0.782
pT3	851	82.9	80.4–85.4		5.7	1.8–17.9	0.003
pT4	174	70.6	63.5–77.7		7.8	2.4–25.6	0.001
pN0	831	93.7	91.9–95.5	<0.001	1.0		
PN1	319	81.1	76.6–85.6		2.1	1.5–2.9	<0.001
pN2	179	50.2	42.6–57.8		5.2	3.6–7.3	<0.001
Stage I	251	99.1	97.7–100	<0.001			
Stage II	580	91.4	89.0–93.8				
Stage III	498	70.2	66 1–74.3				
Low grade	1079	87.9	85.9–89.9	<0.001	1.0		
High grade	249	72.0	66.1–77.9		1.1	0.8–1.6	0.398
Grade unknown	1						
EVI –	1092	89.6	87.6–91.6	<0.001	1.0		

TABLE 34.1   Cancer-Related Survival M0 R0 1978–2002 (5-year rates, n = 1329)

	n	Univariate Analysis			Multivariate Analysis		
		5-Year Survival	95% CI	p	Relative Risk	95% CI	p
EVI +	177	61.9	54.5–69.3		1.7	1.2–2.3	0.003
EVI unknown	60						
No intraoperative TCD	1300	85.2		0.057			
Intraoperative TCD	29	75.0					
≥28 rln examined	824	86.1	83.7–88.5		1.0		
<28 rln examined	505	83.1	79.8–86.4	0.144	1.9	1.4–2.5	<0.001
Elective surgery	1219	86.8	84.8–88.8	<0.001	1.0		
Emergency presentation		83.6	74.0–93.2		1.9	1.3–2.7	<0.001
1995–2002	404	89.1	86.0–92.2		1.0		
1985–1994	514	84.1	80.8–87.4		1.2	08–1.8	0.414
1978–1984	411	82.1	78.4–85.8	0.039	1.2	0.8–1.7	0.285

Source: EVI, extramural venous invasion; TCD, tumor cell disseminations; rln, regional lymph nodes.

TABLE 34.2   Locoregional Recurrence M0 R0 1978–2002 (5-year rates, n = 1329)

	n	5-Year-LR	95% CI
All	1329	4.9	3.7–6.1
pT1	118	0.9	0–2.7
pT2	186	1.2	0–2.8
pT3	851	5.2	3.6–6.8
pT4	174	10.7	5.8–15.6
pN0	831	1.5	0.7–2.3
pN1	319	6.5	3.6–9.4
pN2	179	20.7	13.8–27.6
Stage I	251	0.4	0–1.2
Stage II	580	2.0	0.8–3.2
Stage III	498	11.1	8.2–14.0
1978–1984	411	6.5	4.0–9.0
1985–1994	514	4.6	2.6–6.6
1995–2002	404	3.6	1.6–5.6

In the same period, the cancer-related 5-year survival rates in patients resected for cure increased from 82.1% to 89.1%. Overall survival of all patients was 85%. Five-year survival rates varied significantly among surgeons. pT, pN, extramural venous invasion, and emergency presentation were found to be independent prognostic factors for cancer-related survival on a univariate analysis.

There was a 20% complication rate, with 4.7% reoperation rate. Anastomotic leak occurred in 2.6% of the patients. The complication rate increased to 34.4% in patients undergoing emergency surgery, which constituted 9.5% of all patients. Postoperative mortality of all causes in hospital, irrespective of patient stay was 3.1%. Additionally, there was significant intersurgeon variability with the rate of complications from 11.7% to 35.5%.

Lymph node harvest was evaluated as a secondary end point. Median number of lymph nodes evaluated was 32. After excluding extended resections, the best cutoff value for number of lymph nodes was analyzed using the Leblanc method and was determined to be 28. Statistically significant improvement in 5-year cancer-related survival from 90.7% to 96.3% was associated with 28 or more lymph nodes harvested.

The authors conclude that their data clearly indicate that, with modification of the technique with sharp dissection along embryologic planes and a standardized approach, quality and outcome indeed improve over time, with up to 97% ability to perform R0 resections.

Study Limitations Despite the limitation to surgeons with more than 25 CME operations performed for curative intent during the recruitment period, there was significant variability among surgeons, with rates of complications ranging from 11.7% to 35.5%. Though this may simply demonstrate variable technical skills among a surgical unit, it may be reflective of a more technical challenging operation with a longer learning curve and higher complication rate, thus affecting its applicability and widespread adoption. Multiple subsequent studies have revealed an increased complication rate associate with CME and with increased incident of SMA and SMV injuries, as well as a dramatic increase in respiratory complications thought to be associated with delayed gastric emptying emanating from a more radical dissection along the gastroepiploic arcade.

The rates of locoregional recurrence and cancer-related survival were analyzed during three time periods of treatment to emphasize improvements in outcome associated with evolution in the standardization, implementation, and auditing of the surgical technique. However, the changes between time intervals are subtle and not defined. One can assume there are a myriad of other confounding factors occurring over time, which could account for some of the improvements throughout three decades of cancer care and which are not attributable to the surgical technique alone.

Lastly, the majority of the patients in the study predated the standard use of adjuvant chemotherapy in Germany (1995), which has significantly increased survival. Modern treatment algorithms including neoadjuvant chemotherapy and immunotherapy may render the effects of more aggressive surgical treatment less applicable.

Relevant Studies   To date, all studies evaluating CME in right-sided colon cancer are retrospective in nature; however, currently five actively recruiting randomized controlled trials intend to compare long-term oncologic outcomes. The landmark paper on CME by Hohenberger reported excellent cancer-specific survival rates after CME surgery (stage I, 99.1%; stage II, 91.4%; and stage III, 70.2%). Historic patient control groups were used for comparison, leaving the possibility of other factors to account for the survival benefits, including significant intersurgeon variability. However, the evidence demonstrating improved survival with superior dissection and intact mesocolic excision is undeniable.

Gao et al. presented 3-year outcomes of a prospective nonrandomized study including 330 patients (220 CME and 110 non-CME). They reported a significant increase in median lymph node yield, area of excised mesentery and distance from vascular tie to tumor in both right-sided and left-sided tumors. Although the 3-year overall survival was similar, CME significantly increased 3-year local recurrence free survival.[1]

In another study from Italy, Zurleni et al. compared their results before and after the implementation of CME for right colon cancer in 2010 (97 CME vs. 95 non-CME patients). Their analyses showed a significant increase in both overall and disease-specific survival at 3 years among patients with stages I, II, and III disease. Multivariate analysis concluded that CME was an independent predictive factor for 3-year disease-free survival. Surgeries were performed by an open approach.[2]

Wang et al. performed a systematic review and meta-analysis of 12 studies and 8586 patients who underwent either CME or conventional surgery for colon cancer. This meta-analysis also reported a significantly increased length of colonic segment, distance from tumor to vascular tie, and resected mesenteric area in favor of CME. Three- and 5-year overall survival and disease-free survival were increased in patients who underwent CME.[3]

Another systematic review and pooled analysis of 14 studies was recently published by Alhassan et al.[4] In their analysis, only two studies showed an increase in overall survival for stages I–III and stage III only, whereas five studies did not show a significant increase in overall survival. Disease-free or disease-specific survival was reported to be higher in 3 of six studies.

In the largest population-based study, Bertelsen et al. evaluated all patients undergoing colonic surgery during a 3.5-year period in validated centers in Denmark for stages I–III colon cancers [Union for International Cancer Control (UICC)], including left-sided tumors. The CME group consisted of 364 patients, and the non-CME group consisted of 1031 patients. The 4-year disease-free survival for patients with UICC stages II and III disease was superior in the CME group compared to the non-CME group (91.9%, 73.5% vs. 77.9%, 67.5%). Further analysis demonstrated disease-free survival was significantly higher after CME irrespective of stage following CME. Furthermore, CME surgery was a significant independent predictive factor for higher disease-free survival for all patients.[5]

Regarding the surgical approach, Negoi et al. performed a systematic review and meta-analysis of 12 studies comparing open versus laparoscopic CME.[6] They showed that laparoscopic surgery was associated with better 3-year overall and disease-free survival, although there was no difference in 5-year outcomes. Lymph node yield and distance from tumor to vascular tie were similar; however, area of resected mesentery was significantly larger in laparoscopic approach.

Potential benefits of CME must be carefully weighted against the potential increased risk of complications. Several series report a significant increase in postoperative complications.[7] In a series of 529 patients operated on in a CME-validated center in Denmark, 9 patients developed vascular injury to the superior mesenteric vein with two mortalities as a result.[8] They also report 1 case of postoperative perforation of the stomach and an additional case of gastric necrosis. However, the authors conclude that, despite the significantly higher risk of lesions in the SMV with CME procedure, there was no significant difference in the consequences of these lesions compared to the conventional right colectomy group that they compared against. Pulmonary complications were the overall most common nonsurgical complication. Bertelsen et al. also found a higher respiratory failure rate in their series, compared to the conventionally operated group (8.1% vs. 3.4%, $p < 0.001$), and overall higher postoperative morbidity with SMV injuries was noted as well.[9]

Bernes et al., from University of Bergen reported complications occurring in 47% of patients with severe complications (grades III and IV) in 15%.[7] Wang performed a meta-analysis including a total of 8586 patients from 12 studies. CME was associated with greater intraoperative blood loss [weighted mean difference (WMD) 79.87, 95% CI 65.88–93.86] and with more postoperative surgical complications. CME consistently results in significantly increased operative time. More unique complications compared to conventional right colectomy have also been described including pancreatic fistula and lymph leak with lymphorrea.[10] It is, therefore, unclear whether the benefits of removing more tissue outweigh the increased operating time and potential morbidity associated with these procedures by some surgeons.

Although CME has demonstrated impressive oncologic results with improved 3- and 5-year survival, its widespread adoption has been slowed by the increased technical challenge and fears of increased morbidity with minimal benefit.

There is no consensus on the routine implementation of CME due to the lack of prospective randomized controlled trials. However, currently, several randomized control trials comparing standard laparoscopic right colectomy to CME are accruing patients. The RELARC (Radical Extent of lymphadenectomy: D2 dissection versus complete mesocolic excision of LAparoscopic Right Colectomy) trial in Beijing, China is a prospective, multicenter, randomized controlled trial that will provide evidence on the optimal extent of lymphadenectomy during laparoscopic right colectomy in terms of better oncological outcome and operation safety. The COLD trial, recruiting patients in Russia, is a multicenter randomized controlled trial assessing the superiority of 5-year overall survival as the primary end point in patients undergoing D3 lymph node dissection versus D2 dissection. The UK is similarly evaluating the technique with the CME versus standard right hemicolectomy trial.

REFERENCES

1. Gao Z, Wang C, Cui Y, et al. Efficacy and safety of complete mesocolic excision in patients with colon cancer: Three-year results from a prospective, nonrandomized, double-blind, controlled trial. Ann Surg. 2018.
2. Zurleni T, Cassiano A, Gjoni E, et al. Surgical and oncological outcomes after complete mesocolic excision in right-sided colon cancer compared with conventional surgery: a retrospective, single-institution study. Int J Colorectal Dis. 2018;33:1–8.
3. Wang C, Gao Z, Shen K, et al. Safety, quality and effect of complete mesocolic excision vs non-complete mesocolicexcision in patients with colon cancer: a systemic review and meta-analysis. Colorectal Dis. 2017;19(11):962–72.
4. Alhassan N, Yang M, Wong-Chong N, et al. Comparison between conventional colectomy and complete mesocolic excision for colon cancer: a systematic review and pooled analysis: A review of CME versus conventional colectomies. Surg Endosc. 2019;33:8–18.
5. Bertelsen CA, Neuenschwander AU, Jansen JE, et al. Disease-free survival after complete mesocolic excision com-pared with conventional colon cancer surgery: a population-based study. Lancet Oncol. 2015;16:161–8.
6. Negoi I, Hostiuc S, Negoi RI, et al. Laparoscopic vs open complete mesocolic excision with central vascular ligation for colon cancer: A systematic review and meta-analysis. World J Gastrointest Oncol. 2017;9:475–91.
7. Storli KE, Sondenaa K, Furnes B, et al. Outcome after introduction of complete mesocolic excision for colon cancer is similar for open and laparoscopic surgical treatments. Dig Surg. 2013;30:317–27.
8. Kirkegaard-Klitbo A, Goegenur I, Bertelsen CA. Severe complications related to central vascular resection: complete mesocolic resection vs traditional resection. J Am Coll Surg. 2015;221(4):e66.

9. Bertelsen CA, Neuenschwander AU, Jansen JE, et al. Short-term outcomes after complete mesocolic excision compared with "conventional" colonic cancer surgery. Br J Surg. 2016;103:581–9.

10. Wang Y, Zhang C, Zhang D, et al. Clinical outcome of laparoscopic complete mesocolic excision in the treatment of right colon cancer. World J Surg Oncol. 2017;15:174.

CHAPTER 35

Prevention of Colorectal Cancer by Colonoscopic Polypectomy

Winawer SJ, Zauber AG, Ho MN, et al. NEJM. 329:1977–1981, 1993

Reviewed by W. Donald Buie and Anthony R. MacLean

Research Question/Objective   Although it was generally accepted that colonic polyps should be removed when detected and the colon should be examined for additional polyps in follow-up, there was no proof of concept that adenomatous polyps were the precursor for colorectal cancer and that removal would prevent colorectal cancer. The aim of this trial was to investigate whether endoscopic polypectomy reduced the incidence of colorectal cancer.

Study Design   A randomized controlled trial regarding the timing of surveillance intervals after colonoscopic polypectomy was conducted in 7 participating centers. Following an index polypectomy, patients were randomized to colonoscopies at years 1 and 3 or to a single colonoscopy at year 3. The primary outcome was the incidence of colorectal cancer over the study period. As it was unethical to randomize patients to colonoscopic removal versus observation, 3 published retrospective cohorts from the precolonoscopy era were used as controls to establish the expected incidence of colorectal cancer: Mayo Clinic (1965–1970), St. Marks Hospital (1957–1980), and general population SEER data (1983–1987). The calculated incidence of colorectal cancer in the study group was compared with the observed incidence in the 3 reference groups matched for age, sex, and polyp size.

Sample Size   A total of 1418 patients were enrolled; 993 were men (70%) with a mean age of 61+/−10 years range (22–88 years). At the time of enrollment, 494 (35%) had adenomas larger than 1 cm and 137 (10%) had adenomas with high-grade dysplasia. Most patients (92%) had been referred for symptoms or a positive screening or diagnostic test.

Follow-Up   Complete follow-up occurred in 97% of patients: 1210 until the end of the study and 169 until death at an average of 5.9 years.

Inclusion/Exclusion Criteria   Inclusion criteria included complete colonoscopy between November 1980 and February 1990 with all identified polyps removed and one or more documented adenoma(s). Exclusion criteria included family or personal history of FAP, IBD, a previous polypectomy, or colorectal cancer. Patients were excluded after index colonoscopy if they

DOI: 10.1201/9780429285714-35

did not have a polyp, had a nonadenomatous polyp, a malignant polyp, a sessile adenoma greater than 3 cm in diameter, or a colorectal cancer.

Intervention or Treatment Received   Following colonoscopic polypectomy, patients were randomized to either colonoscopy at year 1 and year 3 (frequent) or once at year 3 (less frequent). All patients had yearly phone contact with the study team, completed a questionnaire, yearly FOBT, and were offered a follow-up colonoscopy at year 6.

Results   Five asymptomatic early-stage cancers (malignant polyps) were detected at follow-up colonoscopy; 3 at 3 years, 1 at 6 years, and 1 at 7 years. No patient had a symptomatic cancer or died of colorectal cancer. The cumulative incidence of colorectal cancer for the study cohort and the reference groups is shown in Figure 35.1. The observed incidence of colorectal cancer per 1000 person-years was 0.6 in the study cohort, whereas the expected incidence was 5.8 (Mayo Clinic), 5.2 (St. Mark's), and 2.5 (SEER).

Regardless of index adenoma size at enrollment, the incidence of colorectal cancer was lower than expected. In the subgroup of patients with large adenomas, the observed and expected numbers of colorectal cancers were 3 and 40.2, respectively, for a standardized incidence of 0.07 (95% CI 0.02 to 0.22). In the subgroup with small to medium-sized adenomas, 2 cancers were observed, and 8.1 were expected for a standardized incidence ratio of 0.25 (95% CI 0.03 to 0.89).

The following conclusions were drawn:

1. CRC could be prevented by colonoscopic removal of all identified adenomatous polyps.

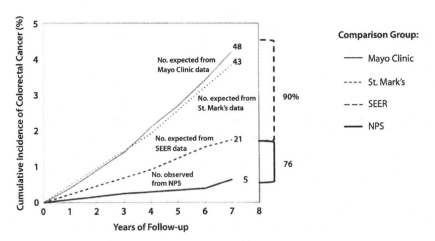

Figure 35.1   Cumulative colorectal cancer incidence in the National Polyp Study (NPS) cohort. (*Source:* From Winawer SJ, Zauber AG, Ho MN, et al. Prevention of colorectal cancer by colonoscopic polypectomy. N Engl J Med 1993;329(27):1977–1981. Reprinted with permission.)

2. The data supported the adenoma to adenocarcinoma sequence.
3. Surveillance intervals following polypectomy could be safely increased from 1 to 3 years as there was no difference in the accumulated percentage of patients with advanced adenomas, whether they were detected with frequent or less frequent surveillance (RR = 1.0; 95% CI 0.5 to 2.2).
4. Following polypectomy, patients with advanced adenomas at baseline had a greater colorectal cancer risk reduction than those with early adenomas (1).

Study Limitations   For ethical reasons, patients were randomized postpolypectomy and compared to a control group made up of 3 retrospective cohorts eliminating the risk conferred to patients in an observation arm. The incidence of cancer in the study cohort was lower than the observed rates in each of the 3 independent control groups, increasing the confidence in the observed results.

The optimum surveillance interval could not be determined, only that it could be lengthened from 1 to 3 years without increasing the incidence of advanced adenomas. Participating endoscopists would not accept an interval longer than 3 years and insisted on yearly FOBT.

The original cohort was not large enough to use death as an outcome measure; thus the question of whether polypectomy could reduce the risk of death from colorectal cancer could not be answered. There was no data on adenoma detection rates or withdrawal time, important quality assurance measures in screening colonoscopy. Serrated adenomas were not yet described and thus could not be used as a measure of quality. Given improvements in techniques and instrumentation, particularly the optical quality of current-generation colonoscopes, one would expect greater risk reductions in the screened population at the present time.

The incidence of missed lesions was not well described in the literature. Technical limitations meant that smaller polyps and some flat adenomas may have been missed, potentially contributing to the misidentification of early polyp growth and possibly to the early cancers that were found. The authors conducted a sensitivity analysis by excluding the total number of at-risk person-years during the first 2 years of follow-up, to account for missed polyps that would develop into early cancers. Although the recalculated differences between the experimental and control groups were smaller (66–86%), they were still significant. Currently, better optics and standardized colonoscopy techniques should result in improved polyp clearance.

Large, advanced adenomas were recognized as higher-risk polyps and were excluded from the trial; so no conclusions could be made regarding an appropriate surveillance interval. In addition, there were not enough data to make any recommendations regarding Lynch syndrome as only 1% of the population had 3 or more first-degree relatives with colorectal cancer.

Relevant Studies   The National Polyp Study (NPS) was the first prospective study to examine the effect of colonoscopic polypectomy on the incidence of colorectal cancer and the efficacy and safety of less intense colonoscopic surveillance. The 75–90% reduction after an average follow-up of 5.9 years supported the concept of the adenoma-to-carcinoma sequence. Consequently, it had a significant influence on clinical practice supporting the safety of a 3-year interval for screening colonoscopy. Subsequent data suggested that low-risk patients could safely undergo surveillance colonoscopy at a 5-year interval and more recently at 5–10 years, conserving resources and reducing the overall costs of screening (2–6).

The NPS data also demonstrated that patients could be categorized into low and high risk for the development of advanced adenomas according to the pathology of their baseline adenoma (1, 7). NPS data were used to support changes to the 2003 screening colonoscopy guidelines, which recommended risk stratification: Patients with low-risk polyps were recommended to have their first surveillance colonoscopy in 5 years (8) based on the low rates of advanced adenomas in subsequent surveillance colonoscopies at 1, 3, and 6 years. Patients with high-risk adenomas were recommended to have surveillance colonoscopy at 3 years based in part on the higher risk of CRC in this population. Recent data suggest that the surveillance interval should be based more on the findings of the first interval colonoscopy in addition to the initial one (6, 9).

Serrated polyps were not described at the time of this study, and it was unclear whether they should be followed like conventional adenomas. Subsequent studies have shown that small serrated polyps (<10 mm) have a low risk of developing into advanced adenomas or CRC and thus do not require close follow-up, whereas larger serrated polyps and those with dysplasia have a higher risk of subsequent high-risk lesions and thus merit closer follow-up, currently a 3-year repeat colonoscopy (10).

While the original study looked at colonoscopy to increase early detection, it also raised the possibility of expanding to prevention. Unfortunately, the original numbers were too small to determine whether screening would prevent death from CRC. However, long-term follow-up with comparison to matched SEER data demonstrated a 53% risk reduction in CRC mortality over a median period of 15.8 years (Figure 35.2) (11).

Randomized controlled trials have confirmed that population screening with colonoscopy is effective (12, 13). An additional question is how much screening is needed and for how long, which has a significant effect on resource utilization and cost-effectiveness (14). The greatest impact now seems to be from the first polypectomy rather than the surveillance itself (15, 16), and screening recommendations are changing to reflect this.

The NPS data also addressed familial risk following adenoma removal in probands. A follow-up retrospective cohort study using NPS data assessed the

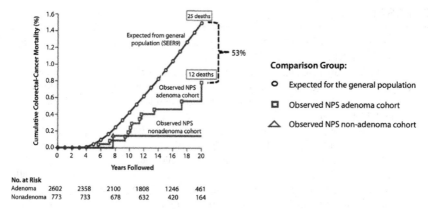

Figure 35.2 Cumulative colorectal cancer mortality of colorectal cancer in the National Polyp Study (NPS) cohort of adenoma patients compared with the incidence-based mortality of the Surveillance, Epidemiology and End Results (SEER) and with a cohort with no adenomas. (*Source:* From Zauber, AG, Winawer SJ, O'Brien MJ, et al. Colonoscopic polypectomy and long-term prevention of colorectal-cancer deaths. N Engl J Med 2012;366:687–696. Reprinted with permission.)

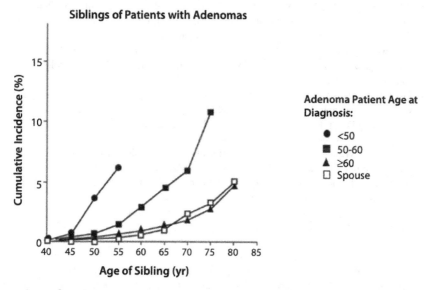

Figure 35.3 Cumulative incidence of colorectal cancer in siblings of adenoma patients by age of diagnosis of adenomas of the national polyp study proband. *Source:* From Winawer SJ, Zauber AG, Gerdes H et al. Risk of colorectal cancer in families of patients with adenomatous polyps. N Engl J Med 1996;334:82–87. Reprinted with permission.

risk of CRC in a cohort of siblings and parents versus a cohort of spouses. The cumulative risk was increased for siblings and parents of the probands compared with spouses (controls), especially when the adenoma was diagnosed in the proband before the age of 60 (Figure 35.3) (17). These data confirmed results from previous studies (18, 19).

REFERENCES

1. Winawer SJ, Zauber AG, Ho MN, et al. Prevention of colorectal cancer by colonoscopic polypectomy. NEJM 1993;329:1977–81.
2. Winawer SJ, Zauber AG, Fletcher RH, et al. Guidelines for colonoscopy surveillance after polypectomy: a consensus updated by the US Multi-society Task Force on Colorectal Cancer and the American Cancer Society. Gastroenterology 2006;130:1872–85.
3. Levin B, Lieberman DA, McFarland B, et al. Screening and surveillance for the early detection of colorectal cancer and adenomatous polyps, 2008; a joint guideline from the American Cancer Society, the US Multisociety Task Force on Colorectal Cancer and the American College of Radiology. CA Cancer J Clin 2008;58:130–60.
4. Lieberman DA, Rex Dk, Winawer S, et al. Guidelines for colonoscopy surveillance after screening and polypectomy: a consensus update by the US Multi-society Task Force on Colorectal Cancer. Gastroenterology 2012:143:844–57.
5. Rex DK, Boland CR, Dominitz JA, et al. Colorectal cancer screening recommendation for physicians and patients from the US Multi Society task Force on Colorectal Cancer. Gastroenterology 2017;153:307–23.
6. Gupta S, Lieberman D, Anderson JC, et al. Recommendations for follow-up after colonoscopy and polypectomy: a consensus update by the US Multi-society Task Force on Colorectal Cancer. Am J Gastroenterol 2020;115:415–34.
7. Winawer SJ, Zauber AG, O'Brien MJ, et al. Randomized comparison of surveillance intervals after colonoscopic removal of newly diagnosed adenomatous polyps. The National Polyp study workgroup. N Engl J Med 1993;328:901–6.
8. Winawer S, Fletcher R, Rex D, et al. Colorectal cancer screening and surveillance: clinical guidelines and rationale-update based on new evidence. Gastroenterology 2003;124:544–60.
9. Jover R, Bretthauer M, Dekker E, et al. Rationale and design of the European polyp surveillance EPoS trials. Endoscopy 2016;48:571–8.
10. He X, Hang D, Wu K, et al. Long-term risk of colorectal cancer after removal of conventional adenomas and serrated polyps. Gastroenterology 2020;158(4):861.
11. Zauber AG, Winawer SJ, O'Brien MJ, et al. Colonoscopic polypectomy and long-term prevention of colorectal-cancer deaths. N Engl J Med 2012;366:687–96.
12. Bretthauer M, Løberg M, Wieszczy P, et al. Effect of colonoscopy screening on risks of colorectal cancer and related death. N Engl J Med 2022;387:1547–56.
13. Dominitz JA, Robertson DJ. Understanding the results of a randomized trial of screening colonoscopy. N Engl J Med 2022;387:1609–11.
14. Aronsson M, Carlsson P, Levin L-A, et al. Cost-effectiveness of high sensitivity fecal immunochemical test and colonoscopy screening for colorectal cancer. BJS 2017;104:1078–86.
15. Zauber A, Winawer S, Loeve F, et al. Effect of initial polypectomy versus surveillance polypectomy on colorectal cancer incidence reduction: microsimulation modeling of National Polyp Study Data. Gastroenterology 2000;A187:1200.
16. Meester RGS, Lansdorp-Vogelaar I, Winawer SJ, et al. High-intensity versus low-intensity surveillance for patients with colorectal adenomas: a cost-effectiveness analysis. Ann Intern Med 2019;171:612–22.
17. Winawer SJ, Zauber AG, Gerdes H. Risk of colorectal cancer in the families of patients with adenomatous polyps. NEJM 1996;334;82–7.
18. Fuchs CS, Giovannucci EL, Colditz GA, et al. A prospective study of family history and the risk of colorectal cancer. N Engl J Med 1994;331:1669–74.
19. St John DJ, McDermott FT, Hopper JL, et al. Cancer risk in relatives of patients with common colorectal cancer. Ann Intern Med 1993;118:785–90.

CHAPTER 36

Survival after Laparoscopic Surgery versus Open Surgery for Colon Cancer: Long-Term Outcome of a Randomised Clinical Trial (COLOR Trial)

Colon Cancer Laparoscopic or Open Resection Study Group, Buunen M, Veldkamp R, Hop WCJ, Kuhry E, Jeekel J, Haglind E, Påhlman L, Cuesta MA, Msika S, Morino M, Lacy A, Bonjer, HJ. Lancet Oncol. 10(1):44–52, 2009

Reviewed by Tarik Sammour

Research Question/Objective   At the time that the study was conducted, the equivalence of laparoscopic surgery for colon cancer had not yet been established. The aim of the COlon cancer Laparoscopic or Open Resection (COLOR) trial was to compare 3-year disease-free survival and overall survival after laparoscopic and open resection of solitary colon cancer (1).

Study Design   This was a randomized controlled multicenter noninferiority trial (not blinded) conducted at 29 participating hospitals in 8 European countries. Randomization was stratified by participating center and type of resection, and analysis was performed as intention-to-treat. Power calculation was based on disease-free survival 3 years after surgery (estimated as 75%). The prespecified noninferiority margin was set at 7% with a *P*-value < 0.025 (one-sided test), requiring accrual of 1200 patients at a power of 80%.

Sample Size   Between March 1997 and March 2003, 1248 patients were randomly assigned to either open surgery (*n* = 621) or laparoscopic surgery (*n* = 627). After randomization, 172 patients were excluded, leaving 1076 patients eligible for analysis, and they were assigned to open surgery (*n* = 542) or laparoscopic surgery (*n* = 534).

Follow-Up   Median follow-up in the laparoscopic group of 52 months (SD 17.0; range 0.03–60) and in the open-surgery group of 55 months (SD 17.0; 0.03–60).

DOI: 10.1201/9780429285714-36

Inclusion/Exclusion Criteria

Inclusion Criteria

- Patients with colon cancer
- Aged 18 years or older
- Provided written informed consent
- Solitary adenocarcinoma
- Localized in the caecum, ascending colon, descending colon, or sigmoid colon above the peritoneal reflection
- Eligible for random assignment to either laparoscopic or open surgery

Exclusion Criteria

- Body mass index (BMI) greater than 30 kg/m²
- Distant metastases
- Acute intestinal obstruction
- Multiple primary tumors of the colon
- Transverse colon or splenic flexure adenocarcinomas
- A scheduled need for synchronous intra-abdominal surgery
- Preoperative evidence of invasion of adjacent structures, as assessed by CT, MRI, or ultrasonography
- Previous ipsilateral colon surgery
- Previous malignancies (except adequately treated basocellular carcinoma of the skin or *in situ* carcinoma of the cervix)
- Absolute contraindications to general anesthesia and a long-term pneumoperitoneum

Intervention or Treatment Received   Laparoscopic-assisted colonic resection in the study arm and open colonic resection in the control arm. All surgical teams had done at least 20 laparoscopically assisted colectomies before entering the trial. An unedited videotape of a laparoscopic colectomy was submitted to the trial investigators for assessment.

Results   The procedure was converted to open surgery in 102 of 534 patients assigned to undergo laparoscopic surgery [19% (95% CI 16–20)]. Laparoscopic surgery took longer than open surgery 202 min (140–315) versus 170 min (113–255), $P < 0.001$ but was associated with less blood loss 100 ml (19–410) versus 175 ml (40–500), $P\ 0.003$. Otherwise, there were no differences in complication rates, cancer stage, resection margins, nodal harvest, adjuvant therapy use, or short-term mortality.

There was no difference in 3-year disease-free or overall survival, but the p-value for noninferiority did not meet the predetermined significance level of 0.025 on intention-to-treat analysis. However, in a per-protocol analysis, laparoscopic surgery was deemed noninferior.

Study Limitations   A limitation of this study is the exclusion of patients with a BMI greater than 30 kg/m² and transverse colon cancers, which limits the generalizability of the results to those patient groups (which are not uncommon). The investigators were also not blinded, which may have introduced some bias in data collection and analysis. Despite the methods focusing on intention to treat, the authors conducted a per-protocol analysis and used this to justify noninferiority in the discussion and conclusion. Due to the multicenter nature of the study, consistency and robustness of enhanced recovery protocols could not be assured. Funding was provided by industry (Ethicon Endo-Surgery, Hamburg, Germany), which represents possible conflict of interest bias as this company could potentially stand to gain financially from the adoption of laparoscopic surgery.

Relevant Studies   The most pertinent study to discuss is the subsequent publication of 10-year outcomes arising from the Dutch subset of this dataset (2). Out of the 1248 patients randomized, 256 Dutch patients were eligible for 10-year analysis. Disease-free survival rates were 45.2% in the laparoscopic group and 43.2% in the open group (CI −10.3 to 14.3, $P = 0.96$). Overall survival rates were 48.4 and 46.7 %, respectively (CI −10.6 to 14.0, $P = 0.83$). This confirmed the long-term oncological safety in this subgroup of patients with high-quality prospective data.

Three other notable large multicenter RCTS were conducted in parallel with the COLOR trial. These were the COST trial (3), MRC-CLASICC (4), and the ALCCaS trial (5) in North America, the UK, and Australasia, respectively. All three trials have published long-term survival data demonstrating equivalence between laparoscopic and open colonic surgery. Furthermore, MRC-CLASICC presented quality of life data showing no difference between groups, while ALCCaS demonstrated some short-term quality of life benefits to laparoscopic surgery out to 2 months postoperatively, including measures of appetite, insomnia, pain, fatigue, bowel, daily living, and overall health (6).

An early meta-analysis, focusing on intraoperative complications and using statistical methods that compensated for a low event rate, raised concern that there was a higher total intraoperative complication rate (OR 1.37, $P = 0.010$) and a higher rate of bowel injury in the laparoscopic group (OR 1.88, $P = 0.020$). However, these small differences in relatively infrequent intraoperative complications did not translate into a higher overall complication rate, which was similar between groups.

A Cochrane review comparing long-term results of laparoscopic versus open colorectal cancer resection was published and last updated in 2008 and included 12 RCTs with 3346 patients (7). No differences were found in cancer-related mortality after laparoscopic surgery compared to open surgery for colon cancer [5 RCTs, 1575 pts, 14.6% vs. 16.4%; OR (fixed) 0.80; CI 0.61–1.06, $P = 0.15$]. There was also no significant difference in recurrence rate (HR 0.86; CI 0.70–1.08). The review concluded that laparoscopic resection colon adenocarcinoma is associated with a long-term outcome no different from that of open colectomy but that further studies are required on incisional hernias and clinically significant adhesions (7). This specific meta-analysis was done and published by Udayasiri et al. in 2020, including 6 randomized studies and 9 nonrandomized comparative studies with a total of 84,172 patients. They showed decreased odds of developing incisional hernia in the laparoscopic group (OR 0.79; CI 0.66–0.95, $P = 0.01$) but no difference in requirement for surgery (OR 1.07; CI 0.64–1.79, $P = 0.79$). Similarly, there were decreased odds of developing adhesional intestinal obstruction in the laparoscopic cohort (OR 0.81; CI 0.72–0.92, $P = 0.001$) but no difference in requirement for surgery (OR 0.84; CI 0.53–1.35, $P = 0.48$). Another updated survival meta-analysis, published in 2014, further supported the results of the Cochrane review (8).

In general, laparoscopic surgery for colon cancer is now accepted standard care for most patients in the absence of contraindications, and, to allow this to happen, the COLOR trial was one major piece of the data generation puzzle by providing robust level 1 evidence in a European cohort.

REFERENCES

1. Colon Cancer Laparoscopic or Open Resection Study G, Buunen M, Veldkamp R, Hop WC, Kuhry E, Jeekel J, et al. Survival after laparoscopic surgery versus open surgery for colon cancer: long-term outcome of a randomised clinical trial. Lancet Oncol. 2009;10(1):44–52.
2. Deijen CL, Vasmel JE, de Lange-de Klerk ESM, Cuesta MA, Coene PLO, Lange JF, et al. Ten-year outcomes of a randomised trial of laparoscopic versus open surgery for colon cancer. Surg Endosc. 2017;31(6):2607–15.
3. Fleshman J, Sargent DJ, Green E, Anvari M, Stryker SJ, Beart RW, Jr., et al. Laparoscopic colectomy for cancer is not inferior to open surgery based on 5-year data from the COST Study Group trial. Ann Surg. 2007;246(4):655–62; discussion 62–4.
4. Green BL, Marshall HC, Collinson F, Quirke P, Guillou P, Jayne DG, et al. Long-term follow-up of the Medical Research Council CLASICC trial of conventional versus laparoscopically assisted resection in colorectal cancer. Br J Surg. 2013;100(1):75–82.
5. Bagshaw PF, Allardyce RA, Frampton CM, Frizelle FA, Hewett PJ, McMurrick PJ, et al. Long-term outcomes of the Australasian randomized clinical trial comparing laparoscopic and conventional open surgical treatments for colon cancer: the Australasian Laparoscopic Colon Cancer Study trial. Ann Surg. 2012;256(6):915–9.
6. McCombie AM, Frizelle F, Bagshaw PF, Frampton CM, Hewett PJ, McMurrick PJ, et al. The ALCCaS Trial: A Randomized Controlled Trial Comparing Quality of Life Following Laparoscopic Versus Open Colectomy for Colon Cancer. Dis Colon Rectum. 2018;61(10):1156–62.
7. Kuhry E, Schwenk WF, Gaupset R, Romild U, Bonjer HJ. Long-term results of laparoscopic colorectal cancer resection. Cochrane Database Syst Rev. 2008;2008(2):CD003432.
8. Theophilus M, Platell C, Spilsbury K. Long-term survival following laparoscopic and open colectomy for colon cancer: a meta-analysis of randomized controlled trials. Colorectal Dis. 2014;16(3):O75–81.

CHAPTER 37

Colon Cancer Survival Is Associated with Increasing Number of Lymph Nodes Analyzed: A Secondary Survey of Intergroup Trial INT-0089

Le Voyer TE, Sigurdson ER, Hanlon AL, et al. Journal of Clinical Oncology. 21(15):2912–2919, 2003

Reviewed by Niket H. Shah, Andrew G. Hill, and Primal P. Singh

Research Question/Objective   The presence of metastases to surrounding regional lymph nodes in colon cancer is one of the most important prognostic factors for overall survival. However, the number of lymph nodes that are recovered during surgical resection and subsequently undergo pathologic examination varies, and it is unclear whether this in itself has an impact on patient survival. The aim of this study was to evaluate whether the number of lymph nodes retrieved and subsequently analyzed for staging from surgical specimens affects survival in patients with colon cancer.

Study Design   This study was a secondary analysis of a large randomized controlled trial (INT-0089) of adjuvant chemotherapy in patients with stages II and III colon cancer. The initial trial enrolled and randomized patients from 1988 to 1992 into four different chemotherapy regimens. There was no difference in survival between the groups, thus allowing for further analyses to be conducted on the trial cohort as one group. This study analyzed the relationship between number of lymph nodes removed at surgical resection and survival. The primary end point was overall survival, with secondary end points being cause-specific survival and disease-free survival.

Sample Size   A total of 3759 patients were entered into the INT-0089 trial, of which 3561 met the inclusion and exclusion criteria. For this study, 3411 patients had relevant data available for analysis.

Follow-Up   Overall median follow-up was 79 months (6.6 years). Follow-up after completion of chemotherapy in the original INT-0089 trial consisted of regular clinical assessment and blood tests. This was 3-monthly in the first year, then 6-monthly for the next 4 years, after which annual assessment was conducted. Routine investigations conducted were a chest radiograph every 6 months, and either proctoscopy and barium enema or a colonoscopy at the 6- and 12-month marks and then subsequently every 2 years.

DOI: 10.1201/9780429285714-37

Inclusion/Exclusion Criteria   To be eligible for the initial trial, patients needed to have histological proof of colon adenocarcinoma and to have undergone curative surgical resection with no evidence of residual disease. Patients had to have nodal involvement (Dukes C) or a Dukes B2 tumor (into or through serosa) with evidence of perforation or obstruction. Exclusion criteria included any evidence of distant metastases, concurrent radiation, or chemotherapy, concurrent second malignancy, or previous malignant tumor within the past 3 years and major medical illness making them ineligible for protocol chemotherapy. Patients were also excluded if the gross inferior margin was at or below the peritoneal reflection as they were considered to have rectal cancer.

Intervention or Treatment Received   Standard surgical resection was carried out for all patients with the type of surgical procedure varying depending on location of primary tumor in the colon (Table 37.1).

Results

Study Demographics   The study population was divided into node-positive and node negative groups. The node-positive group consisted of 2763 patients, and as per the AJCC tumor node metastases (TNM) classification system, 1857 patients were classified as N1 and 906 patients as N2 disease. There were no significant differences in baseline demographics of age, gender, and median number of lymph nodes between the node-positive and node-negative groups.

Overall Survival   Overall survival improved as the number of lymph nodes recovered increased in the node-positive group, for both N1 and N2 disease, and also in the node-negative group. In N2 patients with more than 35 lymph nodes recovered, overall survival was shown to improve by 20% at 5 years and by 28% at 8 years compared to N2 patients with a lower number of lymph nodes recovered. For N1 patients with more than 40 lymph nodes recovered, there was an absolute survival improvement of 16% at 5 years and 26% at 8 years compared

TABLE 37.1 Operations Performed for Node-Positive and Node-Negative Groups

Operation Performed	Node-Positive (*n* = 2763)	Node-Negative (*n* = 648)
Right hemicolectomy	1199 (43%)	276 (42%)
Left hemicolectomy	375 (14%)	106 (16%)
Anterior resection	368 (13%)	47 (7%)
Segmental resection	583 (21%)	134 (21%)
Subtotal colectomy	83 (3%)	41 (6%)
Total colectomy	42 (2%)	5 (1%)
Other	113 (4%)	39 (6%)

to patients in whom 11–40 lymph nodes were recovered, and an improvement of 23% at 5 years and 34% at 8 years compared to when 1–10 lymph nodes were recovered. In the node-negative group, more than 20 lymph nodes recovered improved overall survival by 14% and 20% at 5 years and 8 years, respectively, compared to when only 1–10 lymph nodes were recovered.

Cause-Specific Survival   Similar to overall survival, cause specific survival also improved significantly in both node-positive and node-negative groups when more lymph nodes were recovered at surgery.

Disease-Free Survival   This was shown to have absolute improvement in the node-positive group, for both N1 and N2 patients; however, there was no significant difference in the node-negative group as lymph nodes recovered at surgery increased.

Study Limitations   By nature of this study being a secondary analysis of the original INT-0089 trial, it was not specifically designed to evaluate the effect that lymph node retrieval has on survival in colon cancer. The surgical procedures undertaken were not standardized across the included centers and variations in operative technique, along with many other potential confounders, may have a significant effect on this study's analyses. Further, it is likely that, with increasing number of lymph nodes examined, a stage migration effect occurred.

The authors of this study discuss multiple techniques pathologists can employ to maximize the number of lymph nodes examined which was another factor not standardized and may be dependent on the individual pathologist. This may lead to differences in the number of nodes examined between patients, independent of the completeness of the surgical excision.

Hence, this study cannot determine whether recovery of more lymph nodes itself improves survival or if it is perhaps a surrogate marker for improved colon cancer care. This encompasses improved quality of surgical resection, which can be related to multiple factors including surgeon and hospital volumes (1, 2), pathologic assessment, and adjuvant chemotherapy.

Finally, this study only evaluated patients that were primarily high-risk and did not include patients without poor prognostic indicators. This limits the generalizability of this study's results, in particular, it is unclear whether lower risk stage 2 patients, that would not usually be offered chemotherapy, also have an improved survival from increased lymph node recovery numbers.

Relevant Studies   The Working Party Report to the World Congresses of Gastroenterology in 1990 made a consensus recommendation that a minimum of 12 lymph nodes should be sampled to allow for adequate staging of colon cancer (3). Numerous studies since have also provided varying recommendations for the minimum number of lymph nodes required for accurate staging, ranging from 6 (4) to 17 (5).

This study's findings have been corroborated by a number of other studies and a systematic review, with some including all Dukes B patients in their analysis (6, 7). However, two studies showed no significant difference in survival as the number of lymph nodes recovered increased, but both these studies had a much lower threshold value for the number of lymph nodes recovered when conducting their analyses (8, 9).

Lymph node ratio (LNR), the ratio of positive nodes to the total number of nodes examined, has also been investigated by numerous studies as an indicator for prognosis and survival in colon cancer (10, 11). Berger et al. evaluated the prognostic significance of LNR in the same population as this study and showed that, as the LNR increases, survival decreases in stage III colon cancer (12).

Multiple studies have evaluated the factors in lymph node recovery and assessment (13, 14). Nathan et al. showed that among the modifiable factors, hospital level factors were the majority variable (74%), contributing to adequate number of lymph nodes assessed when compared to surgeon (8%) and pathologist factors (18%). Hospital-level factors included hospital volume, teaching hospitals, and treatment at a comprehensive cancer center (14).

REFERENCES

1. Harmon JW, Tang DG, Gordon TA, et al. Hospital volume can serve as a surrogate for surgeon volume for achieving excellent outcomes in colorectal resection. Ann Surg. 1999;230:403–4.
2. Ko CY, Chang JT, Chaudhry S, Kominski G. Are high-volume surgeons and hospitals the most important predictors of in-hospital outcome for colon cancer resection? Surgery. 2002;132:268–73.
3. Fielding LP, Arsenault PA, Chapuis PH, et al. Working report to the World Congresses of Gastroenterology, Sydney 1990. J Gastroenterol Hepatol. 1991;6:325–44.
4. Hernanz F, Revuelta S, Redondo C, Madrazo C, Castillo J, Gómez-Fleitas M. Colorectal adenocarcinoma: Quality of the assessment of lymph node metastases. Dis Colon Rectum. 1994;37:373–7.
5. Goldstein NS, Sanford W, Coffey M, Layfield LJ. Lymph node recovery from colorectal resection specimens removed for adenocarcinoma: Trends over time and a recommendation for a minimum number of lymph nodes to be recovered. Am J Clin Pathol. 1996;106:209–16.
6. Chang GJ, Rodriguez-Bigas MA, Skibber JM, Moyer VA. Lymph node evaluation and survival after curative resection of colon cancer: Systematic review. J Natl Cancer Inst. 2007;99:433–41.
7. Vather R, Sammour T, Zargar-Shoshtari K, Metcalf P, Connolly A, Hill A. Lymph node examination as a predictor of long-term outcome in Dukes B colon cancer. Int J Colorectal Dis. 2009;24:283–8.

8. Prandi M, Lionetto R, Bini A, et al. Prognostic evaluation of stage B colon cancer patients is improved by an adequate lymphadenectomy: Results of a secondary analysis of a large scale adjuvant trial. Ann Surg. 2002;235:458–63.
9. Caplin S, Cerottini JP, Bosman FT, Constanda MT, Givel JC. For patients with Dukes' B (TNM stage II) colorectal carcinoma, examination of six or fewer lymph nodes is related to poor prognosis. Cancer. 1998;83:666–72.
10. Vather R, Sammour T, Kahokehr A, Connolly AB, Hill AG. Lymph node evaluation and long-term survival in stage II and stage III colon cancer: A national study. Ann Surg Oncol. 2009;16:585–93.
11. Sjo OH, Merok MA, Svindland A, Nesbakken A. Prognostic impact of lymph node harvest and lymph node ratio in patients with colon cancer. Dis Colon Rectum. 2012;55:307–15.
12. Berger AC, Sigurdson ER, LeVoyer T, et al. Colon cancer survival is associated with decreasing ratio of metastatic to examined lymph nodes. J Clin Oncol. 2005;23:8706–12.
13. Moro-Valdezate D, Pla-Martí V, Martín-Arévalo J, et al. Factors related to lymph node harvest: Does a recovery of more than 12 improve the outcome of colorectal cancer? Color Dis. 2013;15:1257–66.
14. Nathan H, Shore AD, Anders RA, Wick EC, Gearhart SL, Pawlik TM. Variation in lymph node assessment after colon cancer resection: Patient, surgeon, pathologist, or hospital? J Gastrointest Surg. 2011;15:471–9.

CHAPTER 38

The Results of Cytoreductive Surgery and Hyperthermic Intraperitoneal Chemotherapy in 1200 Patients with Peritoneal Malignancy

Moran B, Cecil K, Chandrakumaran K, et al. Colorectal Dis. 17(9):772–778, 2015

Reviewed by Christopher T. Aquina

Research Question/Objective   While randomized controlled trial data supported the use of cytoreductive surgery (CRS) and hyperthermic intraperitoneal chemotherapy (HIPEC) for appendiceal and colorectal cancer compared with systemic therapy alone in appropriately selected patients, concerns remained regarding perioperative morbidity and long-term survival. The primary aim of this study was to evaluate the outcomes of 1200 consecutive patients who underwent laparotomy for peritoneal surface malignancy at a single high-volume center over a 20-year period.

Study Design   This study was a retrospective cohort study of prospectively collected data at a single English National Peritoneal Malignancy Center that included consecutive patients who underwent a primary laparotomy based on a goal of CRS and HIPEC for a presumed or confirmed peritoneal malignancy between March 1994 and January 2014. Outcome measures included completeness of cytoreduction, postoperative hospital morbidity and mortality, overall survival, and disease-free survival. The rates of completeness of cytoreduction, morbidity, and mortality were compared over time, and overall survival and disease-free survival were compared by histopathological diagnosis.

Sample Size   This study identified 2956 patients referred for a suspected or confirmed diagnosis of peritoneal malignancy. Of these patients, a consecutive series of 1200 patients who underwent a laparotomy were selected. Patients were taken for surgery if complete macroscopic tumor removal was considered likely or for palliation of symptoms.

Follow-Up   The patients were followed up to 5 years with annual computed tomography imaging and tumor marker assessment or at shorter intervals if clinically indicated. Short-term outcomes included completeness of cytoreduction, postoperative morbidity, and postoperative mortality, and long-term outcomes included overall and disease-free survival.

DOI: 10.1201/9780429285714-38

Inclusion/Exclusion Criteria   The study included the first 1200 consecutive patients to undergo a laparotomy for presumed or confirmed peritoneal malignancy of appendiceal, colorectal, mesothelial, ovarian, or other origin with a goal of complete macroscopic tumor removal. No patients were excluded.

Intervention or Treatment Received   For patients in which complete cytoreduction of macroscopic tumors or maximal tumor debulking was achieved, HIPEC was administered at 42° C for 1 hour utilizing an open abdominal perfusion technique with mitomycin C for appendiceal or colorectal peritoneal metastases or a combination of doxorubicin and cisplatin for peritoneal mesothelioma or ovarian cancer. For those in which maximal tumor debulking was not possible, laparotomy and biopsy were performed.

Results

Histopathological Diagnosis   The proportion of patients by primary cancer site and quartile of the study period were recorded. There was an increase in the proportion of patients with colorectal cancer peritoneal metastases from the first quartile (3%) to the fourth quartile (12.3%), while there were decreases in the proportion of patients with appendiceal cancer (82.3% vs. 75.3%), peritoneal mesothelioma (6.7% vs. 5.7%), and other malignancies (8% vs. 6.7%).

Completeness of Cytoreduction   There were 2956 patients referred for proven or suspected peritoneal malignancy between March 1994 and January 2014. Of the 1200 patients who underwent a laparotomy during that time period, 863 (71.9%) achieved complete cytoreduction, 294 (24.5%) underwent maximal tumor debulking, and 43 (3.6%) had a laparotomy and biopsy. There was an increase in the rate of complete cytoreduction from the first quartile to the fourth quartile of the study period from 60.7% to 80.3% with concomitant decreases in the rate of maximal tumor debulking from 32.9% to 18.4% and the rate of laparotomy and biopsy only from 6.4% to 1.3%.

Postoperative Morbidity and Mortality   The rate of a grade III/IV Clavien–Dindo complication decreased from 13.7% to 6.7% in the first quartile compared with the fourth quartile, and the mortality rate decreased from 3% to 0.7%.

Overall and Disease-Free Survival   While no statistical analyses comparing survival by histopathological diagnosis were performed, overall survival and disease-free survival graphs were presented as figures. Among patients that underwent complete cytoreduction, it appears that overall and disease-free survival were similar among patients with appendiceal cancer or peritoneal mesothelioma with long-term overall survival achieved in approximately 70% of patients, whereas patients with colorectal cancer peritoneal metastases who underwent complete cytoreduction had worse overall and disease-free survival. Among those that underwent maximal tumor debulking, approximately 10% of patients with peritoneal metastases from appendiceal cancer achieved long-term overall survival of ≥10 years, whereas no patients with peritoneal mesothelioma or colorectal cancer peritoneal metastases survived beyond 72 months and 36 months, respectively.

Study Limitations   The retrospective design is a limitation of the study. Important patient factors that may affect outcomes, such as age, sex, race, comorbidity burden, socioeconomic status, peritoneal carcinomatosis index (PCI), and receipt of systemic therapy, were not reported. While the study included the largest series of patients with peritoneal malignancy who underwent surgery to date, there have been improvements in the efficacy of systemic therapy over the 20-year study period that have likely affected long-term overall and disease-free survival. Furthermore, the study was limited to a single, high-volume peritoneal surface malignancy center in England. Therefore, the study results may not be generalizable to patient populations treated at other centers or in other regions. Finally, no statistical analyses comparing outcomes between groups were performed.

Relevant Studies   Prior to this study, the landmark randomized clinical trial by Verwaal et al. published in 2003 demonstrated a median overall survival benefit for CRS and HIPEC compared with systemic therapy alone (22.3 months vs. 12.6 months, $p = 0.03$) in the treatment of appendiceal and colorectal cancer peritoneal metastases [1]. However, CRS and HIPEC remained controversial given the high morbidity and mortality of the operation. This study by Moran et al. demonstrated that CRS and HIPEC can be performed safely with a low rate of morbidity and mortality and can confer long-term survival in patients who achieve complete cytoreduction at an experienced, high-volume center. These findings are similar to that of a study by Foster et al. in which the authors compared the morbidity and mortality of CRS/HIPEC with other high-risk surgical oncology procedures using data from the American College of Surgeons National Surgical Quality Improvement Program [2]. Morbidity, including return to the operating room, superficial incisional infection, deep incisional infection, and organ space infection, was similar or lower following CRS/HIPEC, and the postoperative 30-day mortality rate was lower for CRS/HIPEC (1.1%) compared with pancreaticoduodenectomy (2.5%), right hepatectomy (2.9%), esophagectomy (3.0%), and trisegmental hepatectomy (3.9%).

While CRS has become the standard of care in appropriately selected patients with peritoneal metastases from appendiceal, colorectal, and ovarian neoplasms and peritoneal mesothelioma where optimal cytoreduction can be achieved, the use of HIPEC remains controversial for colorectal cancer. The recent PRODIGE-7 trial attempted to answer the question regarding the efficacy of HIPEC for colorectal cancer peritoneal metastases following cytoreduction to <1 mm residual tumor tissue [3]. Patients with a PCI ≤ 25 were randomly assigned to CRS alone or to CRS and HIPEC with a bidirectional approach utilizing intravenous fluoruracil followed by intraperitoneal oxaliplatin at 43° C for 30 minutes. The authors observed no difference in overall survival between the two groups. However, the study had several major limitations. First, the choice of perfusing intraperitoneal oxaliplatin for 30 minutes for HIPEC was questionable as the standard duration for HIPEC perfusion at most centers is 90–100 minutes, and many institutions utilize mitomycin C rather than oxaliplatin. Second, the study population was heavily pretreated, with 83% of patients having received preoperative systemic therapy, and many of the patients had already received oxaliplatin-based systemic therapy, raising concerns regarding selection bias and oxaliplatin resistance in the study population. While the study suggests that CRS and HIPEC with intraperitoneal oxaliplatin administered over 30 minutes is not beneficial, the question regarding the efficacy of HIPEC with other intraperitoneal chemotherapy agents and/or perfused over a longer duration of time in combination with optimal cytoreduction remains unanswered in the treatment of colorectal cancer peritoneal metastases. However, given the median overall survival of >41 months for patients who underwent CRS ± HIPEC in the PRODIGE-7 trial compared with 12–16 months for those who received systemic therapy alone in other clinical trials, the combination of CRS ± HIPEC and modern systemic therapy is clearly efficacious and is the only treatment strategy that currently offers the possibility of long-term survival for patients with colorectal cancer peritoneal metastases (1, 4).

REFERENCES

1. Verwaal VJ, van Ruth S, de Bree E, et al. Randomized trial of cytoreduction and hyperthermic intraperitoneal chemotherapy versus systemic chemotherapy and palliative surgery in patients with peritoneal carcinomatosis of colorectal cancer. J Clin Oncol. 2003;21(20):3737–43.
2. Foster JM, Sleightholm R, Patel A, et al. Morbidity and mortality rates following cytoreductive surgery combined with hyperthermic intraperitoneal chemotherapy compared with other high-risk surgical oncology procedures. JAMA Netw Open. 2019;2(1):e186847.
3. Quenet F, Elias D, Roca L, et al. Cytoreductive surgery plus hyperthermic intraperitoneal chemotherapy versus cytoreductive surgery alone for colorectal peritoneal metastases (PRODIGE 7): a multicenter, randomised, open-label, phase 3 trial. Lancet Oncol. 2021;22(2):256–66.
4. Franko J, Shi Q, Meyers JP, et al. Prognosis of patients with peritoneal metastatic colorectal cancer given systemic therapy: an analysis of individual patient data from prospective randomised trials from the Analysis and Research in Cancers of the Digestive System (ARCAD) database. Lancet Oncol. 2016;17(12):1709–19.

Genetic Alterations during Colorectal-Tumor Development

Vogelstein B, Fearon ER, Hamilton SR, et al. N Engl J Med. 319(9):525–532, 1988

Reviewed by Fadwa Ali and Emina Huang

Research Question/Objective The development of colorectal cancer is a multistep process that entails the accumulation of genetic mutations resulting in the transition from adenomas to carcinomas. Several studies have identified mutations that are common in colorectal carcinomas. However, the sequence of genetic alterations that results in tumor progression is not well understood. The authors aim to study colorectal tumors of different stages including adenomas, advanced adenomas, and carcinomas to identify genetic alterations that result in development of colorectal cancer.

Study Design This was a retrospective analysis of colorectal tumor specimen representing various stages of neoplastic development. DNA samples were analyzed for 4 genetic alterations (ras gene mutations and allelic deletions of chromosomes 5, 17, and 18). Allelic deletions in chromosome 5 have been previously linked to familial adenomatous polyposis.

Sample Size The authors analyzed 172 colorectal tumor specimens. Of that total, 167 of the specimens were obtained from surgical resections performed at the Johns Hopkins Hospital through the Bowel Tumor Working Group, and 5 from hospitals in Atlanta, Georgia, through the National Disease Research Interchange. The specimens consisted of 40 predominantly early-stage adenomas from 7 patients with familial adenomatous polyposis, 40 adenomas (19 without associated foci of carcinoma and 21 with such foci) from 33 patients without familial polyposis, and 92 carcinomas resected from 89 patients.

Classification of Adenomas The adenomas were divided into 3 distinct classes. The first group (class I) consists of 40 adenomas from 7 patients with familial adenomatous polyposis. These were small tubular adenomas with low-grade dysplasia. The other two groups came from patients without familial adenomatous polyposis. Class II adenomas consisted of 19 lesions that had not progressed to invasive cancer. Class III adenomas consisted of 21 or more adenomas with foci of adenocarcinomas. The three classes of adenomas represent different stages of neoplasia with size, villous component, and dysplasia increasing from class I to class III.

Follow-Up Not applicable.

DOI: 10.1201/9780429285714-39

Inclusion/Exclusion Criteria   Not applicable.

Intervention or Treatment Received   Not applicable.

Results

Ras Gene Mutations Mutations in the ras protooncogene were found in 47% of carcinomas. About 88% of these mutations were in the K-ras gene. Class II and III adenomas contained ras mutations as frequently as did carcinomas. Only 13% of class I adenomas contained mutations in the ras gene. Of the adenomas larger than 1 cm in size, 58% had mutations in the ras gene compared to only 9% of smaller adenomas.

Allelic Deletions on Chromosome 5q, Spanning the Region Linked to Familial Adenomatous Polyposis In class I adenomas from patients with polyposis, none had an allelic loss from chromosome 5q. Allelic loss of several probes from chromosome 5q were observed more commonly in more advanced tumors: 29% in class II or III adenoma. Of carcinomas, 36% had lost a chromosome 5 allele.

Allelic Deletions on Chromosome 18 Allelic deletions within chromosome 18 were seen in 73% of carcinomas. Deletions were also frequently seen in class III adenomas (47%). Deletions on chromosome 18 were less frequently seen in class I and II adenomas (13% and 11%, respectively).

Allelic Deletions on Chromosome 17 Allelic deletions of chromosome 17 were seen in 75% of 60 colorectal carcinomas. These deletions were uncommon in adenomas.

Timing and Interrelations of Genetic Alterations Unlike mutations in ras gene and 5q allelic deletions, there was a statistically significant difference in the prevalence of chromosome 17p allelic deletion between colorectal carcinomas and any class of adenoma. Allelic deletions of chromosomes 17p and 18q were uncommon in class I and II adenomas. Allelic loss of chromosome 18 occurred in almost half of class III adenomas. Allelic deletions of chromosome 17p were relatively uncommon even in these advanced adenomas. These results suggest that ras gene mutations and allelic deletion on chromosome 5q occur in the early stages of neoplasia. They often occurred earlier than allelic deletions of chromosome 18, which in turn preceded allelic deletions of chromosome 17p. When looking collectively at the 4 genetic alterations tested in the study (ras gene mutation or allelic deletion on chromosome 5, 17, or 18), the progressive accumulation of genetic limitations becomes apparent. Only 9% of class I adenomas had more than 1 of the 4 somatic genetic alterations that were tested in the study. This is in striking contrast to carcinomas, where 90% of them had undergone two or three genetic alterations. Class II and III adenomas had an intermediate level of alterations where 24% of class II adenomas and 43% of class III adenomas accumulated two or more of the four alterations.

Study Limitations   The main limitation of the study is the relatively small sample size. The heterogeneity of the polyps in size, villous component, and dysplasia can cause confounding. Detection of allelic deletions from small adenomas can also be challenging.

Relevant Studies   Various tumors have been linked to allelic deletions of one specific gene or chromosome. This includes the RB-1 gene in retinoblastoma, chromosome 11 in Wilms tumor, BRCA-1, or BRCA-2 mutations in breast cancer. In contrast, this study shows that allelic deletions occur on 2 or more chromosomes in most colorectal cancers. In fact, a comprehensive analysis of mutations of colorectal tumors by the Cancer Genome Atlas Network has revealed that colorectal tumors have one of the highest tumor mutational burdens.[1] This is the first study to investigate genetic alteration at various stages of colorectal tumor development and provides a model for colorectal tumorigenesis in which sequential genetic mutations result in progression of adenomas to carcinomas.[2] In this model, the mutational activation of an oncogene, ras gene, coupled with mutational inactivation of tumor suppressor genes that reside on chromosomes 5, 17, and 18 result in tumorigenesis. While these genetic alterations happen in a sequential fashion, the summation of changes is more important than the order at which these genetic changes occur.

An interesting finding from the study is that adenomas from patients with familial adenomatous polyposis did not harbor allelic deletions on the long arm in chromosome 5, which has been linked to the disease. This contrasts with class II and III adenomas where 29% of tumors in patients without polyposis harbored allelic deletions in chromosome 5. This led to an alternate hypothesis for tumorigenesis different from the hypothesis that inherited neoplastic syndromes are the result of mutations in tumor suppressor genes, where the two alleles must be inactivated before a tumor arises. The authors propose that the fap gene locus on chromosome 5 plays a role in negative regulation of cell proliferation. When the gene is inactivated via the loss of one allele, this results in accelerated cell proliferation even if the other allele is normal. The result is the epithelial hyperproliferation that precedes the formation of adenomas. Allelic loss or loss of heterozygosity in the APC gene has been shown to increase in frequency from early adenomas to carcinomas.[3] Mutations in the APC gene have been seen in adenomas as small as 5 mm, which verifies their demonstration early in the adenoma-to-carcinoma sequence.[4]

The authors conclude that mutations in the ras oncogene occur early in the process of colorectal tumorigenesis. However, mutations in the ras gene may not be the first genetic alterations as small and early-stage adenomas often do not harbor mutations in this gene. In one study of genetic alterations in adenomatous polyps, the APC gene was found to be highly associated with dysplasia, and mutations in the APC gene were present in over 80% of polyps with dysplasia.[5] K-ras mutations were present equally in dysplastic and nondysplastic polyps. All dysplastic polyps that harbored a K-ras mutation also had an APC mutation, which shows that K-ras mutations are not sufficient to induce dysplasia.[5]

In this study, allelic deletions in the short arm of chromosome 17 were seen frequently in carcinomas but infrequently in earlier tumors. We now know the p53 gene is on the short arm of chromosome 17 and is the gene most altered in all human cancers. Mutations in p53 gene have been identified in 4–26% of adenomas, 50% of adenomas with foci of invasive carcinoma, and 50–75% of invasive cancer.[6] These cumulative results have led to the belief that inactivation of the p53 gene is responsible for the transition from adenoma to carcinoma.

Allelic loss on the long arm of chromosome 18 is very common in colorectal carcinomas. It is present in about 70% of colorectal cancers.[7] Numerous efforts have been made to try to identify target genes on chromosome 18q, and 2 potential genes were detected.[6,7] The initial candidate for the tumor suppressor gene was the DCC gene, deleted in the colorectal cancer gene. However, there have been several cases with 18q deletions and no inactivation of the DCC gene, implying the involvement of another gene. Another candidate gene is the SMAD4 gene, which was detected on 18q21.1 and which is mutated in about 35% of colorectal cancers. Allelic deletions of 18q and SMAD mutations are more common in stage IV colon cancer compared to other stages. They have also been associated with worse prognosis in stage III patients.[7]

The chromosomal instability model of colorectal carcinogenesis has been verified in different studies.[8] Understanding the adenoma-to-carcinoma sequence in colorectal cancer has been key in establishing colonoscopy screening guidelines that aim to decrease risk of colorectal cancer by detection and elimination of adenomatous/precancerous polyps. Identification of the molecular pathway to colorectal cancer can lead to development of new diagnostic tools. The Cologuard test combines detection of K-ras mutations and hypermethylation of promotor regions, in addition to detecting blood in the stool using an immunological assay to screen for colorectal cancer.[9] Blood assays for tumor-associated DNA markers are currently being developed and validated. Quantification of circulating tumor cells or cell-free tumor DNA (ctDNA) can be used to monitor treatment response and to detect recurrence and is a promising area of investigation.[10] Understanding genetic alterations can also provide some prognostic information and can also aid in the development of targeted therapy. Knowledge of the mutational status of KRAS, NRAS, and BRAF genes has been essential in determining choice and sequence of therapy in patients with stage IV disease. More evidence has emerged since the publication of the study to support another alternative pathway to colorectal tumorigenesis that includes mutations in mismatch repair genes resulting in microsatellite instability. The interplay between different mechanisms of tumorigenesis and the coexistence of genetic abnormalities can explain the heterogeneity of colorectal cancer. Understanding the interaction between genomic instability, tumor microenvironment, and other external environmental factors needs to be advanced. As we continue to learn more about the pathogenesis of colorectal cancer, more diagnostic and therapeutic approaches will arise.

REFERENCES

1- Cancer Genome Atlas Network. Comprehensive molecular characterization of human colon and rectal cancer. Nature. 2012;487(7407):330–7.
2- Vogelstein B, Fearon ER, Hamilton SR, Kern SE, Preisinger AC, Leppert M, et al. Genetic alterations during colorectal-tumor development. N Engl J Med. 1988;319(9):525–32.
3- Miyaki M, Konishi M, Kikuchi-Yanoshita R, Enomoto M, Igari T, Tanaka K, et al. Characteristics of somatic mutation of the adenomatous polyposis coli gene in colorectal tumors. Cancer Res. 1994;54(11):3011–20.
4- Powell SM, Zilz N, Beazer-Barclay Y, Bryan TM, Hamilton SR, Thibodeau SN, et al. APC mutations occur early during colorectal tumorigenesis. Nature. 1992;359(6392):235–7.
5- Jen J, Powell SM, Papadopoulos N, Smith KJ, Hamilton SR, Vogelstein B, et al. Molecular determinants of dysplasia in colorectal lesions. Cancer Res. 1994;54(21):5523–6.
6- Leslie A, Carey FA, Pratt NR, Steele RJ. The colorectal adenoma-carcinoma sequence. Br J Surg. 2002;89(7):845–60.
7- Tanaka T, Watanabe T, Kazama Y, Tanaka J, Kanazawa T, Kazama S, et al. Chromosome 18q deletion and Smad4 protein inactivation correlate with liver metastasis: A study matched for T- and N- classification. Br J Cancer. 2006;95(11):1562–7.
8- Nguyen LH, Goel A, Chung DC. Pathways of colorectal carcinogenesis. Gastroenterology. 2020;158(2):291–302.
9- Imperiale TF, Ransohoff DF, Itzkowitz SH, et al. Multitarget stool DNA testing for colorectal-cancer screening. N Engl J Med. 2014;370:1287–97.
10- Church TR, Wandell M, Lofton-Day C, et al. Prospective evaluation of methylated SEPT9 in plasma for detection of asymptomatic colorectal cancer. Gut. 2014;63:317–25.

CHAPTER 40

Hereditary Factors in Cancer: Study of Two Large Midwestern Kindreds

Lynch HT, Shaw MW, Magnuson CW, Larsen AL,
Krush AJ. Arch Intern Med. 117(2):206–212, 1966

Reviewed by David B. Stewart

Research Question/Objectives   At the time this manuscript was published, knowledge of human genetics and the genetic basis of cancer were in their infancy. The medical community was aware of familial clustering of various benign and malignant conditions prior to this report, but at the time of this paper's publication the mode of inheritance for Lynch Syndrome was not clear. In their own words, the authors' purpose was "to present the findings in two large midwestern kindreds in which a high frequency of particular histological types of malignant neoplasms involving a large variety of anatomical sites was found."

Study Design   This was a case series involving two large families that cancer researchers were aware of, given their high incidence of various malignancies. One family was in Nebraska (referred to as "Kindred N") and the other family was located in Michigan (referred to as "Kindred M"). While in both families the propositus (the initial subject presenting with the condition of interest) was studied, questionnaires were also sent to all adult members of each family to inquire about their personal cancer histories. Questionnaires also included requests for permission to contact family members' primary and consulting providers, hospitals, and local and state departments for retrieving vital statistics and other health information. When feasible, complete histories and physicals were performed and, when appropriate, pelvic and proctosigmoidoscopic examinations were undertaken. Histology slides were reviewed, and blood typing was performed when possible.

Sample size   The Kindred N pedigree included 40 cases of cancer, while the Kindred M pedigree revealed 18 individuals with cancer.

Follow-Up   The information was collected by the authors over the unspecified time during which they contacted members of each kindred. Family members were not followed longitudinally.

Inclusion/Exclusion Criteria   None were stated by the authors, consistent with a methodology that involved pedigree construction and retrospective records reviewed to identify all malignancies associated with two large families.

DOI: 10.1201/9780429285714-40

Intervention or Treatment Received   None.

Results   Kindred N was characterized by a 44-year-old proband with adrenocortical carcinoma. This family demonstrated a total of 40 cases of cancer distributed over 4 generations. The proband had 12 siblings, of which 6 developed cancers involving the lip, stomach, colon, endometrium, and kidney. Four family members developed multiple primary cancers involving combinations of colon and skin, uterus and ovary, stomach and colon, and cervix and colon. This family was also noted to have a strong history of diabetes, hypertension, obesity, arthritis, and anemia.

Kindred M was characterized by a 36-year-old proband who died from metastatic breast cancer. Their family was noted to have 18 members with cancer through three generations. Four members developed multiple primary cancers involving combinations of colonic, uterine, and ovarian malignancies, three primary colonic cancers, cancers of the pancreas and uterus, and cancers of the lip and colon. This family had a strong history of diabetes, hypertension, obesity, and rheumatoid arthritis.

Study Limitations   Case series are descriptive, and the information provided was limited to data provided by questionnaires completed by family members as well as the incomplete records regarding these kindreds.

Relevant Studies   This publication is the seminal report demonstrating that the hereditary condition that came to be known as Lynch Syndrome (after the first author) has a genetic basis and that the inheritance fits an autosomal dominant pattern. The methods of this manuscript are simple and straightforward; in a day predating electronic transmission of medical data, the effort required to gather family history and medical and health department data was a tour de force for its time.

From this initial recognition of a genetic basis for Lynch Syndrome, the medical community can trace two subsequent developments:

1. Investigations into the genetic variations associated with Lynch Syndrome, and the development of genetic testing that has expanded our understanding[1,2] of this syndrome.
2. Of the many arguments in favor of universal genetic testing,[3,4] the ability to provide genetic testing for Lynch Syndrome, the changes that a positive test introduces into a patient's screening and treatment, and the ability to test family members for the same genetic variant stem from the initial discovery in this manuscript.

REFERENCES

1. Maratt JK, Stoffel E. Identification of lynch syndrome. Gastrointest Endosc Clin N Am. 2022;32(1):45–48.

2. Buza N, Ziai J, Hui P. Mismatch repair deficiency testing in clinical practice. Expert Rev Mol Diagn. 2016;16(5):591–604.
3. O'Shea R, Rankin NM, Kentwell M, Gleeson M, Tucker KM, Hampel H, Taylor N, Lewis S. Stakeholders' views of integrating universal tumour screening and genetic testing for colorectal and endometrial cancer into routine oncology. Eur J Hum Genet. 2021;29(11):1634–1644.
4. Kim MH, Kim DW, Lee HS, Bang SK, Seo SH, Park KU, Oh HK, Kang SB. Universal screening for lynch syndrome compared with pedigree-based screening: 10-year experience in a Tertiary Hospital. Cancer Res Treat. 2022. doi:10.4143/crt.2021.1512.

CHAPTER 41

HPV Vaccine against Anal HPV Infection and Anal Intraepithelial Neoplasia

Palefsky JM, Giuliano AR, Goldstone S, et al.
N Engl J Med. 365(17):1576–1585, 2013

Reviewed by Timothy J. Ridolfi and Kirk A. Ludwig

Research Question/Objective   While it is known that the quadrivalent HPV (qHPV) vaccine is efficacious in preventing persistent cervical infection with HPV-6, -11, -16, or -18 and high-grade dysplasia associated with these infections, at the time of this study it was unclear whether this relationship would be maintained for anal dysplasia. Therefore, the authors evaluated the efficacy of a qHPV vaccine in preventing anal intraepithelial neoplasia (including condyloma) and anal cancer related to HPV-6, -11, -16, or -18 infection in men who have sex with men (MSM).

Study Design   This was a subset analysis of a larger multi-institutional double-blind placebo-controlled trial, designed and sponsored in collaboration with Merck. The primary efficacy objective was prevention of anal intraepithelial neoplasia or anal cancer related to infection with HPV-6, -11, -16, or -18. Efficacy was analyzed in both the intention-to-treat group (those receiving at least one dose of placebo or qHPV) and per-protocol group (those who were HPV 6, -11, -16, and -18 negative on day 1 through month 7 and did not have any protocol violations).

Sample Size   A subset of 602 subjects were identified from a cohort of 4065 men enrolled from September 3, 2004, to August 29, 2008. Men were enrolled in 7 countries (Australia, Brazil, Canada, Croatia, Germany, Spain, and the United States).

Follow-Up   Study participants were followed for a period of 36 months. HPV serologic samples were obtained on day 1 and month 7. At approximately 6-month intervals, anal examinations were completed, including anal cytology, HPV analysis, digital rectal examinations, and standard anoscopy. Any abnormal findings prompted a high-resolution anoscopy with biopsy. All participants underwent high-resolution anoscopy and biopsy of any visible lesions at the exit visit.

Inclusion/Exclusion Criteria   Inclusion to the study was limited by an age of 16 to 26 years, five or fewer lifetime sexual partners, and engagement in insertive or receptive anal intercourse or oral sex with another male within the past year. Exclusion criteria included a history or presence of clinically detectable anogenital warts or

206

DOI: 10.1201/9780429285714-41

genital lesions suggesting other sexually transmitted diseases or an intra-anal lesion on anoscopy consistent with anal intraepithelial neoplasia or condyloma. Participants found to be HIV-positive before the first day of the study were excluded from the trial. Participants diagnosed with HIV during the study were not withdrawn from the trial.

Intervention or Treatment Received Participants were randomized to either placebo or the qHPV vaccine in a 1:1 ratio.

Results Of the 602 men enrolled, 299 were vaccinated with qHPV and 299 with placebo. In total, 432 men completed the 36-month follow-up period. There were no significant demographic differences between the qHPV and placebo groups. Of the 598 participants who received at least 1 dose of vaccine or placebo, 194 qHPV-vaccine recipients and 208 placebo recipients were eligible for the per-protocol efficacy analysis. In the intention-to-treat population, vaccine efficacy against anal intraepithelial neoplasia due to any HPV type was 25.7% (95% CI −1.1 to 45.6). Efficacy against HPV-6, -11, -16, or -18–related anal intraepithelial neoplasia was 50.3% (95% CI 25.7 to 67.2). Significant reductions in both anal intraepithelial neoplasia of grade 1 (49.6%; 95% CI 21.2 to 68.4) and anal intraepithelial neoplasia of grade 2 or 3 (54.2%; 95% CI 18.0 to 75.3) were seen in the intention-to-treat population. Within the per-protocol group HPV-6, -11, -16, or -18–related anal intraepithelial neoplasia developed in 29 participants, five in the vaccine group and 24 in the placebo group, with an observed efficacy of 77.5% (95% CI 39.6 to 93.3). The vaccine was efficacious against both anal intraepithelial neoplasia of grade 1 (including condyloma) (73.0%; 95% CI 16.3 to 93.4) and anal intraepithelial neoplasia of grade 2 or 3 (74.9%; 95% CI 8.8 to 95.4). In summary, the qHPV vaccine is efficacious in reducing the anal intraepithelial neoplasia associated with HPV-6, -11, -16, or -18.

Study Limitations The study is limited by the narrow range of ages of the participants and the relatively short follow-up time. The study participants had limited sexual activity as compared with males of similar age or older.

Relevant Studies Anal cancer is biologically similar to cervical cancer, including a causal relationship with human papillomavirus (HPV) infection. Just as cervical cancer is preceded by cervical intraepithelial neoplasia, anal cancer is preceded by high-grade anal intraepithelial neoplasia.[1] In light of the similarities between anal cancer and cervical cancer, anal cancer prevention strategies have mirrored those of cervical cancer prevention. Rates of cervical cancer incidence and mortality have dramatically decreased in countries with programmatic screening for cervical cancer with cytology. As HPV infection is found in over 90% and 75% anal carcinoma cases among women and men, respectively,[2] there is interest in evaluating the effectiveness of HPV vaccination strategies in preventing anal cancer. The study highlighted in this chapter was the first to demonstrate that AIN, a precursor to anal cancer, was less common in those receiving qHPV vaccine in an MSM population. Additional work has been done investigating additional at-risk populations.

The population at highest risk for anal cancer is HIV+ MSM, and studies of the qHPV vaccine in this population are of great importance. Wilkin et al. evaluated 112 HIV+ men (ages 27+ with no evidence of AIN2+) with the 3-dose course of qHPV vaccine and found that all of these HIV+ men seroconverted.[3] Thus it appears that the qHPV vaccine is both immunogenic and safe in HIV+ men.

The effectiveness of the qHPV vaccine in preventing recurrent AIN2+ in older HIV-negative MSM was demonstrated by a retrospective nonconcurrent cohort study by Swedish et al.[4] Two-hundred and two patients over the age of 18 years, with a history of previously treated AIN2+, were divided into two groups: (1) vaccinated (88 patients; 44%), identified by 3 qHPV doses on their medical and billing records after treatment of AIN2+; and (2) unvaccinated (114; 56%), identified by a lack of qHPV vaccination in their medical and billing records. Among vaccinated patients, during 117.6 person-years of follow-up, 12 developed recurrent AIN2+ (95% CI 5.3–17.8/100 person-years), and among the unvaccinated patients during 222.8 person-years of follow-up, 35 developed recurrent AIN2+ (95% CI 10.9–21.0/100 person-years). According to a multivariate hazards model, qHPV vaccination was associated with a statistically significant decreased risk of recurrent AIN2+ regardless of oncogenic HPV status (HR 0.47; 95% CI 22–1.00; P D 0.5) for at least 3 years following vaccination.

Deshmukh et al. found that qHPV vaccination of HIV-negative MSM age 27+ treated for AIN2+ reduced the lifetime risk of anal cancer by 60.77% at an incremental increase of cost-effectiveness ratio of US$87,240 per quality-adjusted life year.[5] The results suggested that qHPV vaccination in HIV-positive MSM aged 27 years who have been diagnosed and treated for AIN2+ decreases the lifetime risk of anal cancer and is a cost-saving strategy as it decreases lifetime costs and increases quality-adjusted life expectancy.

Studies for AIN/anal cancer prevention were conducted with the qHPV vaccine as the nonavalent HPV (9vHPV) vaccine was not yet available. Joura et al. evaluated the safety and efficacy of the 9vHPV vaccine through a double-blind international multicenter trial of 14,215 young women randomized to 9vHPV vaccine or qHPV vaccine.[6] The investigators found that the 9vHPV vaccine prevented infection and disease related to HPV-31, -33, -45, -52, and -58 in a susceptible population and generated an antibody response to HPV-6, -11, -16, and -18 that was noninferior to that generated by the qHPV vaccine. From this data, it is assumed that the 9v HPV vaccine will provide the same degree of protection from persistent HPV infections and development of AIN2+ in patients without evidence of prior vaccine type HPV infection.

Recommendations for the timing of vaccine administration have varied since vaccine approval in 2007. Vaccination for men 9–26 years was approved by the CDC in 2009. In 2019, the United States Advisory Committee on Immunization

Practices guidelines were changed to include vaccination catchup for those up to age 26 and shared decision making for adults up to age 45 who have not had previous adequate vaccination, with a focus on those at risk for exposure.[7] The recommendation for catchup vaccinations for those 27–45 is not endorsed by the American Cancer Society citing low effectiveness and cancer prevention potential in this age group, the burden of decision making on patients and clinicians, and the lack of sufficient guidance on the selection of individuals who might benefit.[8] There is no specific guidance regarding HPV vaccination and the MSM population, although some would consider this group at risk for exposure.

REFERENCES

1. Hoots BE, Palefsky JM, Pimenta JM, Smith JS. Human papillomavirus type distribution in anal cancer and anal intraepithelial lesions. Int J Cancer 2009; 124:2375–83.
2. De Vuyst H, Clifford GM, Nascimento MC, Madeleine MM, Franceschi S. Prevalence and type distribution of human papillomavirus in carcinoma and intraepithelial neoplasia of the vulva, vagina and anus: a meta-analysis. Int J Cancer 2009; 124:1626–36.
3. Wilkin T, Lee JY, Lensing SY, Stier EA, Goldstone SE, Berry JM, Jay N, Aboulafia D, Cohn DL, Einstein MH, et al. Safety and immunogenicity of the quadrivalent human papillomavirus vaccine in HIV-1-infected men. J Infect Dis 2010; 202:1246–53.
4. Swedish KA, Factor SH, Goldstone SE. Prevention of recurrent highgrade anal neoplasia with quadrivalent human papillomavirus vaccination of men who have sex with men: a nonconcurrent cohort study. Clin Infect Dis 2012; 54:891–8.
5. Deshmukh AA, Chhatwal J, Chiao EY, Nyitray AG, Das P, Cantor SB. Long-term outcomes of adding HPV vaccine to the anal intraepithelial neoplasia treatment regimen in HIV-positive men who have sex with men. Clin Infect Dis 2015; 61:1527–35.
6. Joura EA, Giuliano AR, Iversen O-E, Bouchard C, Mao C, Mehlsen J, Moreira ED Jr, Ngan Y, Petersen LK, Lazcano-Ponce E, et al. A 9-valent HPV vaccine against infection and intraepithelial Neoplasia in Women. N Engl J Med 2015; 372(8):711–23.
7. Meites E, Szilagyi PG, Chesson HW, Unger ER, Romero JR, Markowitz LE. Human papillomavirus vaccination for adults: updated recommendations of the Advisory Committee on Immunization Practices. MMWR Morb Mortal Wkly Rep 2019; 68:698–702.
8. Saslow D, Andrews KS, Manassaram-Baptiste D, Smith RA, Fontham ETH, American Cancer Society Guideline Development Group. Human papillomavirus vaccination 2020 guideline update: American Cancer Society guideline adaptation. CA Cancer J Clin 2020; 70:274–80.

CHAPTER 42

Combined Preoperative Radiation and Chemotherapy for Squamous Cell Carcinoma of the Anal Canal

Nigro ND, Seydel HG, Considine B, Vaitkevicius VK, Leichman L, Kinzie, JJ. Cancer. 15:51(10):1826–1829, 1983

Reviewed by John T. Jenkins and Elaine M. Burns

Research Question/Objective   Prior to the publication of this seminal paper, patients diagnosed with anal squamous cell carcinoma (SCC) were managed surgically with abdominoperineal resection; a management strategy that was associated with high locoregional recurrence rates and poor 5-year survival. This paper shifted the paradigm of primary management of anal SCC, moving away from surgery to primary oncological treatment with chemoradiotherapy with surgery reserved for those patients requiring salvage following treatment. This paper reported the authors' expanded experience of patients managed with radiotherapy and chemotherapy.

Study Design   This was a retrospective single center cohort study of patients with anal SCC who underwent chemoradiation followed by abdominoperineal resection or excision of the scar.

Sample size   A total of 28 patients were included with no *a priori* sample size calculation.

Follow-Up   Patients had follow-up recorded to 9 years.

Inclusion/Exclusion Criteria   Biopsy-proven SCC of the anal canal involving the dentate line with no evidence of distant disease on physical examination, chest X-ray, laboratory studies, radioisotope scan of the liver and bones and CT head, abdomen and pelvis. All patients were considered candidates for abdominoperineal resection.

Intervention   Preoperative chemoradiation with intravenous 5-fluorouracil in 2 infusions lasting 96 hours each. The first infusion coincided with the start of radiotherapy, and the second infusion was 1 month later. Intravenous mitomycin C was included as a bolus. Radiotherapy was given at 2 Gy per day over 15 sessions (30 Gy total).

DOI: 10.1201/9780429285714-42

Results

Demographics   Lesions varied in size from 3 to 8 centimeters with most patients having a 4 centimeter lesion (11/28). Most patients had poorly differentiated tumors (12/28 patients), with a further 9 and 7 patients having well and moderately differentiated tumors, respectively. No further demographics are described.

Interventions   All patients underwent chemoradiation. The dose of chemotherapy was reduced after the first 5 patients owing to toxicity.

Outcome   Of the 28 patients, 24 patients had no gross evidence of tumor in the anal canal following chemoradiation. Four patients had clinical evidence of persistent tumor. Twelve patients underwent abdominoperineal resection. Fourteen patients had wide excision of the scar, and 2 patients had no interventions. Twenty-one of the 26 patients (81%) who underwent surgery had no identifiable tumor in the specimen. One patient had microscopic tumor only, and 4 had macroscopic tumor present in the specimens. The 2 patients who did not have surgery had no clinical evidence of tumor and refused surgery. One patient developed bilateral inguinal lymph node disease, which was treated at 1 year with further radiotherapy leading to clinical remission of the disease. One patient had inguinal lymph node metastasis at the time of diagnosis and underwent inguinal lymph node dissection with no evidence of disease on subsequent histopathology.

Six patients died during follow-up. Of these, 5 patients appeared to be related to squamous cell carcinoma. One patient died of cardiovascular causes. All patients who died had undergone abdominoperineal resection.

Study Limitations   This was a retrospective, nonrandomized cohort study amounting to a large case series. There were few data on the selection and exclusion criteria. Limited demographics of the included patients were described. Compliance with treatment was not reported. The impact of the change in chemotherapy regime that occurred during the study was also not described. Neither follow-up regimes nor the role of surveillance imaging was explained. Outcome was limited to mortality. There were no data on completeness of resection, morbidity, quality of life, or bowel, bladder, or sexual dysfunction. Data on local and distant recurrences were not described. The paper was published in 1983, and, as such, the limitations likely reflect the editorial style at the time of publication. Similar publications would now be subject to STROBE guidelines (1) and be expected to include a core outcome set such as CORMAC (2).

Relevant Studies   The earlier smaller study by Nigro and colleagues (3), alongside this paper published in 1983, prompted a paradigm shift in the management of anal SCC (4). This shift signified a move from primarily surgical treatment to reserving salvage surgery for those patients with persistent or recurrent disease following chemoradiation. With modification of chemoradiation protocols, randomized control trials have corroborated these initial cohort studies and demonstrated the safety and superiority of first employing a combined chemotherapy and radiation approach (5).

Randomised control trials comparing radiotherapy to combination chemotherapy and radiotherapy alongside the Nigro studies have established a chemoradiation first approach as the treatment gold standard (6, 7). The UKCCCR Anal Cancer Trial (ACT I) randomized 577 patients to receive radiotherapy alone or radiotherapy combined with 5-fluorouracil and mitomycin C (5). The addition of chemotherapy resulted in a significant reduction in locoregional relapse and improved relapse-free survival over radiotherapy alone. This management strategy has immensely improved outcomes for patients with anal SCC (8).

The next frontier in anal cancer management is to personalize treatment with escalation and de-escalation based upon the individual tumor. The results of ACT3, ACT4, ACT5 as part of the PLATO study are awaited (9). These studies aim to optimize treatment and reduce overtreatment in care. In addition, there is much excitement around the role of immunotherapy, having shown promising results in the management of other squamous cell cancers, for example, those that arise in the head and neck, in the management of squamous cell carcinoma. Although the response rates have not mirrored the exceptional results in mismatch repair-deficient rectal cancers (10), there have been encouraging findings in the management of programmed death-ligand 1 (PD- L1)–positive advanced tumors (11).

Without the change in mindset driven by the work of Nigro and colleagues, none of these advances would have been possible, and therefore this paper must be acknowledged for entirely changing the paradigm in anal squamous cell carcinoma management. This change has vastly improved the outcome for these patients over the last 50 years.

REFERENCES

1. von Elm E, Altman DG, Egger M, Pocock SJ, Gotzsche PC, Vandenbroucke JP, et al. The Strengthening the Reporting of Observational Studies in Epidemiology (STROBE) statement: guidelines for reporting observational studies. *Lancet*. 2007;370(9596):1453–7.
2. Fish R, Sanders C, Adams R, Brewer J, Brookes ST, DeNardo J, et al. A core outcome set for clinical trials of chemoradiotherapy interventions for anal cancer (CORMAC): a patient and health-care professional consensus. *Lancet Gastroenterol Hepatol*. 2018;3(12):865–73.
3. Nigro ND, Vaitkevicius VK, Considine B, Jr. Combined therapy for cancer of the anal canal: a preliminary report. *Dis Colon Rectum*. 1974;17(3):354–6.
4. Nigro ND, Seydel HG, Considine B, Vaitkevicius VK, Leichman L, Kinzie JJ. Combined preoperative radiation and chemotherapy for squamous cell carcinoma of the anal canal. *Cancer*. 1983;51(10):1826–9.
5. Epidermoid anal cancer: results from the UKCCCR randomised trial of radiotherapy alone versus radiotherapy, 5-fluorouracil, and mitomycin. UKCCCR Anal Cancer Trial Working Party. UK Co-ordinating Committee on Cancer Research. *Lancet*. 1996;348(9034):1049–54.

6. Stewart DB, Gaertner WB, Glasgow SC, Herzig DO, Feingold D, Steele SR, et al. The American society of colon and rectal surgeons clinical practice guidelines for anal squamous cell cancers (revised 2018). *Dis Colon Rectum.* 2018;61(7):755–74.

7. Rao S, Guren MG, Khan K, Brown G, Renehan AG, Steigen SE, et al. Anal cancer: ESMO clinical practice guidelines for diagnosis, treatment and follow-up(☆). *Ann Oncol.* 2021;32(9):1087–100.

8. Kim E, Kim JS, Choi M, Thomas CR, Jr. Conditional survival in anal carcinoma using the national population-based survey of epidemiology and end results database (1988–2012). *Dis Colon Rectum.* 2016;59(4):291–8.

9. Available from: www.isrctn.com/ISRCTN88455282.

10. Cercek A, Lumish M, Sinopoli J, Weiss J, Shia J, Lamendola-Essel M, et al. PD-1 blockade in mismatch repair-deficient, locally advanced rectal cancer. *N Engl J Med.* 2022;386(25):2363–76.

11. Marabelle A, Cassier PA, Fakih M, Kao S, Nielsen D, Italiano A, et al. Pembrolizumab for previously treated advanced anal squamous cell carcinoma: results from the non-randomised, multicohort, multicentre, phase 2 KEYNOTE-158 study. *Lancet Gastroenterol Hepatol.* 2022;7(5):446–54.

CHAPTER 43

Internal Sphincterotomy Is Superior to Topical Nitroglycerin in the Treatment of Chronic Anal Fissure: Results of a Randomized, Controlled Trial by the Canadian Colorectal Surgical Trials Group

Richard CS, Gregoire R, Plewes EA, Silverman R, Burul C, Buie D, Reznick R, Ross T, Burnstein M, O'Connor BI, Mukraj D, McLeod RS. Dis Colon Rectum. 43(8):1048–1058, 2000

Reviewed by William C. Cirocco

Research Question/Objective   This was a multicenter randomized, controlled trial comparing the effectiveness of topical nitroglycerin (NTG) versus lateral internal sphincterotomy (LIS) for the treatment of chronic anal fissure [1].

Study Design   Patients with symptomatic chronic anal fissure recruited from 9 Canadian university hospitals, from February 1997 to October 1998, were randomly assigned to 0.25% NTG applied 3 times daily versus LIS. Both groups received stool softeners and fiber supplements and were assessed at 6 weeks and 6 months. Healing was defined as complete re-epithelialization as determined by the surgeon. Continence was assessed by use of the Continence Index by Jorge and Wexner [2].

Sample Size   A total of 90 patients were accrued, but 8 were excluded from the analysis: 6 patients refused LIS after randomization; the anal fissure healed before operation in 1 patient; and anal fissure was not found at operation in 1 patient. Of 82 total patients, 44 patients (15 men) were in the NTG group, and 38 patients (22 men) in the LIS group.

Follow-Up   Both groups were assessed at 6 weeks, 6 months, and finally in a separate follow-up study at 6 years [3].

Inclusion/Exclusion Criteria   Patients with a painful chronic anal fissure located in the anterior or posterior midline location of the anus were included. Chronic

DOI: 10.1201/9780429285714-43

anal fissure was defined as exhibiting at least one of the following: fibrosis at the base of the fissure with exposed internal sphincter muscle fibers; hypertrophied anal papilla proximal to the fissure; or a sentinel pile (skin tag) distal to the fissure. On average, the fissure had been present for more than 2 years. Patients were excluded for the practice of anal intercourse, evidence of sepsis, underlying Crohn's disease, immunosuppression, or contraindication to the use of NTG.

Intervention or Treatment Received   Nonoperative treatment included NTG applied in a standardized fashion with a vaginal applicator 3 times daily (8 a.m., 12 p.m., and 5 p.m.) for 6 weeks. The topical NTG consisted of hydrous lanolin BP, white petroleum jelly BP, and 2% NTG ointment at a concentration of 0.5% for the first 11 patients, decreased to 0.25% for the remaining 33 patients because of headaches (using 0.25% NTG, nearly 80% of patients developed headaches and 20% had to discontinue use). Within 2 weeks of patient assignment to operation, LIS was performed by an experienced colorectal surgeon using the standard closed technique described by Notaras [4], without restriction as to type of anesthesia (local, regional, or general) or site of operation (office, clinic, or operating room).

Patients in both groups took psyllium seed and sodium docusate 100 mg twice daily for 6 weeks, starting on postoperative day 1 or the first day of nonoperative treatment for the topical NTG group. Both groups were assessed at 6 weeks, 6 months, and finally at 6 years in a separate follow-up study [3].

Results   At 6 weeks follow-up, 34 patients in the LIS group (89.5%) versus only 13 patients in the NTG group (29.5%) had complete healing of the anal fissure ($P = 5 \times 10^{-8}$). At 6 months follow-up, 35 patients in the LIS group (92.1%) versus only 12 patients in the NTG group (27.3%) had healed completely ($P = 3 \times 10^{-9}$). One patient in the LIS group (2.6%) required further surgery for a superficial fistula versus 20 patients in the NTG group (45.5%) who required LIS for persistent symptoms ($P = 9 \times 10^{-6}$). Nine patients discontinued NTG (20.5%) because of headaches (8 patients), and 1 patient for a severe syncopal episode (postural hypotension).

At 6 years follow-up, 51 (24 LIS patients, 27 NTG patients) of the original 82 patients (62%) completed a telephone survey at a mean follow-up of 79 (+/−1) months. LIS patients were less likely to have experienced fissure symptoms within the last year (0 vs. 41%, $P = 0.0004$) and were less likely to require subsequent surgical treatment (0 vs. 59%, $P < 0.0001$) than topical NTG patients. LIS patients were more likely than topical NTG patients to say that they were "very" or "moderately" satisfied with treatment (100 vs. 56%, $P = 0.04$), and more likely to choose the same treatment again (92 vs. 63%, $P = 0.02$).

Fecal Incontinence (FI) scores [2] deteriorated slightly from baseline to 6 years follow-up after both LIS and topical NTG. The FI score and Fecal Incontinence Quality of Life (FIQL) scale [5, 6] at 6-year follow-up were similar for both groups, even when considering the topical NTG for patients who subsequently underwent LIS for cure.

At 6 years follow-up, LIS provided a more durable cure for chronic anal fissure compared with topical NTG without compromise of long-term fecal continence resulting in a higher rate of patient satisfaction. Nearly 60% of patients randomized to topical NTG required LIS for cure, and nearly 40% would not undergo topical NTG treatment again. Considering the higher cure rate and superior overall patient satisfaction, LIS may appropriately be offered as first-line therapy for patients with chronic anal fissure.

Study Limitations   The study is limited by small sample size and the incomplete follow-up of patients originally enrolled in the trial. For instance, postoperative altered fecal continence, estimated conservatively at 5% for LIS, may not be demonstrable with a sample size of only 38 LIS patients. Indeed, FI was not encountered in the LIS group. Furthermore, only 16 of the 38 original LIS patients were women, a higher-risk group for postoperative FI following LIS, perhaps contributing to the insignificant difference in FI between the 2 groups. The limited length of follow-up of 6 months in the original study could have been a source of contention regarding the durability of results, however, the separate publication at 6 years follow-up allowed plenty of time for further assessment of FI to dispel these concerns [3].

Relevant Studies   The distinction between acute and chronic anal fissure is important without general consensus on the time range for symptoms (e.g., <8 weeks for acute anal fissure) as the sole determinant [7]. However, the stigmata of chronic anal fissure (hypertrophied anal papilla, external skin tag, and exposed internal sphincter fibers at the base of the fissure) are *de facto* evidence and conclusive of chronic anal fissure. Patients with chronic anal fissure are less likely to respond to nonoperative interventions, and LIS may be offered as first-line therapy. Of course, untreated patients with evidence of chronic anal fissure struggling with chronic constipation should have this addressed first, and topical agents during this period may be helpful. Also, patients at higher risk for FI and/or looking to avoid an operation should be offered, and may well prefer, nonoperative interventions.

Topical NTG may allow healing in nearly 50% of chronic anal fissures; however, the side-effect of headache is almost universal [8]. Furthermore, up to 50% of patients managed with topical NTG will have a persistent/recurrent anal fissure [9]. Topical calcium channel blockers have similar rates of healing to topical NTG [9] but with a superior side effect profile [10]. A double-blind, randomized clinical trial found that topical diltiazem patients had equivalent healing (43%) and pain relief to botulinum toxin (BT) after 3 months of treatment [11].

BT therapy is not yet standardized and still in evolution, with only modest healing rates (37–43%). Healing with BT is universally defined as resolution of pain rather than observed healing of the fissure, with studies limited by the variety of dosing and variation in the number of injections and injection sites, which prevent generalization and limit comparison [7]. A Cochrane review suggested that BT was only marginally superior to placebo despite being more costly with few adverse events reported [12]. However, BT is a viable alternative for patients at "high risk for future incontinence" (postoperative FI following LIS) such as patients with preexisting sphincter compromise (e.g., women with obstetric injury) [13].

Multiple randomized clinical trials have established the superiority of LIS compared to topical agents and BT with healing rates at or above 90% but with variable rates of FI. A randomized clinical trial of combined BT and topical diltiazem versus LIS, found LIS patients had a significantly higher cure rate [14]. Because long-term FI and FIQL are preserved in the vast majority of patients, LIS may be safely offered as first-line therapy for patients without preexisting FI [7].

Given the potential for FI following LIS, the concept of a "tailored" approach to the extent of division of the internal sphincter, rather than dogmatic division to the dentate line, was developed in efforts to preserve fecal continence. A retrospective study of division of the internal sphincter to the proximal extent of the fissure resulted in only minor FI (imperfect control of flatus, urgency, and minor "staining") with a 1.7% incidence of treatment failure requiring repeat LIS [15]. A prospective, randomized clinical trial found 100% cure of chronic anal fissure with a significant increase in FI with internal sphincter division to the dentate line versus division to the proximal extent of the fissure ("fissure apex") with insignificant treatment failure (13.2%) in the latter group [16]. In a postoperative study of women who underwent LIS using three-dimensional ultrasound, it was recommended to limit the extent of LIS to <25% of total internal sphincter length (<1cm in women) to avoid FI [17]. A prospective, randomized clinical trial of open versus closed LIS (Notaras technique) did not find a difference in FI between the 2 surgical techniques [18].

For those patients who do not respond to nonoperative management and are deemed to be at high risk for FI and not suitable for LIS, advancement flaps have been described. Anoplasty using a Y-V flap was first described in 1970 [19] followed by a rhomboid flap approach [20]. A prospective, randomized study of LIS versus rhomboid advancement flap revealed 3/20 flaps (15%) failed to heal, 2 patients underwent LIS with cure, and the third flap eventually healed at 3 months follow-up. No patient in either group developed FI [20].

LIS provides a durable cure for chronic anal fissure and may be offered to patients as first-line therapy; however, internal sphincter muscle division may result in postoperative FI, described as the "Achilles Heel" of the operation [18]. The length of internal sphincter muscle division has not been standardized and may be tailored (<25% of length or <1 cm) in order to limit postoperative FI. Chronic anal fissure patients deemed to be at high risk for postoperative FI who fail nonoperative treatment may be offered advancement flap repair as an alternate surgical option to LIS.

REFERENCES

1. Richard CS, Gregoire R, Plewes EA, et al. Internal sphincterotomy is superior to topical nitroglycerin in the treatment of chronic anal fissure: results of a randomized, controlled trial by the Canadian Colorectal Surgical Trials Group. Dis Colon Rectum 2000; 43(8):1048–1058.
2. Jorge JM, Wexner SD. The etiology and management of fecal incontinence. Dis Colon Rectum 1993; 36(1):77–97.
3. Brown CJ, Dubreuil D, Santoro L, Liu M, O'Connor BI, McLeod RS. Lateral internal sphincterotomy is superior to topical nitroglycerin for healing chronic anal fissure and does not compromise long-term fecal continence: six-year follow-up of a multicenter, randomized, controlled trial. Dis Colon Rectum 2007; 50(4):442–448.
4. Notaras MJ. The treatment of anal fissure by lateral subcutaneous sphincterotomy: a technique and results. Br J Surg 1971; 58:96–100.
5. Rockwood TH, Church JM, Fleshman JW, et al. Fecal Incontinence Quality of Life Scale: quality of life instrument for patients with fecal incontinence. Dis Colon Rectum 2000; 43 (9):9–16.
6. Rullier E, Zerbib F, Marrel A, Amouretti M, Lehur PA. Validation of the French version of the Fecal Incontinence Quality-of-Life (FIQL) scale. Gastroenterol Clin Bio 2004; 28:562–568.
7. Stewart DB, Gaertner W, Glasgow S, Migaly J, Feingold D, Steele SR. Clinical practice guideline for the management of anal fissures. Dis Colon Rectum 2017; 60(1):7–14.
8. Berry SM, Barish CF, Bhandari R, et al. Nitroglycerin 0.4% ointment vs placebo in the treatment of pain resulting from chronic anal fissure: a randomized, double-blind, placebo-controlled study. BMC Gastroenterol 2013; 13:106.
9. Nelson RL, Thomas K, Morgan J, Jones A. Non-surgical therapy for anal fissure. Cochrane Database Syst Rev 2012; 2:CD003431.
10. Sanei B, Mahmoodieh M, Masoudpour H. Comparison of topical glyceryl nitrate with diltiazem ointment for the treatment of chronic anal fissure: a randomized clinical trial. Acta Chir Belg 2009; 109:727–730.
11. Samim M, Twigt B, Stoker L, Pronk A. Topical diltiazem cream versus botulinum toxin a for the treatment of chronic anal fissure: a double-blind randomized clinical trial. Ann Surg 2012; 255:18–22.
12. Nelson R. Non-surgical therapy for anal fissure. Cochrane Database Syst Rev 2006;4:CD003431.
13. Mentes BB, Irkorucu O, Akin M, Leventoglu S, Tatlicioglu E. Comparison of botulinum toxin injection and lateral internal sphincterotomy for the treatment of chronic anal fissure. Dis Colon Rectum 2003; 46(2):232–237.
14. Gandomkar H, Zeinoddini A, Heidari R, Amoli HA. Partial lateral internal sphincterotomy versus combined botulinum toxin A injection and topical diltiazem in the treatment of chronic anal fissure: a randomized clinical trial. Dis Colon Rectum 2015; 58(2):228–234.
15. Littlejohn DRG, Newstead GL. Tailored lateral sphincterotomy for anal fissure. Dis Colon Rectum 1997;40(12):1439–1442.
16. Mentes BB, Ege B, Leventoglu S, Oguz M, Karadag A. Extent of lateral internal sphincterotomy: up to the dentate line or up to the fissure apex? Dis Colon Rectum 2005; 48(2): 365–370.
17. Murad-Regadas SM, Fernandes GO, Regadas FS, et al. How much of the internal sphincter may be divided during lateral sphincterotomy for chronic anal fissure in women? Morphologic and functional evaluation after sphincterotomy. Dis Colon Rectum 2013; 56(5):645–651.

18. Wiley M, Day P, Rieger N, Stephens J, Moore J. Open vs. closed lateral internal sphincterotomy for idiopathic fissure-in-ano: a prospective, randomized, controlled trial. Dis Colon Rectum 2004; 47(6):847–852.
19. Samson RB, Stewart WR. Sliding skin grafts in the treatment of anal fissures. Dis Colon Rectum 1970; 13(5):372–375.
20. Leong AF, Seow-Choen F. Lateral sphincterotomy compared with anal advancement flap for chronic anal fissure. Dis Colon Rectum 1995; 38(1):69–71.

CHAPTER 44

A Randomised, Prospective, Double-Blind, Placebo-Controlled Trial of Glyceryl Trinitrate Ointment in Treatment of Anal Fissure

Lund JN, Scholefield JH. Lancet. 4:349(9044):11–14, 1997

Reviewed by Rory F. Kokelaar and Manish Chand

Research Question/Objective   Fissure in ano (FIA) is a common proctological condition characterized by pain on defecation, rectal bleeding, and spasm of the internal anal sphincter (IAS). Traditional treatment strategies for FIA involved stretching or dividing the internal anal sphincter, thus reducing maximal anal (sphincter) resting pressure (MARP) and facilitating healing by improving blood flow to the anoderm. These procedures are, however, associated with a short- and long-term impairment of continence in up to 30% of patients. This paper hypothesized that topical application of nitric oxide (NO) in the form of glyceryl trinitrate (GTN) could also reduce MARP in a transitory fashion and thus effect fissure healing without the risk of long-term incontinence.

Study Design   This paper was the first randomized, prospective, double-blind, placebo-controlled trial examining the efficacy of GTN in chronic fissure healing. Consecutive patients were recruited at 2 hospitals with chronic FIA (>6 weeks of symptoms with evidence of prior healing) to receive an ointment of either 0.2% GTN or placebo. Computerised randomisation was utilised, and both trial and control interventions were prepared by the hospital pharmacy. Patients were instructed to apply the ointment twice daily for 8 weeks. No specific dietary modification or laxatives were stipulated. At first assessment, all patients underwent anal manometry over 20 minutes to record baseline MARP and then again over 40 minutes following application of either trial or placebo intervention. Concurrent measurements of anodermal blood flow adjacent to the FIA were made using a laser Doppler flowmeter.

Sample Size   The study was powered to give a 90% chance of demonstrating a 40% difference in healing rate between the two arms of the trial at the 5% level. In total, 80 patients were recruited, 39 of whom were randomized to GTN and the remaining 41 to the control arm. At manometry, 1 patient from each arm was found not to have FIA and was excluded. One patient in the control arm was lost to follow-up.

DOI: 10.1201/9780429285714-44

Follow-Up   Patients were followed up every 2 weeks over the 8-week trial period. At each review, the anus was inspected, and fissure healing assessed visually. Any side effects were noted. Patients were also asked to indicate on an unmarked scale how much pain they were experiencing; where one end of the scale represented no pain and the other represented the worst pain. Logistic regression was employed to assess independent predictors of healing, χ^2, Mann–Whitney tests, and ANOVA for repeat measures to compare pain scores between the trial and control groups. Student's paired t-test was used to compare MARP and laser Doppler flowmetry before and after application of trial ointment. The Wilcoxon Matched Pairs Signed-Rank test was used to compare pretreatment pain score with pain scores.

Inclusion/Exclusion Criteria   Other than the clinicians' diagnosis of FIA and assessment of chronicity, no other inclusion or exclusion criteria were specified. Notably, 10 patients (5 in each arm) had previously undergone surgery for FIA.

Intervention or Treatment Received   Patients were randomized 1:1 to 0.2% glycerin trinitrate ointment diluted 1 in 5 with white soft paraffin or to placebo (white soft paraffin).

Results   The primary finding of this study was that fissure healing was observed in 68% of patients randomized to GTN (median time to healing was 6 weeks) but only 8% in the control arm ($p < 0.001$, χ^2 test). However, 22 patients in the treatment arm reported significant headache compared to only 7 in the control arm ($p < 0.05\%$, χ^2 test). One patient in the treatment arm discontinued treatment and was counted as a treatment failure on an intention-to-treat basis, although the other patients reporting headaches in this group reported symptoms typically of less than 30 minutes, which were manageable with oral analgesia. There were no differences between groups based on baseline patient characteristics, including MARP and anodermal blood flow.

ANOVA and linear regression analysis indicated that the linear analogue pain score was significantly reduced in the GTN group but not in the placebo group following only 2 weeks of treatment. MARP was significantly reduced from 115.9 cm H_2O to 75.9 cm H_2O in the treatment arm ($p < 0.001$, Student's paired t-test), and laser Doppler flowmetry was correspondingly increased from 21.4 units to 42.8 units ($p < 0.05$, Student's paired t-test). There was no appreciable difference in MARP or flowmetry in the control group (both $p > 0.05$).

Three patients in the treatment arm relapsed within 4 months, all of whom were treated successfully with a further 8-week application of GTN. All remaining patients with persistent fissures after treatment or those unable to tolerate treatment were offered surgical sphincterotomy.

Study Limitations   The primary limitation of this study is that the measured end points do not address one of the significant clinical issues raised in the hypothesis: namely, that treatment with GTN will not result in the short- or long-term impairment in continence. Continence, assessed either subjectively or objectively, is not included as an end point in the trial protocol, and it is assumed that the intervention will have no long-term impact on the measured MARP beyond that observed in the trial. Despite this, it is assumed that if the intervention had resulted in significant impairment of continence it would have been reported in much the same way as the headaches were reported. Long-term and dedicated follow-up would be required to assess long-term healing rates and effect on continence.

Relevant Studies   In balance this is an elegant, if small, randomized, double-blind, placebo-controlled trial that demonstrates the clinical efficacy of GTN both in chronic FIA healing and in developing the understanding of the pathophysiology of the condition (1). The authors allude to the challenge of impaired continence following sphincterotomy, which are reported (in an admittedly old study) as approximately 35, 22, and 5% for incontinence to flatus, soiling of underwear, and incontinence to stool, respectively (2). The same studies do, however, demonstrate that the healing efficacy of sphincterotomy approaches 100%, and the procedure thus remains the gold standard to definitive surgical treatment of chronic FIA. Although now dated, this landmark paper has spawned numerous further studies and should be considered the gateway to the contemporary management of fistula in ano and modern techniques in "chemical sphincterotomy" (3).

Since the publication of this paper, over 148 trials have been conducted to determine the efficacy of different treatment modalities for FIA, describing 14 different surgical interventions and 29 nonsurgical interventions (4). Following the success of GTN, other drugs that induce smooth muscle relaxation and increased blood flow have been trialed in the treatment of FIA with success. Diltiazem, as well as its fellow calcium-channel blocker nifedipine, have both been successful in the management of chronic FIA and are recommended by the American Society of Colon and Rectal Surgeons (ASCRS) and Association of Coloproctology of Great Britain and Ireland (ACPGBI) for first-line management of chronic FIA (5–7). In comparison to GTN, diltiazem has a marginally lower healing rate (typically 60–65%) but avoids the side effect profile and is therefore better tolerated by patients and is therefore considered equally effective by virtue of better compliance [8]. Potassium channel opener minoxidil, although demonstrating effectiveness in increasing vascular smooth muscle relaxation and improved blood flow in treatment for male and female pattern baldness, has proved ineffective for treatment of chronic FIA [9].

The relative newcomer to nonsurgical treatment for FIA is botulinum toxin A (BT). By preventing acetylcholine release and thus neural transmission, smooth muscle relaxation in the internal anal sphincter can be reduced with an effect durable for approximately 3 months (10)]]. In this first small randomized trial, BT was employed following failure of GTN and demonstrated only 43% absolute fissure healing, although 73% of patients reported symptom improvement and avoided surgery. BT was, however, associated with short-term impaired continence. These results have been borne out in further trials of BT versus topical nitrites; in a meta-analysis of 393 patients (1:1) there was no difference in fissure healing or recurrence between groups, although there was a higher rate of transitory incontinence in the BT group (OR = 2.53 (5% CI 0.98–6.57, p = 0.06), although total side effects and headaches were significantly fewer (11). Currently, BT is recommended as an equivalent first-line therapy to topical treatments for chronic FIA by ASCRS and may offer modest improvements in healing rates as a second-line strategy. This recommendation is, however, made on the basis of low- and very-low quality evidence. BT is recommended only as a second-line therapy by the ACPGBI (7, 8).

Ultimately, the intervention with the highest chance of successful healing and lowest chance of recurrence (6.7%) is internal lateral sphincterotomy (12). Some evidence suggests that incontinence rates have fallen as techniques have improved (up to 30% in the 1980s, 10% before 2000, and 3.4% in recent series), although uptake and patient selection, along with better nonoperative options, have contributed to avoiding poor outcomes (13). While LIS is associated with increased incontinence when compared with medical therapy, the absolute risk in low-risk groups is still low.

REFERENCES

1. Gibbons CP, Read NW. Anal hypertonia in fissures: cause or effect? The British journal of surgery. 1986;73(6):443–5.
2. Khubchandani IT, Reed JF. Sequelae of internal sphincterotomy for chronic fissure in ano. The British journal of surgery. 1989;76(5):431–4.
3. Loder PB, Kamm MA, Nicholls RJ, Phillips RKS. 'Reversible chemical sphincterotomy' by local application of glyceryl trinitrate. British journal of surgery. 2005;81(9):1386–9.
4. Nelson RL, Manuel D, Gumienny C, Spencer B, Patel K, Schmitt K, et al. A systematic review and meta-analysis of the treatment of anal fissure. Techniques in coloproctology. 2017;21(8):605–25.
5. Knight JS, Birks M, Farouk R. Topical diltiazem ointment in the treatment of chronic anal fissure. The British journal of surgery. 2001;88(4):553–6.
6. Carapeti EA, Kamm MA, Phillips RK. Topical diltiazem and bethanechol decrease anal sphincter pressure and heal anal fissures without side effects. Diseases of the colon and rectum. 2000;43(10):1359–62.
7. Cross KLR, Massey EJD, Fowler AL, Monson JRT. The management of anal fissure: ACPGBI position statement. Colorectal disease. 2008;10(s3):1–7.
8. Stewart DB, Sr., Gaertner W, Glasgow S, Migaly J, Feingold D, Steele SR. Clinical practice guideline for the management of anal fissures. Diseases of the colon and rectum. 2017;60(1):7–14.
9. Boland PA, Kelly ME, Donlon NE, Bolger JC, Larkin JO, Mehigan BJ, et al. Management options for chronic anal fissure: a systematic review of randomised controlled trials. International journal of colorectal disease. 2020;35(10):1807–15.
10. Lindsey I, Jones OM, Cunningham C, George BD, Mortensen NJ. Botulinum toxin as second-line therapy for chronic anal fissure failing 0.2 percent glyceryl trinitrate. Diseases of the colon and rectum. 2003;46(3):361–6.

11. Sahebally SM, Meshkat B, Walsh SR, Beddy D. Botulinum toxin injection vs topical nitrates for chronic anal fissure: an updated systematic review and meta-analysis of randomized controlled trials. Colorectal disease. 2018;20(1):6–15.
12. Nelson RL, Chattopadhyay A, Brooks W, Platt I, Paavana T, Earl S. Operative procedures for fissure in ano. The Cochrane database of systematic reviews. 2011;2011(11):Cd002199.
13. Menteş BB, Ege B, Leventoglu S, Oguz M, Karadag A. Extent of lateral internal sphincterotomy: up to the dentate line or up to the fissure apex? Diseases of the colon and rectum. 2005;48(2):365–70.

CHAPTER 45

A Comparison of Botulinum Toxin and Saline for the Treatment of Chronic Anal Fissure

Maria G, Cassetta E, Gui D, Brisinda G, Bentivoglio AR, Albanese A. N Engl J Med. 338(4):217–220, 1998

Reviewed by Sonia L. Ramamoorthy

Research Question/Objective Chronic anal fissure treatment remains a clinical challenge as the gold standard surgical treatment is associated with high rates of anal sphincter dysfunction. Botulinum toxin (BT) has been reported to promote fissure healing without associated long-term complications. The aim of this study was to compare botulinum toxin treatment with placebo to determine its efficacy in the management of chronic anal fissures (1).

Study Design The study was designed as a double-blind, placebo-controlled study of botulinum toxin for the treatment of chronic anal fissure in 30 consecutive symptomatic adults. All patients underwent pretreatment assessments consisting of clinical evaluation, anoscopy, and anorectal manometry. Eligible patients were randomly assigned to either the study arm or the placebo arm. All the patients underwent similar posttreatment evaluations (clinical, anoscopy, and manometry) regardless of their treatment and outcome at 1 and 2 months after the injections. If the fissure persisted at the 2-month evaluation, the patients in both arms were offered "rescue" treatment. The retreated patients always received botulinum toxin; patients in the control group received 20 U, and patients in the treated group received 25 U. Retreated patients were then evaluated with the same protocol 1 month and 2 months after retreatment. At each visit, the patients could choose to be treated with anal sphincterotomy or to drop out of the study.

Sample Size From June 1994 to December 1995, 30 consecutive outpatients with CAF were enrolled; 15 received botulinum toxin, and 15 received placebo.

Follow-up The enrollment of the study began in June 1994 and went on through December 1995. Patients underwent similar posttreatment evaluations (clinical, anoscopy, and manometry) regardless of their treatment arm, and outcome at 1 and 2 months after the injections. All patients were followed until September 1996 (10–26 months).

DOI: 10.1201/9780429285714-45

Inclusion/Exclusion Criteria   Patients with signs and symptoms of chronic anal fissures (CAF) were included in the study. Patients with acute fissures, those with anal fissures of various causes (i.e., hemorrhoids, fistula in ano, inflammatory bowel diseases) and those who had previously undergone anal surgical procedures were excluded.

Intervention or Treatment Received   Treating physicians were blinded to randomization. Once randomized, patients received 2 injections into the internal anal sphincter; the treated group (15 patients) received 20 U of BT, and the control group (15 patients) received normal saline. Without sedation or local anesthetic, each of the 30 participants received 0.4 cc of solution divided into 2 injections of equal volume. The internal anal sphincter was palpated and injected with a 27-gauge needle; the solution was placed close to the fissure on each side. All patients received dietary counseling and prescriptions for laxatives.

Results

Pretreatment   The two groups were demographically similar with regard to age, sex, duration of symptoms, and resting anal sphincter pressures. Both study arms suffered similar CAF symptoms of severe anal pain after defecation and physical exam findings of a posterior anal fissure with a hallmark sentinel tag and exposure of the internal anal sphincter fibers. Pretreatment manometry demonstrated no difference in the resting sphincter pressures of the two groups; however, there was a statistically significant difference in the maximal voluntary pressure with the treated group (102 +/−13 treated vs. 71 +/−8 control).

Posttreatment Control Group   At 2 months, resting anal pressure and the maximal voluntary pressure were similar to baseline and 1-month values. At 2 months posttreatment, 2 patients had healed fissures, and 13 patients had persistent fissures. Three patients refused rescue treatment and opted for surgical sphincterotomy. The remaining 10 received a "rescue" treatment of 20 U of BT per the study protocol. At 3 months (1 month post-rescue), 4 patients had healed fissures. Three of the remaining 6 had reduced/no pain but persistent fissures, and three opted for surgical sphincterotomy. Of the patients who received rescue treatment, the mean resting anal pressure at 3 months was 20.7% lower than before receiving the BT. At the end of the follow-up period, 6 of 15 had undergone sphincterotomy, and 9 had healed fissure and symptomatic relief (Figure 45.1).

Posttreatment Study Group   At 1 month, 8 patients in the study group had healed fissures with symptomatic relief. As compared with baseline values, the resting anal pressure was reduced by 27%; the maximal voluntary pressure was not significantly changed. After 2 months, the number of patients with healed fissures increased to 11. Of the 4 patients with persistent fissures, nocturnal pain was resolved, and all 4 opted to receive a 25U "rescue" dose per the study

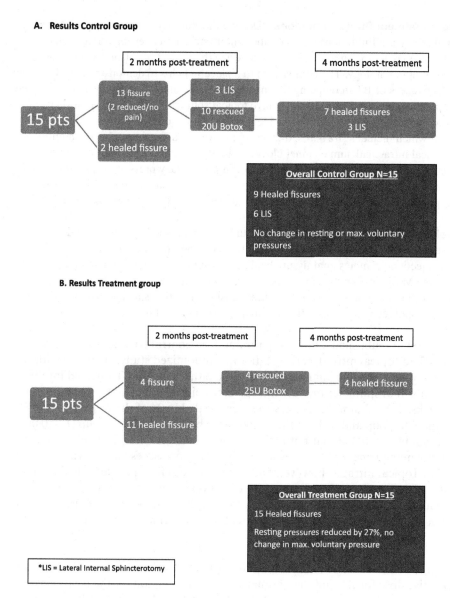

Figure 45.1 (a) Results of control group (b) and treatment group.

protocol. Three months posttreatment and 1 month post-rescue injection, 2 additional patients had healed fissures and resolution of symptoms. At 4 months (2 months after the rescue treatment), the remaining 2 patients also had healing scars, and their postdefecatory pain had resolved. The resting anal pressure and the maximal voluntary pressure in the retreated patients remained similar to their 1-month, and 2-month values (Figure 45.1).

Posttreatment Study Limitations   Despite the simplicity of the study by Maria et al., there are limitations based on the sample size. Thirty evenly randomized patients may be too small to fully characterize the impact of BT on fissure healing and symptomatology. The comparison to a placebo helps to demonstrate the baseline effectiveness of BT in reducing resting anal pressure and fissure symptoms, however, in practice, most patients would receive topical sphincter relaxant in addition to bowel and dietary counseling. The ideal comparison would be to the standard of care, which includes sitz baths, dietary and bowel modifications, plus the addition of a topical nitrate/calcium channel blocker. Finally, patients in the control arm had a statistically significant difference in maximum voluntary pressure as previously noted. In a small study such as this, this discrepancy could impact pain symptoms and the response to more conservative measures such as dietary and bowel modifications.

Relevant Studies   A year before this study was published, Jost published a series of 100 patients with anal fissure that corroborated the finding that BT injection promotes anal fissure healing and symptom relief (2). Both this and the Maria et al. publications, however, left practitioners to ponder more technical considerations such as accurate dosing, injection site, and where topical sphincter relaxants fall in the management of anal fissures.

Maria et al. published a follow-up randomized control trial in 1999, comparing BT to topical nitroglycerin (3). In this randomized study, 50 adults with symptomatic chronic anal fissures received either 20 U of BT injected into the internal anal sphincter or 0.2% nitroglycerin ointment applied twice daily for 6 weeks. After 2 months, the fissures were healed in 24 of the 25 patients (96%) in the BT group and in 15 of the 25 (60%) in the nitroglycerin group ($P = 0.005$). The study concluded that both BT and topical nitrates are effective treatments for the management of CAF by lowering resting pressures and alleviating symptoms. Topical nitrates, however, had a greater side effect profile with almost 20% of patients experiencing moderate to severe headaches. In this study, only 1 patient in the topical nitroglycerin group underwent surgical sphincterotomy indicating the effectiveness of either treatment to reduce the need for surgical intervention.

Over the years, several studies have attempted to further delineate the minimum effective dose for BT and the optimal site for BT injection for the treatment of CAF. A pooled meta-analysis by Vitoopinyoparb et al. compared BT dose and injection sites in chronic anal fissure patients (4). The pooled evidence from RCTs suggests that injections of BT in a different location from the fissure site offered improved outcomes in the short term compared to injections on both sides of the fissure for the treatment of CAF. The analysis also showed no difference in fissure healing between patients who received low-dose BT (<20 U) and those who received high-dose BT (>20 U). There was, however, a higher risk of short-term incontinence in patients who received high-dose BT. Interestingly, a national survey of colorectal surgeons in the United States completed in 2020

(N = 216) showed that 90% of respondents stated that they inject 50 U to 100 U of BT as a matter of practice. A majority of respondents (64%) inject into the internal sphincter and a majority (53%) inject into 4 quadrants in the anal canal circumference (5).

In 2022, the American Society of Colon and Rectal Surgeons published clinical practice guidelines on anal fissure management supporting first-line therapies of sitz baths, fiber (bulking agent) supplementation, and establishment of bowel regularity. For CAF, topical agents such as calcium channel blockers and nitrates are as effective as the use of BT injection. Success rates for both remedies range from 60% to 80% without the additional risk of incontinence seen with the gold standard therapy of the lateral sphincterotomy (8%–30%) (6).

Chronic anal fissure management remains an evolving field. In this study by Maria et al., botulinum toxin was shown to be an effective treatment for patients with CAF by promoting fissure healing, alleviating symptoms, and reducing the need for surgical sphincterotomy when compared with placebo.

REFERENCES

1. Maria G, Cassetta E, Gui D, Brisinda G, Bentivoglio AR, Albanese A. A comparison of botulinum toxin and saline for the treatment of chronic anal fissure. N Engl J Med. 1998;338(4):217–220.
2. Jost WH. One hundred cases of anal fissure treated with botulin toxin. Dis Colon Rectum. 1997;40:1029–1032.
3. Brisinda G, Maria G, Bentivoglio A, Cassetta E, Gui D, Albanese A. A comparison of injections of botulinum toxin and topical nitroglycerin ointment for the treatment of chronic anal fissure. N Engl J Med. 1999;341(2):65–69.
4. Vitoopinyoparb K, Insin P, Thadanipon K, Rattanasiri S, Attia J, McKay G, Thakkinstian A. Comparison of doses and injection sites of botulinum toxin for chronic anal fissure: a systematic review and network meta-analysis of randomized controlled trials. Intern J Surgery. 2022;104:1.
5. Borsuk DJ, Studniarek A, Park JJ, Marecik SJ, Mellgren A, Kochar K. Use of botulinum toxin injections for the treatment of chronic anal fissure: results from an American Society of Colon and Rectal Surgeons Survey. Am Surg. 2023;89(3):346–354.
6. Davids JS, Hawkins AT, Bhama AR, Feinberg AE, Grieco MJ, Lightner AL, Feingold DL, Paquette IM. The American Society of Colon and Rectal Surgeons clinical practice guidelines for the management of anal fissures. Dis Colon Rectum. 2022;66:190–199.

CHAPTER 46

Maintenance Therapy with Unprocessed Bran in the Prevention of Acute Anal Fissure Recurrence

Jensen SL. J R Soc Med. 80(5):296–298, 1987

Reviewed by Kyle G. Cologne

Research Question/Objective   This study investigates the effect of different doses of unprocessed dietary bran fiber on the recurrence rates of anal fissures. Five g 3 times daily (total 15 g fiber) was compared to 2.5 g 3 times daily (7.5 g/day total). There was also a placebo group with no bran (lactulose). The primary outcome was fissure recurrence.

Study Design   This study was a randomized, double-blind triple arm prospective study. Patients were randomized by an independent observer. Sealed packets of a 1-year supply of fiber were given to patients; the packets were centrally packaged (blinded to patients and treating providers). Patients were evaluated in the office at 3-month intervals to determine whether there was any evidence of recurrence (exam and questionnaire).

Sample Size   No power calculations were done prior to the study, which enrolled 25 patients in each of 3 arms (15 g fiber daily, 7.5 g fiber daily, placebo). Five patients were withdrawn from each group (total of 15 patients) for a variety of reasons (colon cancer with recurrence, refusal to follow protocol, other diagnoses).

Follow-Up   Study follow-up occurred at q3-month intervals postoperatively. Compliance based on dietary cards of fiber pack consumption was evaluated, along with recurrence and overall bowel symptoms.

Inclusion/Exclusion Criteria   Eligible patients had a first episode of constipation-induced posterior fissure treated (and healed) initially with 3 weeks of lignocaine ointment, hydrocortisone ointment, or warm sitz baths. Exclusion criteria included chronic fissure, use of bran products prior to initial treatment, fissure etiology thought to be anything other than constipation, pregnancy, or inflammatory bowel disease.

DOI: 10.1201/9780429285714-46

Intervention or Treatment Received   Patients were given sealed, prepackaged fiber supplements according to 3 doses: 15 g fiber daily (5 g TID mixed with 200 mL water); 7.5 g fiber daily (2.5 g TID mixed with 200 mL water), placebo (lactulose supplement mixed with 200 mL water).

Results   Compliance with prescribed regimen was 81.2% in the 15 g bran group, 77% in the 7.5 g group, and 83.8% in the placebo group. These were not statistically different. Bowel habits differed according to group. Straining decreased from 100% to 72% in the placebo group, from 100% to 60% in the 7.5 g group, and from 100% to 8% in the 15 g group. Daily stools changed from 12% to 32% in the placebo group, 20% to 47% in the 7.5 g group, and 16% to 72% in the 15 g group.

Anal fissure recurrence was less common with 15 g fiber (16%, 95% CI: 4.54–36.08) than with 7.5 g fiber (60%, 95% CI: 38.67–78.87) and placebo (60%, 95% CI: 46.50–85.05), all $p < 0.01$. No difference was found between recurrence rates between 7.5 g and placebo. Nine of 17 recurrences in the placebo group showed signs of chronicity and were resistant to further conservative management (all resolved after lateral internal sphincterotomy). Twenty-five percent of patients developed recurrence after fiber was stopped (28% in the 15 g group and 24% in both the 7.5 g and the placebo groups). the side effects of bloating and distention were seen in 64% in the 15 g group versus 20% in the 7.5 g group.

Study Limitations   Overall, this study represents a small group of patients. However, the results seem to corroborate what we have long known: Avoidance of constipation with good dietary and stool management will prevent recurrence of fissure. What has long been lacking is what type and how much fiber is the best to accomplish this goal. More often, especially since every patient is different, it requires a trial-and-error approach.

Relevant Studies   Many of the studies examining this issue are not new. Another randomized, blinded study enrolling 75 patients with similar methodology examined the effect of maintenance fiber therapy versus placebo. Just as with this study, fiber was associated with lower rates of recurrence (16% vs. 60%, $p < 0.01$).[1] Similarly, fiber supplementation seems to have beneficial effects over topical ointments such as hydrocortisone and lidocaine.[2] Finally, signs of chronicity are detrimental to the overall chance of success. This was seen in this study, as patients who developed signs of chronic fissure (particularly in the placebo group) required lateral internal sphincterotomy. Another prospective study of $n = 60$ patients observed 100% healing rates if symptom duration was <1 month, though this dropped to 33.3% with symptoms present for 6 months.[3]

REFERENCES

1. Jensen SL. Maintenance therapy with unprocessed bran in the prevention of acute anal fissure recurrence. J R Soc Med. 1987;80:296–298.
2. Jensen SL. Treatment of first episodes of acute anal fissure: prospective randomised study of lignocaine ointment versus hydrocortisone ointment or warm sitz baths plus bran. Br Med J (Clin Res Ed). 1986;292:1167–1169.
3. Emile SH, Elgendy H, Elfeki H, et al. Does the duration of symptoms of anal fissure impact its response to conservative treatment? A prospective cohort study. Int J Surg. 2017;44:64–70.

CHAPTER 47

Perianal Abscesses and Fistulas: A Study of 1023 Patients

Ramanujam PS, Prasad M, Abcarian H, Tan AB.
Dis Colon Rectum. 27(9):593–597, 1984

Reviewed by Christopher J. Steen and Raymond J. Yap

Research Objectives The primary objective was to anatomically classify each abscess (perianal, ischiorectal, intersphincteric, supralevator, or submucous) and note the location (posterior, lateral, or anterior), as well as note any concurrent fistula tract. Secondary objectives examined the relationship of fistula tracts based on anatomical classification of the abscesses, the management modality used to treat each abscess and fistula (unroofing and drainage of abscess with or without primary fistulotomy or staged fistulotomy with seton), and lastly to investigate recurrence rates with respect to the type of surgical management undertaken.

Study Design This was a retrospective case series, performed by a tertiary-level North American hospital, analyzing patients presenting with anorectal abscesses and fistulas over a 5.5-year period from 1977 to 1982. Demographics recorded included sex, age, associated diseases (comorbidities), distribution, and duration of symptoms.

Sample Size The study included 1023 patients who were admitted to the single hospital over the inclusive period.

Follow-Up Patients were seen in the outpatient clinic every 2 weeks until their wounds were healed. The average follow-up was 36 months, with a range of 12–60 months. During this period any abscess or fistula recurrence was documented.

Inclusion/Exclusion Criteria All patients who presented and were admitted to hospital, during the aforementioned period, were included in the study. There was no comment on exclusion criteria.

Intervention Received All patients underwent examination under regional anesthetic in the prone jackknife position. Antibiotics were used in select cases of toxic, systemic sepsis or diabetic patients. All abscess cavities were carefully explored for a concurrent fistula tract, drained, and necrotic tissue was debrided. Drains were used if the abscess cavity had horseshoe extension. A fistulotomy was performed if the entire fistula tract was identified below the dentate line. Whereas if a complex (e.g., suprasphincteric) tract was identified, a staged fistulotomy was performed by dividing the proximal half of sphincter and placing a seton, followed by division of the distal half of the sphincter 6–8 weeks later. All abscess cavities were packed, with the packing removed the following day. Patients were discharged after 2–4 days. All patients were instructed to take 4 or more sitz baths per day.

Results

Demographics Of the 1023 patients presenting with abscesses and fistulas, 672 (65.7%) were male, with most patients between the ages of 20 and 40 years (65.5%). Hypertension was the most common comorbidity recorded (9.2%), followed by diabetes (4.7%), heart disease (2.2%), and inflammatory bowel disease (0.9%). All patients presented with pain. Other symptoms reported included swelling (95.6%), fever (18.6%), and drainage (12.5%).

Abscess Classification Of the 1023 abscess presentations, the majority were classified as perianal (42.7%), followed by ischiorectal (22.8%), intersphincteric (21.4%), supralevator (7.3%), and submucous (5.8%). Additionally, most were located posteriorly (52.7%), followed by laterally (35.2%) and anteriorly (12.1%).

Abscess with Fistula Classification Of the 1023 abscess presentations, 355 (34.7%) had concurrent fistulas identified. Fistulas occurred in 47.4% of intersphincteric abscesses, followed by 42.6% of supralevator, 34.5% of perianal, 25.3% of ischiorectal, and 15.2% of submucous abscesses.

Abscess and Fistula Intervention Of those 668 (65.3%) abscesses where no fistula was identified, unroofing and drainage of the abscess were done. Where a fistula was identified, 323 (31.6%) of abscesses underwent unroofing, drainage, and primary fistulotomy. The remaining 32 (3.1%) of abscesses with fistula were unroofed and drained, and a staged fistulotomy with seton was done.

Intervention Results Of the 668 patients with abscesses unroofed and drained, 25 (3.7%) had recurrence of anorectal abscess and fistula. Of those who had a fistula identified and underwent primary fistulotomy (323), 6 (1.8%) patients were found to have had disease recurrence. Lastly, only 1 of 32 (3.1%) patients who had a staged fistulotomy, presented with recurrence.

Study Limitations   In total, 1023 patients who were admitted with anorectal abscess and fistulas were included in this study. However, there was no mention of any exclusion criteria and whether any of these included patients had any previous anorectal abscess and fistula disease. Additionally, there was no mention of any patients being lost to follow-up. Furthermore, it would have been prudent to do a subgroup analysis on those 18.6% patients who received antibiotics in order to ascertain abscess and fistula classification, as well as surgical intervention, and to establish whether antibiotics played a role in disease recurrence rates, especially if those patients were discharged from hospital on oral antibiotics. Moreover, all patients were instructed to undertake at least 4 sitz baths per day; however, it is unclear which patients complied with this and if this had any impact on abscess and fistula recurrences. Lastly, this was a single-center retrospective study, which could account for bias and an increased treatment effect.

Relevant Studies   This landmark paper, along with that of McElwain et al. (1975), were the first studies to demonstrate that management of the fistula tract, at time of abscess drainage, led to a reduced risk of recurrence (1). This study exhibited a remarkable 1.8% recurrence rate after primary fistulotomy, compared to a 3.7% recurrence after abscess drainage alone, representing an over 50% decrease in recurrence rates. It is noted that the rate of recurrence of staged fistulotomy was 3.1%, although this was with a low event occurrence (1 of 32) and these were more complex fistulae. Similarly, McElwain et al. (1975) published a 3.6% rate of recurrence following primary fistulotomy (1). Subsequent randomized controlled trials (RCTs) were able to mimic these low recurrence rates following fistulotomy (2, 3).

However, despite low recurrence rates following successful fistula management at the time of abscess drainage, critics were soon to point out that fistula management potentially increased the risk of adverse events, like flatus or fecal incontinence (4, 5), and that primary drainage alone was sufficient (4–6). After examining 5 RCTs with 406 patients, Quah et al. (2005) found that sphincter-cutting for fistula management during the abscess drainage was associated with a significant decrease (83%) in risk of disease recurrence (7). There was concern regarding higher rates of minor fecal incontinence to flatus and soiling, although this was not significant (7). Despite this, the authors concluded that abscess drainage alone is adequate, regardless of the increased risk of recurrence and that staged fistulotomy should be only be carried out on those presenting with fistula recurrence (7). They further suggested that there was no conclusive evidence that either procedure was better for treatment of anorectal abscess with fistula and that a large RCT, powered with 1176 patients, would be required to address recurrence and risk of incontinence in abscess drainage with fistulotomy (7). To date, no such trial exists.

In stark contrast to this viewpoint, a Cochrane review in 2010 examined and expanded upon findings by Quah et al. (2005) and concluded that there is strong enough evidence to suggest that fistula surgery at the time of abscess drainage results in a significant decrease in the risk of persistent fistula (8). Furthermore, significant incontinence, following a single-stage fistulotomy approach, is not a major concern in low anal fistula (8).

More recent guidelines, however, tend to err on the side of caution and recommend careful probing for fistula tract only, assuming that many internal openings heal spontaneously and that fistulotomy should only be done if the tract is superficial (without sphincter involvement) and carried out by experienced surgeons (9–11).

In summary, since publication of this study almost 40 years ago, there is still ongoing debate surrounding the fistula management at the time of anorectal abscess drainage. Proponents argue a lower recurrence rate, while critics highlight increased trends in incontinence sustained from fistulotomy, or the need for a second operation if a fistula tract is established with seton.

REFERENCES

1. McElwain JW, MacLean MD, Alexander RM, et al. Anorectal problems: experience with primary fistulectomy for anorectal abscess, a report of 1,000 cases. *Dis Colon Rectum.* 1975 Nov–Dec;18(8):646–9.
2. Ho YH, Tan M, Chui CH, et al. Randomized controlled trial of primary fistulotomy with drainage alone for perianal abscesses. *Dis Colon Rectum.* 1997 Dec;40(12):1435–8.
3. Oliver I, Lacueva FJ, Pérez Vicente F, et al. Randomized clinical trial comparing simple drainage of anorectal abscess with and without fistula track treatment. *Int J Colorectal Dis.* 2003 Mar;18(2):107–10.
4. Hebjørn M, Olsen O, Haakansson T, et al. A randomized trial of fistulotomy in perianal abscess. *Scand J Gastroenterol.* 1987 Mar;22(2):174–6.
5. Schouten WR, van Vroonhoven TJ. Treatment of anorectal abscess with or without primary fistulectomy. Results of a prospective randomized trial. *Dis Colon Rectum.* 1991 Jan;34(1):60–3.
6. Tang CL, Chew SP, Seow-Choen F. Prospective randomized trial of drainage alone vs. drainage and fistulotomy for acute perianal abscesses with proven internal opening. *Dis Colon Rectum.* 1996 Dec;39(12):1415–7.
7. Quah HM, Tang CL, Eu KW, et al. Meta-analysis of randomized clinical trials comparing drainage alone vs primary sphincter-cutting procedures for anorectal abscess-fistula. *Int J Colorectal Dis.* 2006 Sep;21(6):602–9.
8. Malik AI, Nelson RL, Tou S. Incision and drainage of perianal abscess with or without treatment of anal fistula. *Cochrane Database Syst Rev.* 2010 Jul 7;(7):CD006827.
9. Ommer A, Herold A, Berg E, et al. German S3 guideline: anal abscess. *Int J Colorectal Dis.* 2012 Jun;27(6):831–7.
10. Amato A, Bottini C, De Nardi P, et al. Evaluation and management of perianal abscess and anal fistula: SICCR position statement. *Tech Coloproctol.* 2020 Feb;24(2):127–143.
11. Tarasconi A, Perrone G, Davies J, et al. Anorectal emergencies: WSES-AAST guidelines. *World J Emerg Surg.* 2021 Sep 16;16(1):48.

CHAPTER 48

Clinical Examination, Endosonography, and MR Imaging in Preoperative Assessment of Fistula in Ano: Comparison with Outcome-Based Reference Standard

Buchanan GN, Halligan S, Bartram CI, Williams AB, Tarroni D, Cohen CR. Radiology. 233(3):674–681, 2004

Reviewed by Rishi Batra and Sean J. Langenfeld

Research Question/Objective Fistula in ano is a common condition with the tendency to recur despite seemingly curative surgery. Preoperative imaging can alert the surgeon to infection that would otherwise be missed. Magnetic resonance (MR) imaging can depict fistulas and any associated secondary tracts or abscesses. It allows physicians to identify features specifically associated with postoperative recurrence and could alter the surgical approach. The benefit of preoperative investigation of fistula in ano with use of anal endosonography remains uncertain. The central aim of this study was to prospectively evaluate the relative accuracy of digital examination, anal endosonography, and magnetic resonance (MR) imaging for preoperative assessment of fistula in ano by comparison with an outcome-derived reference standard.

Study Design This was a prospective, single-institution cohort study from St. Mark's Hospital in London, England. Consecutive patients suspected of having fistula in ano from 1998 to 2002 were recruited from outpatient clinics. All patients underwent 3 sequential assessments: (1) office exam by consultant colorectal surgeons or senior colorectal trainees, including digital exam and proctosigmoidoscopy, (2) anal endosonography (AES) performed by either experienced gastrointestinal radiologists or 2 dedicated surgical research fellows using a 10-MHz transducer, and (3) 1.0-T pelvic MR imaging interpreted by experienced gastrointestinal radiologists who were blinded to AES results. Fistula classification was determined with each modality using a standardized sheet, including muscle involvement and the presence of abscesses and/or accessory tracts. Examination under anesthesia was performed by colorectal consultants and experienced colorectal trainees. Based on clinical outcome and findings of MR imaging and examination under anesthesia, an outcome-derived reference standard for each fistula classification was determined. This method was first described by Schwartz et al.,[1] who found that a combination of at least two modalities was necessary to be confident that classification

DOI: 10.1201/9780429285714-48

was correct. The authors wanted to determine the value of anal endosonography and therefore did not use it in the outcome-derived reference standard.

Sample Size   This study screened 108 consecutive patients who were suspected of having a fistula in ano and who gave appropriate informed consent prospectively from outpatient clinics. Overall, the study included 104 patients for analysis.

Follow-Up   Patients were followed postoperatively in clinic to detect fistula healing or recurrence for a mean of 23 months (range 3–46 months).

Inclusion/Exclusion Criteria   To avoid selection bias, all patients with a suspected possible fistula were eligible for inclusion in this study, regardless of presumed complexity or underlying systemic diseases.

Intervention/Treatment Received   All patients underwent examination under anesthesia performed by colorectal consultants and experienced colorectal trainees. During surgery, their fistulas were further defined and treated as necessary, including fistulotomy and/or seton placement.

Results

Sampling This study evaluated 108 consecutive patients with fistula in ano. Three patients were excluded for declining AES, and a fourth was excluded due to intolerance of clinical exam due to severe pain. Therefore, 104 patients were included in the final analysis.

Cohort Demographics The cohort included 74 male patients with a median age of 42.5 (range 21–66 years) and 30 female patients with a median age of 42 years (range 17–61 years). With this group, 27% of fistulas were primary and 73% were recurrent. Crohn's disease was present in 8.7% of patients with the remainder believed to have cryptoglandular fistulas.

Cohort Interventions A significant linear tread was noted in the proportion of tracks correctly classified with office exam (61%), AES (81%), and MR imaging (90%). Similarly, correct classification of abscesses ($P < 0.001$), horseshoe extensions ($P = 0.003$), and internal openings ($P < 0.001$) were best identified with MR imaging. AES correctly predicted the internal opening in 91% of patients compared to 97% for MR imaging. AES identified fewer extensions than MR imaging. When abscesses and horseshoe extensions were analyzed together, digital exam currently identified only 36% compared to 70% with AES and 88% with MR imaging. The authors concluded that AES is likely to be a worthwhile test when MR imaging is unavailable or expertise in its interpretation is lacking. As the authors hypothesized, MR imaging was the most accurate modality in all comparisons made.

Study Limitations   This study was performed at a tertiary referral center where the majority of the cases were for recurrent fistula in ano. AES is operator dependent, and results may have differed in less experienced hands. AES was also done without hydrogen peroxide, which has been suggested as a useful adjunct in identification of fistula tracts and internal openings. During examination under anesthesia, surgeons had access to MR images, which may have led to a higher concordance between MR and surgical assessments. Most importantly, this study was conducted more than 20 years ago using a nonstandardized definition of fistula anatomy, and changes in fistula definitions, along with improvements in the resolution of both AES and pelvic MR, may limit the study's relevance to modern-day practice.

Relevant Studies   MR use had been steadily increasing since a small 1992 case series demonstrated its ability to correctly classify fistulas in 88% (14/16) of patients,[2] but it would still be several years until subsequent studies would confirm the utility of pelvic MR in fistula classification.[3,4] Benefits of MR imaging include accuracy, reproducibility, and overall patient tolerance.[5] Early use of pelvic MRI included endoanal coils, but they were poorly tolerated by patients and provided limited views.[6] With improvements of MR imaging technology with both 1.5 Tesla and 3.0 Tesla magnets, body coil MRI findings are now used routinely and preferred over endoanal coils.[7,8] The use of pelvic MR should be determined on a case-by-case basis, and it has more utility for longer, more complex fistulas compared to simple and superficial tracts.[9]

Prior to this study, the utility of anal endosonography remained uncertain with some studies reporting superior,[10] equivalent,[1,11] and inferior[12,13] results compared to MR imaging. AES is now know to be a useful adjunct to clinical exam in the assessment of anal fistulas, especially in environments where pelvic MR is not readily available or affordable.

In 2023, pelvic MR and AES are both widely used to define the anatomy of complex fistulas.[14,15] It was studies like this that helped popularize the techniques and validate them as highly-accurate supplements to the surgeon's clinical exam.

REFERENCES

1. Schwartz, D. A. *et al.* A comparison of endoscopic ultrasound, magnetic resonance imaging, and exam under anesthesia for evaluation of Crohn's perianal fistulas. *Gastroenterology* **121**, 1064–1072 (2001).
2. Lunniss, P. J., Armstrong, P., Barker, P. G., Reznek, R. H. & Phillips, R. K. Magnetic resonance imaging of anal fistulae. *Lancet* **340**, 394–396 (1992).
3. Joyce, M., Veniero, J. C. & Kiran, R. P. Magnetic resonance imaging in the management of anal fistula and anorectal sepsis. *Clin. Colon Rectal Surg.* **21**, 213–219 (2008).
4. Halligan, S. Magnetic resonance imaging of fistula-in-ano. *Magn. Reson. Imaging Clin. N. Am.* **28**, 141–151 (2020).
5. Williams, G. *et al.* The treatment of anal fistula: second ACPGBI position statement—2018. *Colorectal Dis.* **20 Suppl 3**, 5–31 (2018).

6. deSouza, N. M., Gilderdale, D. J., Coutts, G. A., Puni, R. & Steiner, R. E. MRI of fistula-in-ano: a comparison of endoanal coil with external phased array coil techniques. *J. Comput. Assist. Tomogr.* **22**, 357–363 (1998).

7. West, R. L. *et al.* Prospective comparison of hydrogen peroxide–enhanced three-dimensional endoanal ultrasonography and endoanal magnetic resonance imaging of perianal fistulas. *Dis. Colon Rectum* **46**, 1407–1415 (2003).

8. Halligan, S. & Bartram, C. I. MR imaging of fistula in ano: are endoanal coils the gold standard? *AJR Am. J. Roentgenol.* **171**, 407–412 (1998).

9. Konan, A., Onur, M. R. & Özmen, M. N. The contribution of preoperative MRI to the surgical management of anal fistulas. *Diagn. Interv. Radiol.* **24**, 321–327 (2018).

10. Orsoni, P. *et al.* Prospective comparison of endosonography, magnetic resonance imaging and surgical findings in anorectal fistula and abscess complicating Crohn's disease. *Br. J. Surg.* **86**, 360–364 (1999).

11. Gustafsson, U. M., Kahvecioglu, B., Aström, G., Ahlström, H. & Graf, W. Endoanal ultrasound or magnetic resonance imaging for preoperative assessment of anal fistula: a comparative study. *Colorectal Dis.* **3**, 189–197 (2001).

12. Maier, A. G. *et al.* Evaluation of perianal sepsis: comparison of anal endosonography and magnetic resonance imaging. *J. Magn. Reson. Imaging* **14**, 254–260 (2001).

13. Hussain, S. M., Stoker, J., Schouten, W. R., Hop, W. C. & Laméris, J. S. Fistula in ano: endo-anal sonography versus endoanal MR imaging in classification. *Radiology* **200**, 475–481 (1996).

14. Iqbal, N. *et al.* Getting the most out of MRI in perianal fistula: update on surgical techniques and radiological features that define surgical options. *Clin. Radiol.* **76**, 784.e17–784.e25 (2021).

15. Mantoo, S., Mandovra, P. & Goh, S. Using preoperative three-dimensional endoanal ultrasound to determine operative procedure in patients with perianal fistulas. *Colorectal Dis.* **22**, 931–938 (2020).

CHAPTER 49

A Classification of Fistula-in-Ano

Parks AG, Gordon PH, Hardcastle JD. Br J Surg. 63(1):1–12, 1976

Reviewed by Ana M. Otero-Piñeiro and Tracy Hull

Research Question/Objective   The aim of this study was to provide a detailed classification of anal fistulas and their variations, based on the analysis of 400 patients treated in the 15 years prior to 1976. There was an emphasis on exact nomenclature and relating fistula tracts to anatomy. Additionally, they sought to discuss pathogenesis. In a historical context, terms to describe anal fistula and abscesses were ambiguous. This study attempted to refine the knowledge and relate fistula tracks to anatomy.

Study Design   This study was a retrospective cohort study conducted in St. Mark's and The London Hospitals (London) reference centers for perianal disease. The primary outcome of this study was to classify the main anal fistulas and their variations. Secondary outcome measures included the pathogenesis of this disease, normal pelvic floor anatomy, and key points to consider in different surgical procedures.

Sample Size   Four hundred patients with fistula in ano. These patients were accumulated over the 15 years prior to publication in 1976.

Follow-Up   Not applicable.

Inclusion/Exclusion Criteria   Consecutive patients with fistula in ano who had been referred to these specialists were analyzed. Exclusion criteria were gross anorectal disease due to carcinoma, ulcerative colitis, or Crohn's disease.

Intervention or Treatment Received   Careful assessment of the relationship of the fistula tract to anal anatomy was performed. Each fistula was classified into 1 of 4 categories (intersphincteric, transsphincteric, suprasphincteric, and extrasphincteric). Treatment options were suggested for each type of fistula.

Results   The authors felt that anal abscess and anal fistula were part of the same disease, which was a novel concept at that time. They felt the anal abscess was the "acute" phase of the disease. The authors also felt the internal sphincter could be divided without alteration in fecal control. The external sphincter and puborectalis were felt to be most important for "maintenance of rectal continence."

The 4 categories of fistula (see Figure 49.1) and subcategories were:

DOI: 10.1201/9780429285714-49

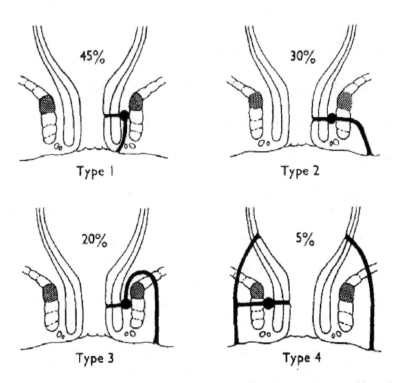

Figure 49.1   Classification of fistula in ano: type 1, intersphinteric; type 2, transsphincteric; type 3, suprasphincteric; type 4 extrasphincteric. (*Source*: From Parks et al., Br J Surg 63;1976, p. 5.)

Type I: Intersphincteric Fistula   There were 183 cases (45%) and 7 subcategories of this type of fistula. The researchers felt that this was the easiest type of fistula to treat. See Table 49.1 for an overview of the 7 subcategories.

Type 2: Trans-Sphincteric Fistula   There were 116 cases (30%) of this type.

1. *Uncomplicated (85 cases)*: Track passes through the internal and external sphincter into the ischiorectal fossa and to the skin. Most are distal in the anal canal, and laying open the track usually only divides the distal portion of the external sphincter. Therefore changes in fecal continence were unlikely to occur.
2. *Transsphincteric fistula with a high blind track (34 cases)*: The authors felt this type of fistula was important to recognize as the track crosses through the external sphincter, then divides into lower and upper components. The lower portion goes to the perineal skin. The upper may pass to the most cephalad aspect of the ischiorectal fossa. At times it may traverse the levator and pass into the pelvic cavity.

TABLE 49.1   Seven Subcategories of Intersphincteric Fistula

	N out of 183	Anatomy	Surgical Treatment	Extra Info
Simple intersphincteric	137	Abscess passes down intersphincteric groove to anal verge.	Division of lower half of internal sphincter	Perianal abscess in acute phase, rarely leads to problems with fecal control
Intersphincteric with high blind tract	15	Track passes upward in intersphincteric groove and ends at rectal wall (still has perineal external opening).	Heals when initial focus of infection dealt with (may also need to divide the entire internal sphincter).	
Intersphincteric with high track opening into lower rectum	9	Track passes upward in intersphincteric groove and has opening into rectum (still has perineal external opening).	Division of entire internal sphincter over the tract	Liable to misdiagnosis due to second internal opening or mistaken for extrasphincteric fistula if rectal opening only detected and not mid-anal canal internal opening
High intersphincteric without perineal opening	5	Track passes in intersphincteric groove cephalad into the pararectal space (no downward extension to anal skin).	Unroof fistula into the rectum.	Acute phase may see an abscess in rectal wall.
High intersphincteric fistula with pelvic extension	15	Infection tracks upward, through the levator plate, into the pelvis.		In acute phase, drain into the rectum. Draining via the ischiorectal fossa will result in suprasphincteric fistula.
Intersphincteric fistula from pelvic disease	2	Infection tracks from source in pelvis through the intersphincteric groove.	Eradicate pelvic sepsis and source.	Not true anal fistula

Type 3: Suprasphincteric Fistula   There were 78 cases (20%) of this type. The fistula starts in the intersphincteric space and tracks cephalad above the puborectalis muscle. It then tracks downward between the puborectalis and the levator ani muscles into the ischiorectal fossa. In the supralevator compartment, it may form a horseshoe-shaped track around the rectum. This is one of the most difficult to treat.

Type 4: Extrasphincteric Fistula   There were 20 cases (5%) of this type. There is a track from the perianal skin through the ischorectal fossa and the levator muscle penetrating the rectal wall. The track is outside the sphincter complex. These are classified according to pathogenesis; see Table 49.2.

Study Limitations   There are several limitations in this study. It is a retrospective study based on a selected series of patients referred to a specialty center and may be prone to selection bias. Hence this may not be representative of the incidence of the

TABLE 49.2   Extrasphincteric Fistula Classified by Pathogenesis

	N out of 20	Anatomy	Surgical Treatment	Extra Info
Extrasphincteric fistula secondary to transsphincteric fistula	10	An internal opening in the mid-anal canal passes through the sphincter and then to the anal skin. There is an extension upward and the track reenters the rectum	Usually requires a colostomy to address the rectal opening. The track through the sphincter is laid open.	Pathogenesis may be spontaneous or from vigorous probing.
Extrasphincteric due to trauma	2	The fistula goes from the rectum to the anal skin totally outside the sphincter.	Remove the foreign body, and establish drainage. Possible colostomy	Due to trauma or penetration from a foreign body
Extrasphincteric due to anorectal disease	Excluded from this study	Fistula tracks that do not follow normal anatomy	Treat underlying disease	Due to Crohn's disease, cancer, or ulcerative colitis
Extrasphincteric due to pelvic inflammation	8	The infection passes from the abdomen or pelvis directly to the anal skin.	Treat cause in pelvis	Recognize early to avoid damage to anal sphincter.

disease in the general population. The authors did not have the advantage of current radiological studies (like magnetic imaging) to assist in classifying these fistula.

Relevant Studies Parks study was the first classification of fistula in -ano ever based on clinical experience (1). It is also one of the first to include exact anatomical terms to describe the fistula tracks. Almost all (>92%) of the fistulas were grouped into the first two categories (types I–II) Extrasphincteric fistulas were assigned a separate category (grade IV). MRI-based studies looking at fistulas in a large number of patients have shown that extrasphincteric fistulas are extremely rare (2, 3). Transsphincteric fistula (type II) were subgrouped into uncomplicated and those with a high blind track. Most likely low transsphincteric fistulas were the majority of the low transsphincteric and are conveniently managed by fistulotomy. Transsphincteric fistula that encompass more anal sphincter have a greater risk of fecal incontinence and currently are typically managed with sphincter-sparing procedures. Therefore, this classification may have certain limitations as a surgical guide.

In 2000, Morris et al. using sophisticated radiological testing proposed the St. James University Hospital (SJUH) classification, attempting to improve on Parks classification (4). SJUH classification was a slight modification of Parks, bifurcating the first two grades I–II into 4 grades and combining grades III and IV into a single grade (grade V). Although this classification was based on MRI, it provided no implications or recommendations for fistula management.

In 2005, the Standard Practice Task Force (SPTF, American Society of Colon and Rectal Surgeons) was published to guide surgeons in anal fistula disease management (5). However, it only discussed two categories: simple fistulas, in which fistulotomy is safe, and complex fistulas, in which fistulotomy is risky, leading to a high incidence of incontinence. This classification was not based on patient data and therefore may not be accurate. Anal fistula disease is felt to be more complex than this two-category system.

In 2017, Garg et al. made a new classification based on clinical findings, magnetic resonance imaging, intraoperative findings, and follow-up. Initially 440 patients were studied (6), and similar results were found in another study with 848 patients (7). Fistulas were divided into 5 grades. Garg grades I–II were simple fistulas and can be safely treated by fistulotomy, while grades III–V are complex fistulas that should be referred to specialized centers. In these cases, sphincter preservation procedures such as anal fistula plug (8), LIFT (ligation of the intersphincteric fistula track) (9), VAAFT (video-assisted anal fistula treatment) (10), PERFACT (proximal superficial cauterization, emptying regularly fistula tracts and curettage of tracts) (11), or TROPIS (transanal opening of intersphincteric space) (12) could be performed. In addition, since it was also based on radiological parameters, this classification allowed radiologists to provide information to assist surgeons in disease management.

In 2021, Emile et al. suggested a modification of the Parks Classification by incorporating predictors of failed healing and impaired continence after surgery (13). Intersphincteric fistula were divided into 2 subgroups. The first subgroup was the simple linear intersphincteric track that can be adequately treated with a fistulotomy with minimal risk of recurrence or incontinence. The second subgroup involved intersphincteric fistula with a higher recurrences risk, such as horseshoe fistula, fistula with extensions, and recurrent fistula after previous surgery that may require alternative intervention. This classification was based on a cohort of 665 patients and was felt to be more useful to accurately predict treatment failure and/or postprocedure incontinence.

Historically, anal fistulas have been classified in many different ways. However, the Parks classification introduced in 1976 is the most comprehensive and widely used. Subsequently, new classifications have emerged to assist surgeons in classifying complex fistula that would not be appropriate for a fistulotomy. The Garg classification seems to be the most complete. Even with these many proposed classification schemes, Parks was truly the first to look carefully at anatomy and use terms that were very specific to describe anal fistula tracks.

REFERENCES

1. Parks AG, Gordon PH, Hardcastle JD. A classification of fistula-in-ano. Br J Surg. 1976;63(1):1–12.
2. Garg P, Singh P, Kaur B. Magnetic Resonance Imaging (MRI): operative findings correlation in 229 fistula-in-ano patients. World J Surg. 2017;41(6):1618–24.
3. Garg P. Supralevator extrasphincteric fistula-in-ano are rare as supralevator extension is almost always in the intersphincteric plane. World J Surg. 2017;41(9):2409–10.
4. Morris J, Spencer JA, Ambrose NS. MR imaging classification of perianal fistulas and its implications for patient management. Radiographics. 2000;20(3):623–35.
5. Whiteford MH, Kilkenny J, Hyman N, Buie WD, Cohen J, Orsay C, et al. Practice parameters for the treatment of perianal abscess and fistula-in-ano (revised). Dis Colon Rectum. 2005;48(7):1337–42.
6. Garg P. Comparing existing classifications of fistula-in-ano in 440 operated patients: is it time for a new classification? A retrospective cohort study. Int J Surg. 2017;42:34–40.
7. Garg P. Assessing validity of existing fistula-in-ano classifications in a cohort of 848 operated and MRI-assessed anal fistula patients—cohort study. Ann Med Surg. 2020;59:122–6.
8. Garg P, Song J, Bhatia A, Kalia H, Menon GR. The efficacy of anal fistula plug in fistula-in-ano: a systematic review. Colorectal Dis. 2010;12(10):965–70.
9. Hong KD, Kang S, Kalaskar S, Wexner SD. Ligation of intersphincteric fistula tract (LIFT) to treat anal fistula: systematic review and meta-analysis. Tech Coloproctol. 2014;18(8):685–91.
10. Garg P, Singh P. Video-Assisted Anal Fistula Treatment (VAAFT) in cryptoglandular fistula-in-ano: a systematic review and proportional meta-analysis. Int J Surg. 2017;46:85–91.
11. Garg P, Garg M. PERFACT procedure: a new concept to treat highly complex anal fistula. World J Gastroenterol. 2015;21(13):4020–9.
12. Garg P. Transanal opening of intersphincteric space (TROPIS)—a new procedure to treat high complex anal fistula. Int J Surg. 2017;40:130–4.
13. Emile SH, Elfeki H, El-Said M, Khafagy W, Shalaby M. Modification of parks classification of cryptoglandular anal fistula. Dis Colon Rectum. 2021;64(4):446–58.

CHAPTER 50

A Clinical Pathway to Accelerate Recovery after Colonic Resection

Basse L, Hjort Jakobsen D, Billesbolle P, Werner M,
Kehlet H. Ann Surg. 232(1):51–57, 2000

Reviewed by Deborah S. Keller and Thais Reif de Paula

Research Question/Objective   The objective of this work was to determine whether
a 48-hour postoperative stay program after elective colonic resection was feasible
using a multimodal rehabilitation program to enhance the recovery of organ function.

The authors had previously reported promising outcomes integrating multimodal pain relief into an accelerated rehabilitation program in 16 consecutive
elective open sigmoid resection patients with a planned discharge 2 days after
surgery (1). They parlayed these initial results into a standardized accelerated
multimodal care program that was introduced and routinely used in the author's
department of surgical gastroenterology from January 1, 1998, onward.

Study Design   The study design was a prospective observational study performed
at a single institution.

Sample Size   The patient population was 60 consecutive patients scheduled for
elective colon resection. The study included 16 historical patients from the author's
preliminary findings designing the standardized protocol for 48-hour discharge
and the next 44 patients from January 1998 to October 1998. The study had no
control group, and the sample size was not powered for hypothesis testing.

Follow-Up   Follow-up visits were performed at 8 and 30 days after discharge.
At postdischarge day 8, patients were seen in the outpatient clinic for removal of
stitches and information about histology; then the final postoperative checkup
was performed on day 30.

Inclusion/Exclusion Criteria   Patients included were adults having an elective
open right, transverse, left, or sigmoid colon resection at a single gastrointestinal
surgery department. The procedures were performed using standardized steps and
incisions. No defined patient demographics for exclusion or surgeon information were
provided. Patients undergoing a low anterior resection, proctectomy, or surgery for

DOI: 10.1201/9780429285714-50

TABLE 50.1   Multimodal Rehabilitation Program

Before Surgery	Day of Surgery (0–24 hours)	During Surgery	Postoperative Day 1 (24–48 hours)	Postoperative Day 2 (48 hours)
• Repeat information about perioperative course, previously given in the outpatient clinic. • Discuss the 2-day program with family. • Fluid nutrition with 4 protein drinks daily for 3 days • Laxatives and oral bowel cleaning.	• Mobilize ~2 hours, initiated 6 hours postoperatively. • Drink 1000 mL with 2 protein drinks. • Acetaminophen 2 g q12h, magnesium 1 g q12 h, and cisapride 20 mg q12h (repeat). • Bupivacaine, ibuprofen, opioid for breakthrough pain • Normal food allowed	• Thoracic epidural catheter was inserted before surgery (morphine and bupivacaine). • Anastomoses were hand-sewn. • Nasogastric tubes were not left after surgery. • General anesthesia with propofol and remifentanil • 1500 mL isotonic saline + 500 mL 6% hydroxyethyl starch fluid given. • Ketorolac and ondansetron given 30 minutes before ending anesthesia. • At closure, peri-incisional 0.25% bupivacaine administered. • Normothermia maintained with a Bair Hugger.	• Urinary bladder catheter removed in the morning. • Mobilization ≥8 hours • Normal food and oral fluid ≥2000 mL, including 4 protein drinks • Plan discharge.	• Remove epidural catheter in morning. • Oral ibuprofen 600 mg q8h • Full mobilization • Normal oral intake • Stop cisapride. • Magnesium × 1 week • Discharge after lunch

Source: Basse L, Hjort Jakobsen D, Billesbolle P, Werner M, Kehlet H. Ann Surg. 232(1):51–57, 2000. The first 16 patients received additional intrathecal anesthesia with lidocaine.

inflammatory bowel disease were excluded. Patients with subjective comorbidities and intraoperative findings deemed to preclude a 2-day hospital stay were also excluded, but this was not done prospectively or using standardized criteria.

Intervention or Treatment Received   The intervention was a standardized multimodal care pathway for preoperative and postoperative nursing care, which later developed into Enhanced Recovery After Surgery programs (Table 50.1). All patients received the intervention; there was no control group.

Results   The patient population had a median age of 74 years and one-third were ASA groups III–IV. The authors stated this was a "high-risk" group with the results, but there was no risk stratification. The preoperative diagnosis was 72% ($n = 43$) cancer and 28% ($n = 17$) benign disease. The procedures performed were 23 right hemicolectomies, 34 sigmoid or left colectomies, 2 transverse colectomies, and 1 subtotal colectomy. The median duration of surgery was 120 minutes (range 70–360) and median intraoperative blood loss was 100 mL (range 50–2450).

Of the 60 consecutive patients, just over half were actually discharged on postoperative day (POD) 2 ($n = 32$). There were 4 patients deemed not appropriate for discharge from the hospital POD 2 for demographic issues; they needed further inpatient care for previous cerebral infarctions and a myocardial infarction, severe depression, severe deconditioning, and a femoral venous thrombosis requiring close postoperative monitoring of anticoagulation. Three patients were deemed impossible during surgery for discharge on POD 2: a tumor invading the duodenum, requiring a gastroenteric anastomosis; previous ileotransverse shunt, requiring a more extensive procedure for continuity; and tumor invasion into the bladder wall, requiring a partial cystectomy and postoperative drainage. If looking only at the 53 patients whom the authors deemed appropriate for discharge POD 2, 30 (57%) were actually discharged POD 2, 13 were discharged POD 3 (25%), 6 on POD 4 (11%), and 2 on POD 5 (4%). These prolonged LOS were due to psychosocial factors (9 patients), delayed return of gastrointestinal function (7 patients), dizziness and fatigue (4 patients), delayed reoperation (1 patient), and pneumonia (1 patient). Pain was not a limiting factor for discharge, and a few patients required supplemental pain medication outside of the pathway.

Clinically, patients tolerated starting a regular diet immediately after surgery; postoperative ileus and nasogastric tube insertion were not described. Return of bowel function was measured with defecation, and 57 patients had defecation in the first 48 hours; flatus was not described. The overall morbidity was not clearly described. For Clavien Class 1–2/minor complication, 7 patients (11%) had urinary retention, 3 had vomiting (5%), 2 (3%) had abdominal distension, and 1 (2%) had a spinal headache and superficial site infection; it is unknown if these complications were in distinct patients or if 1 patient had multiple complications. For Clavien Class 3–5/serious complications, there were 2 anastomotic leaks, 1 case of bowel ischemia requiring reoperation, 1 case of incision bleeding requiring repair, and 1 wound dehiscence. Nine patients (15%) needed readmission; 7 of the 9 were readmitted before the first follow-up visit. Three patients (5%) required reoperation, and there were 2 deaths (3%).

Study Limitations   The greatest limitation was the study design, using a consecutive case series with no control or comparative group. As such, the authors cannot draw conclusions on the relationship of their multimodal rehabilitation regimen to postoperative complications, readmissions, or other outcome measures. The lack of clear reporting of postoperative complications was another limitation, as the actual morbidity rate remains unclear. Furthermore excluding high-risk patients was a limitation of the study. While the authors described the 53 patients they deemed appropriate for discharge on POD 2 as at very high risk, it was the 7 patients they excluded as impossible to discharge on POD 2 that were actually high-risk and could benefit the most from an enhanced recovery protocol.

Relevant Studies   This work is a key paper in the ERAS literature, as it sparked the length of stay revolution. Multimodal rehabilitation pathways had been introduced more than a decade earlier, but the benefits of application were not widely demonstrated from a quality standpoint (2, 3). The authors used the critical concept of multimodal rehabilitation pathways and showed their potential for further improving the postoperative course and specifically the length of hospital stay.

These findings served as the catalyst for further work on the benefits of ERAS for reducing complications and improving postoperative outcomes. Perioperative complications are a main driver of LOS (4), and numerous studies have demonstrated ERAS protocols led to substantial reductions in LOS and complications, as well as improving costs and patient satisfaction (5, 6). Similar results are seen in high-risk groups, including the elderly and cancer patients, where ERAS protocols were safe, showed improved recovery, and allowed better maintenance of independence (7–10). As protocols became well implemented, readmissions also were reduced (11, 12).

This paper's results questioned the proposed advantages of laparoscopic-assisted colonic resection in the setting of a multimodal rehabilitation program. The randomized controlled multicenter LAFA-trial (LAparoscopy and/or FAst track multimodal management versus standard care) trial, developed to determine whether laparoscopic surgery, fast track care, or a combination of both was preferred over open surgery with standard care in colectomy for cancer, showed that the optimal perioperative treatment is laparoscopic resection embedded in a fast track program (13, 14).

ERAS protocols are now standard of care, and guidelines are published to aid education and implementation (15, 16). The implementation process of ERAS protocols is critical, as increased adherence to ERAS components is directly associated with improvement in postoperative complications (17). Implementation requires a coordinated multimodal team effort with top-down support and buy-in from all stakeholders, including patients (18). To aid successful implementation, programs such as the American College of Surgeons Enhanced Recovery in National Surgical Quality Improvement Program (ERIN) have been created, with promising outcomes (19). As programs continue to adjust for changing patient needs, we look forward to seeing ongoing development of the multimodal rehabilitation pathway.

REFERENCES

1. Kehlet H, Mogensen T. Hospital stay of 2 days after open sigmoidectomy with a multimodal rehabilitation programme. Br J Surg. 1999;86:227–230.
2. Kehlet H. Surgical stress: the role of pain and analgesia. Br J Anaesth. 1989;63:189–195.
3. Kehlet H. The stress response to surgery: release mechanisms and the modifying effect of pain relief. Acta Chir Scand Suppl. 1989;550:22–28.
4. Cohen ME, Bilimoria KY, Ko CY, Richards K, Hall BL. Variability in length of stay after colorectal surgery: assessment of 182 hospitals in the national surgical quality improvement program. Ann Surg. 2009;250:901–907.
5. Thiele RH, Rea KM, Turrentine FE, et al. Standardization of care: impact of an enhanced recovery protocol on length of stay, complications, and direct costs after colorectal surgery. J Am Coll Surg. 2015;220:430–443.
6. Greco M, Capretti G, Beretta L, Gemma M, Pecorelli N, Braga M. Enhanced recovery program in colorectal surgery: a meta-analysis of randomized controlled trials. World J Surg. 2014;38:1531–1541.
7. Ostermann S, Morel P, Chalé JJ, et al. Randomized controlled trial of enhanced recovery program dedicated to elderly patients after colorectal surgery. Dis Colon Rectum. 2019;62:1105–1116.
8. Wang Q, Suo J, Jiang J, Wang C, Zhao YQ, Cao X. Effectiveness of fast-track rehabilitation vs conventional care in laparoscopic colorectal resection for elderly patients: a randomized trial. Colorectal Dis. 2012;14:1009–1013.
9. van Rooijen S, Carli F, Dalton S, et al. Multimodal prehabilitation in colorectal cancer patients to improve functional capacity and reduce postoperative complications: the first international randomized controlled trial for multimodal prehabilitation. BMC Cancer. 2019;19:98.
10. Keller DS, Lawrence JK, Nobel T, Delaney CP. Optimizing cost and short-term outcomes for elderly patients in laparoscopic colonic surgery. Surg Endosc. 2013;27:4463–4468.
11. Shah PM, Johnston L, Sarosiek B, et al. Reducing readmissions while shortening length of stay: the positive impact of an enhanced recovery protocol in colorectal surgery. Dis Colon Rectum. 2017;60:219–227.
12. Lawrence JK, Keller DS, Samia H, et al. Discharge within 24 to 72 hours of colorectal surgery is associated with low readmission rates when using enhanced recovery pathways. J Am Coll Surg. 2013;216:390–394.
13. Vlug MS, Wind J, Hollmann MW, et al. Laparoscopy in combination with fast track multimodal management is the best perioperative strategy in patients undergoing colonic surgery: a randomized clinical trial (LAFA-study). Ann Surg. 2011;254:868–875.
14. Wind J, Hofland J, Preckel B, et al. Perioperative strategy in colonic surgery; LAparoscopy and/or FAst track multimodal management versus standard care (LAFA trial). BMC Surg. 2006;6:16.
15. Carmichael JC, Keller DS, Baldini G, et al. Clinical practice guidelines for enhanced recovery after colon and rectal surgery from the American Society of Colon and Rectal Surgeons and Society of American Gastrointestinal and Endoscopic Surgeons. Dis Colon Rectum. 2017;60:761–784.
16. Gustafsson UO, Scott MJ, Hubner M, et al. Guidelines for perioperative care in elective colorectal surgery: Enhanced Recovery After Surgery (ERAS') society recommendations: 2018. World J Surg. 2019;43:659–695.

17. Ripollés-Melchor J, Ramírez-Rodríguez JM, Casans-Francés R, et al. Association between use of enhanced recovery after surgery protocol and postoperative complications in colorectal surgery: the Postoperative Outcomes Within Enhanced Recovery After Surgery Protocol (POWER) study. JAMA Surg. 2019;154:725–736.

18. Aloia TA, Keller DS, Kowalski RB, et al. Enhanced recovery program implementation: an evidence-based review of the art and the science. Surg Endosc. 2019.

19. Berian JR, Ban KA, Liu JB, et al. Association of an enhanced recovery pilot with length of stay in the national surgical quality improvement program. JAMA Surg. 2018;153:358–365.

Index

Note: Page numbers in *italics* indicate a figure and page numbers in **bold** indicate a table on the corresponding page.